TORBAY HOSPITAL MEDICAL LIBRARY

Childhood Diabetes
and its Management

POSTGRADUATE PAEDIATRICS SERIES

Under the General Editorship of

JOHN APLEY
CBE, MD, BS, FRCP

Emeritus Consultant Paediatrician,
United Bristol Hospitals

Childhood Diabetes
and its Management

Second Edition

OMAN CRAIG
FRCP (Edin)

Consultant Paediatrician, Royal Hospital for Sick Children, Glasgow

BUTTERWORTHS
London - Boston
Sydney - Wellington - Durban - Toronto

United Kingdom London	**Butterworth & Co (Publishers) Ltd** 88 Kingsway, WC2B 6AB
Australia Sydney	**Butterworths Pty Ltd** 586 Pacific Highway, Chatswood, NSW 2067 Also at Melbourne, Brisbane, Adelaide and Perth
Canada Toronto	**Butterworth & Co (Canada) Ltd** 2265 Midland Avenue, Scarborough, Ontario, M1P 4S1
New Zealand Wellington	**Butterworths of New Zealand Ltd** T & W Young Building, 77–85 Customhouse Quay, 1, CPO Box 472
South Africa Durban	**Butterworth & Co (South Africa) (Pty) Ltd** 152–154 Gale Street
USA Boston	**Butterworth (Publishers) Inc** 10 Tower Office Park, Woburn, Massachusetts 01801

All rights reserved. No part of this publication may be reproduced or transmitted in any form or by any means, including photocopying and recording, without the written permission of the copyright holder, application for which should be addressed to the Publishers. Such written permission must also be obtained before any part of this publication is stored in a retrieval system of any nature.

This book is sold subject to the Standard Conditions of Sale of Net Books and may not be re-sold in the UK below the net price given by the Publishers in their current price list.

First published 1981

© **Butterworth & Co (Publishers) Ltd, 1981**
ISBN 0 407 00209 X

British Library Cataloguing in Publication Data

Craig, Oman
  Childhood diabetes and its management. - 2nd ed.
  - (Postgraduate paediatrics series).
  1. Diabetes in children
  I. Title   II. Series
  618.9'24'62   RJ420.D5   80-41760

ISBN 0-407-00209-X

Set, printed and bound in Great Britain
by Billing and Sons Limited,
Guildford, London, Oxford, Worcester

Dedicated to Dr Margaret Methven

Foreword

This is not just a book about syringes and their contents; it is about children. So refreshingly personal a book could have been written only by a paediatrician. This is clear from the very first chapter, with its discussion of differential diagnosis; it becomes even more obvious when the author turns to childhood problems of behaviour, of communication and of development. No adult-oriented or biochemically dominated physician could comprehend them so perceptively or so brilliantly illuminate them. The descriptions give full weight to the important biochemical aspects, as for ketoacidosis, yet maintain a commendable breadth and comfortable balance. In addition, the author maintains a long-term perspective through the childhood years to adult life.

To watch a greatly experienced children's doctor move on from theory to practice, going through real cases in detail and with vivid descriptions, is an experience that enriches the reader. The author's sharp and sensitive thinking is matched by his writing, which remains kindly though pungent. The language sparkles, and indeed I cannot remember a medical book that has charmed me more and given me greater enjoyment in the reading.

The keenness of Dr Craig's observation, matched by the keenness of his descriptions, is apparent throughout. A broad sketch of the whole patient is amplified by those many details that are so essential in clinical practice 'for Art and Science cannot exist but in minutely organised Particulars' (Blake). His clinical experience and sharp eye are displayed by the descriptions of transient oedema, skin lesions, and perhaps especially by his work on hepatomegaly. Although far from dogmatic, the author gives unmistakably clear and practical advice; like a good cook, he gets his ingredients from far and wide and blends them with his own experience, then presents the complete dish as a tasty and nutritious meal.

Diabetes is stuffed with controversial problems, as we may see by the perennial arguments between permissive and rigid treatment. The author willingly takes them up, discusses them broad-mindedly and objectively, then says in effect 'This is what I do and why'. I was left with the impression that long encrusted opinions have been gently scraped clean; that the subject discussed has been spring-cleaned and freshened up. The author's own reasonableness enables the reader to come to his own equally reasonable conclusions, and is likely to be instrumental in modifying both attitudes and practice. Certainly that is what the book has done for me. I hope other readers will get as much practical help, wisdom and sheer enjoyment from it as I have done.

JOHN APLEY

Preface to Second Edition

The stress in this book is laid on the management of the diabetic child, from the first talks with him and his parents to later difficulties such as recurrent acidosis and rejection of the diabetic state. There is no one set of rules which applies to all diabetic children, nor is there a set of rules for their families. 'Doctor and patient together form one "system" and the functioning of the system for the benefit of the patient's health depends just as much on the "compliance" (or cooperation) of the doctor as of the patient' (Groen, 1979). In managing a diabetic child there are *three* components in the system; the child, his family and the doctor.

Our knowledge of the physiology of diabetes is increasing rapidly and, fortunately, so is our interest in the clinical application of that knowledge. Since the first edition of this book more has been written about somatostatin, glucagon, glycosylated haemoglobin and so forth; but more has also been written about diet, over-treatment, overnight hypoglycaemia and the place of the diabetic child in the family. In this second edition it has therefore been possible to maintain, without strain, the balance between diabetes in the home and diabetes in the laboratory.

I remain indebted to many of my colleagues in the Royal Hospital for Sick Children, Glasgow. Dr R. A. Shanks and Professors J. H. Hutchison, G. C. Arneil and F. Cockburn have allowed me to undertake much of the management of their patients. Dr R. W. Logan has read Chapter 7. Professor Fred Stone and his staff in the Department of Child and Family Psychiatry have helped greatly with some of the more difficult cases. Mr J. Devlin and the staff of the Department of Medical Illustration have supplied most of the diagrams and illustrations. Drs Myron Genel, Donnell Etzwiler and

PREFACE TO SECOND EDITION

James Farquhar have allowed me to transplant some flowers of their labours. I am particularly indebted to Dr Joyce Richardson who shares the diabetic clinic with me and gives me invaluable advice and to Mrs Fiona House, our dietitian, who has supplied the last chapter in the book.

OMAN CRAIG

Ref.: Groen, J. J. (1979). Nutrition and the Diabetic Child. *Pediat. adolesc. Endocr.*, **7**, 175 (in a discussion). Karger; Basel

SI Units

The change to SI (Système International) Units in Europe is not yet complete in that some older physicians still find it easier to think in the older units. Two readings are therefore often given, particularly when referring to blood glucose. The changes are:

Plasma glucose in mmol/1×18.02 = plasma glucose in mg per cent
Plasma urea in mmol/1×6.01 = plasma urea in mg per cent
On the other hand, the readings for sodium, potassium, chloride and bicarbonate remain identical.

Contents

1	The History and Differential Diagnosis	1
2	Strictness, Liberality and Control	20
3	The First Admission	37
4	Behaviour	58
5	Communication and Education	72
	Appendix	89
6	The Outpatient Clinic	93
7	Insulin and Metabolism	138
8	Ketoacidosis, Pre-coma and Coma	160
9	The Course of Childhood Diabetes	193
10	The Aetiology of Diabetes	209
11	Diabetes Associated with Other Diseases	233
12	Complications	248
13	Food for the Diabetic	273
14	Notes on Diabetic Diet—Fiona House	286
	Appendix	297
	Index	303

CHAPTER 1

The History and Differential Diagnosis

LENGTH OF HISTORY

Seldom does the juvenile form of diabetes mellitus appear as gradually as the adult form. This means that if diabetes is suspected in a child it is an emergency: he should be referred to hospital at once, without waiting for a routine outpatient appointment, as delay may lead to his admission in severe ketoacidosis.

Pond (1971) states that roughly 20 per cent of children with diabetes are admitted with a history going back two weeks or less, 60 per cent with a history of two to six weeks and 20 per cent with a history of more than six weeks. Recent figures derived from 100 cases admitted to the Royal Hospital for Sick Children, Glasgow are similar and are shown in *Table 1.1*.

TABLE 1.1

The length of history at time of admission in 100 cases of diabetes

	1 week or less	8–14 days	3 weeks	4 weeks	Duration of history 5 weeks	6 weeks	7 weeks	8 weeks	More than 8 weeks
Numbers	12	13	25	23	0	4	1	8	14
Percentage		25			52			23	

(It will be seen from this table that parents seem to have an aversion to certain periods of time, such as five and seven weeks. Their estimate of time seems fairly accurate up to a month, but thereafter goes in for even numbers.)

The short history

Some newly diabetic children deteriorate at great speed, reaching hospital within three or four days of the onset of clinical diabetes. It seemed of interest to determine what relationship, if any, existed between the length of history and the blood sugar. The cases in *Figure 1.1* were all untreated prior to admission.

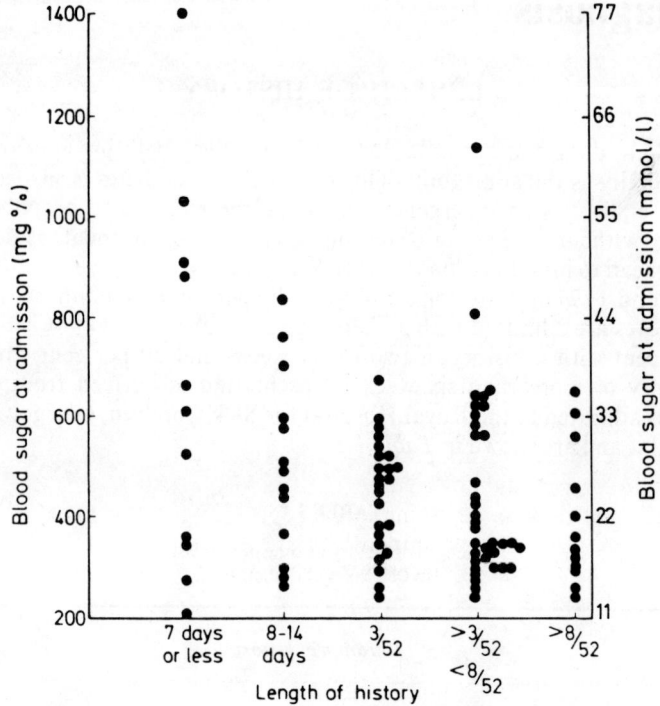

Figure 1.1. *Height of the blood sugar in relation to the duration of the history. Based on 100 consecutive cases (blood sugar on admission not recorded in three)*

Four out of the 11 with a history of a week or less had a blood sugar of more than 44 mmol/l (800 mg per cent). Only three of the other 86 with longer histories had blood sugars over 44 mmol/l.

Thirty-three of 37 with histories from eight days to three weeks had blood sugars below 33 mmol/l (600 mg per cent), only 13 of them below 22 mmol/l (400 mg per cent). Thirty-nine of 49 with histories longer than three weeks had blood sugars below 33 mmol/l, but 30 of them were below 22 mmol/l.

The general impression is that the longer the history, the lower the blood sugar at admission, although there are many exceptions and much overlapping.

It is a pity that the numbers involved in the table are relatively small, enough to raise questions but not enough to supply answers. The questions posed are:

(1) With a history of one week or less, is it true that there is a wide scatter of blood sugars, with a definite tendency for some to be high?
(2) When the history is longer than one week, is it true that there is a tendency for sugars to become concentrated at a lower level, say below 33 mmol/l (600 mg per cent).
(3) Can we say that such a tendency is established at three weeks, and changes only slightly thereafter?

If we could answer 'Yes' to these questions, we would be left wondering whether the three to four week history is part of the 'basic' chronology of juvenile diabetes, sometimes accelerated and sometimes slowed down by additional factors. The actual length of history found, clustered around three or four weeks *(Table 1.1)* is in keeping with the hypothesis just stated, a hypothesis derived originally from blood sugar levels only. What the 'additional factors' might be is uncertain. From the records themselves there is no definite evidence of infection, but infection may play a part. The length of history did not seem related to age.

Whether there be anything in this hypothesis or not, there is one fact that stands out prominently from *Figure 1.1*. Children can suffer high blood sugar levels within days of the onset of diabetes. The child with the blood sugar of over 66 mmol/l (1200 mg per cent) had a four-day history, was admitted in non-ketotic hyperglycaemic coma, and died within two hours of admission. It is hoped that *Figure 1.1* will be a warning to those whose only previous experience of diabetes has been with adults.

The long history

When the history is long it is often difficult to decide when diabetes began.

4 THE HISTORY AND DIFFERENTIAL DIAGNOSIS

One boy of nine years had a history of thirst and polyuria 'from birth'. His general health was good apart from obesity. His random blood sugar was 13.3 mmol/l (240 mg per cent) and there was no ketosis. This appeared to be an 'adult-onset' type of diabetes, and enquiries were made about his diet. These got off to a slow start, as his mother, a restaurant proprietrix of Italian origin, seemed to regard the house officer as an industrial spy whose main aim was to set up a rival business of his own. It eventually emerged that the boy was on a very high carbohydrate intake in the form of food such as pasta. His urine became sugar-free on small doses of insulin and he was maintained for several months on diet alone. So much for his 'adult onset'. Thereafter he became a typical juvenile diabetic, requiring the usual doses of insulin. He is now thought to be developing diabetes insipidus as well, and has early optic atrophy (see p. 243).

A more usual type of 'long history' concerned a girl of five and three-quarter years.

For rather more than two months there had been thirst, polyuria and nocturia. Her appetite was increased. Her parents were doubtful about weight loss, but her general health had been excellent. Investigation of her polyuria showed glycosuria. Her blood sugar at admission was 16 mmol/l (291 mg per cent) with a trace of ketones in the urine, blood pH 7.41, base excess − 3; Na, 130; K, 3.9; Cl, 101; and urea 5 mmol/l (30 mg per cent). There was no metabolic upset apart from her hyperglycaemia, but she has needed insulin ever since.

We debate on what causes the difference between ketoacidotic coma and non-ketotic hyperglycaemic coma, but we could well extend this debate to include many less dramatic, run-of-the-mill cases which show minor but similar differences.

Maturity onset diabetes in the young (MODY)

When writing about the long history, mention must be made of 'maturity onset diabetes in the young' (MODY), an unfortunate term which has caused confusion. All that is usually meant is that the diabetes has been of gradual onset and has been observed as chemical diabetes ('latent' in American usage) for months or years before overt diabetes appears. Fajans *et al.* (1969) followed 15 patients aged nine to 17 years, all of whom had abnormal glucose tolerance tests (GTT), low insulin responses and strong family histories, for periods averaging 7.6 years. Three of these developed diabetes, one after four months, two after two years, but all three became insulin-dependent and one was readmitted many times in coma. Once diabetes has appeared it is a swift goodbye to the maturity onset type, a term usually taken to apply to non-ketotic, non-insulin-dependent diabetes. In the author's opinion it would be better to talk of 'slow onset' diabetes sometimes happening in children. Pildes (1973) described an obese girl of 12 years who had been under observation for two years because of polyuria, polydipsia and glycosuria, without showing systemic upset or weight loss, and mention is made elsewhere in this book (p. 47) of a girl who has gone through her diabetic career, including puberty, without needing insulin, but these two cases are exceptional. They, indeed, could be labelled 'MODY', but the wider use of the term encourages the false belief, in those who are not well acquainted with diabetes in childhood, that many diabetic children must behave like elderly adults, which is not true.

There is a 'true' form of MODY (Tattersall, 1974; Tattersall and Fajans, 1975). Tattersall described three families in which there were 37 diabetics. Nine of these were aged 14 or under at the time of diagnosis, which in most was based on polyuria, polydipsia or pruritus, but in some the diagnosis was made as the result of routine investigation. They were followed for several years, but did not become insulin-dependent, thus resembling the adult type. This familial form of diabetes appears to be inherited as an autosomal dominant.

TAKING THE HISTORY

Diabetes mellitus is an easy diagnosis to make if one has it in mind. Many years ago the correct diagnosis was hardly ever made in a child before admission to hospital. This was probably due in part to the smaller numbers of children with diabetes, so that the family doctor did not have the same reason to be on the alert, and in part to the relative difficulty of testing urine for sugar in those days. Fehling's solution and Benedict's solution had to be heated and when they were they had a habit of spurting over the wall. Urine was therefore seldom tested for sugar, and diabetic children were most often admitted after a course of sulphonamide for an imagined urinary infection. The overbreathing of ketosis sometimes led to a diagnosis of pneumonia, and a few who had reached pre-coma were sent to fever hospitals as tuberculous meningitis which was all too common at the time. The advent of the dipstick has changed all that. Urine can now easily be tested in the child's home. The commonest cause of delay in diagnosis at present is the failure to take an adequate history.

The diagnosis of diabetes mellitus is there for the asking, but the right questions may not be asked. Parents may forget the preceding polyuria and polydipsia and volunteer information only on the signs that seem to them more important—lethargy, anorexia, weight loss and diminished consciousness. The family doctor will have the parent and child with him during history-taking and examination, but in hospital, particularly if the child is being admitted, the history may be taken from the parent while the child is being put to bed and the parent may be allowed to go before the child is examined. The parent should always be present at the initial examination so that subsidiary questions can be asked. If I am seeing a child with a wheezy chest I often forget to ask about the urine while taking the history, but I remember when I am prodding the kidney areas during the general examination. The presenting signs of diabetes in childhood are polyuria and polydipsia, and the history is there if one asks for it.

SIGNS AND SYMPTOMS

Polyuria and polydipsia

Polyuria and polydipsia, as has just been said, are the first signs of the disease. Occasionally a case is picked up at a routine medical examination even before symptoms have appeared, but when they do appear they are polyuria and polydipsia. In the very young patient in nappies the parent may not have recognized the presence of polyuria, in the slightly older child they may be more concerned with the resultant enuresis than with what is happening by day, and in the schoolchild nocturia may be the presenting complaint. Nocturia is much more likely to indicate physical disease than enuresis.

There are, of course, many causes of polyuria and polydipsia.

(1) If one considers the field of childhood as a whole, the commonest cause is probably *compulsive water drinking*. This is usually a disorder of the pre-school child and may be associated with signs of regression to infancy. It is rare in the child of school age though it may occur if the child is handicapped, for example by mental defect or near-blindness. It has even been known to produce coma in the presence of underlying renal disease (Kohn *et al.*, 1976).

(2) *Diabetes insipidus* can be very like diabetes mellitus. The child with diabetes insipidus is much more likely to become severely distressed by withholding fluids overnight than is the child with the early case of diabetes mellitus, but a test for sugar should give the answer (a patient with diabetes insipidus may have had a bottle of Lucozade just before the test). Diabetes mellitus and diabetes insipidus may co-exist (p. 244) but mellitus comes first.

(3) *Urinary infection* tends to be diagnosed because it is more common than diabetes mellitus. With a urinary infection the picture is dominated by frequency and dysuria, rather than by the true polyuria and polydipsia of diabetes. *Chronic renal failure* may imitate diabetes mellitus, but there may be a preceding history of renal disease.

Anorexia

The anorexia which is often seen in diabetic children may mislead those who concentrate on the adult patient with his 'eating diabetes'. I have previously informed students that anorexia is a cardinal sign of diabetes, but it is in fact variable. Of our 100 patients, appetite was mentioned in 56; 31 were reported to be anorexic, 19 were eating normally and six showed increased appetite. The failure to take notes on appetite in 44 cases is not quite as incompetent as it seems at first sight, because one tends not to ask the mother of a hyperventilating child if he is eating well. Five of the six with increased appetite were mild cases with minimal ketosis and moderate blood sugars, but one was still eating well with a blood sugar of 33 mmol/l (594 mg per cent) and a blood pH of 7.18. One suspects that anorexia indicates the appearance of ketosis, but one would have to take a more detailed history of variations in appetite throughout the history to be sure of this.

Lethargy and weight loss

Lethargy and weight loss are common to so many disorders and diseases that they are of little value in making a diagnosis of diabetes mellitus. Again one must stress the need for taking an adequate history. Although not presenting symptoms they may be the symptoms of which the parents first complain, and the finding of a preceding history of polyuria and polydipsia makes the diagnosis of diabetes mellitus probable.

Alimentary signs and symptoms

Alimentary signs and symptoms, such as vomiting, abdominal pain, abdominal distension and even diarrhoea are of relatively late onset in the history of diabetes, and usually mark the onset of ketosis. The abdominal pain may be severe, and the physician may suspect an acute abdomen. In the past year we have taken over from the surgical side two diabetics admitted as '? appendicitis'. The situation has been described by Valerio (1976). The clues to diagnosis are not so much in the abdominal findings as in the hyperventilation and dehydration, backed up by a history suggesting diabetes. The symptoms are associated with gastric dilatation and partial ileus, but the underlying cause is uncertain (Katz and Spiro, 1966): some believe that an enlarging liver stretches its capsule, causing pain and reflex ileus. A recent editorial (*Br.med.J.*, 1979) reviews the effects of diabetes on the gut. Diarrhoea must be a very uncommon presentation of diabetes in childhood, but I have come across it as the presenting complaint in a teenager with diabetes.

Skin sepsis

Skin sepsis has a time-honoured role as a presenting symptom of diabetes in adults, but is uncommon in children. Only one child in our series showed it. She had been admitted to the Eye Infirmary because of styes, and glycosuria was found on routine examination, with no history to suggest diabetes. On the other hand, monilial infection of the vulva and perineum is relatively common.

Hypoglycaemia

Hypoglycaemia seems to precede the diabetic state in many adult patients judging from episodes of weakness, irritability, trembling and hunger. Such patients may show a quick rise in blood sugar during a glucose tolerance test, with a subsequent fall to very low levels. This state of affairs has been described in childhood (Lloyd, 1964) but it is very rare in that age group. Lloyd discussed two cases, in whom the diagnosis of diabetes was based on the finding of synalbumin antagonist in the plasma, one of them also having an abnormal glucose tolerance test. Too often are attempts made to attribute any preceding psychological disorder in a diabetic child to hypoglycaemia. I have seen one child with a clear-cut history of hypoglycaemia preceding diabetes, but only one.

Myopia

Myopia may be present when a child is first admitted with diabetes. It is attributed to dehydration affecting the lens and the vitreous humour, but is very rare as a complaint in childhood. Whether it commonly exists or not, I do not know: routine refraction would be necessary to decide.

THE DIFFERENTIAL DIAGNOSIS

Certain conditions which have been confused with diabetes have already been discussed while considering the history. These were:

Urinary infection
Pneumonia
Meningitis
Diabetes insipidus
Compulsive drinking
'Acute abdomen'

Before turning to the differential diagnosis of glycosuria one must first consider the validity of tests for glycosuria.

Validity of tests for glycosuria

The colour change produced by a Clinitest tablet in a diabetic urine represents the oxidation of cupric sulphate to cuprous oxide, and any reducing agent may do it. Salicylates, homogentisic acid and ascorbic acid can do it (Feldman and Lebovitz, 1973) and so can many sugars, pentoses (for example xylose), hexoses (fructose, galactose) and disaccharides (lactose, maltose). A weak reaction to Clinitest is therefore not diagnostic of diabetes.

The enzyme tests (Clinistix, Diastix) contain a system of glucose oxidase, peroxidase and chromogen which responds specifically to glucose. However, the ingestion of aspirin or L-dopa, or the presence of alcaptonuria, can interfere with this reaction and give false negatives. Clinistix is also a very sensitive test, giving a positive with only about 30 mg per cent of sugar in the urine, whereas Clinitest 'turns' at about 150 mg per cent. As a normal human may excrete up to 15 mg per cent of sugar in the urine, it might appear that false positives with Clinistix would be common. In practice they are much more common with Clinitest, due to traces of substances referred to above. A weak positive to Clinitest coupled with a negative to Clinistix almost certainly is a negative result.

DIFFERENTIAL DIAGNOSIS OF GLYCOSURIA

Some causes of glycosuria need little more than a mention here. It is well known that glycosuria may occur with Cushing's syndrome or with steroid therapy and its associated Cushingoid state. It may occur with phaeochromocytoma, thyrotoxicosis and haemochromatosis. The 'piqure' diabetes of intracranial disorder has been known for 100 years. The drug diazoxide causes glycosuria, but the glycosuria which sometimes followed general anaesthesia is disappearing as chloroform and ether fall into desuetude. Shock, burns and hypoxia may show glycosuria, particularly if the shock has affected a young child who has been vigorously treated with intravenous glucose.

A girl of nine was admitted with a one-day history of illness. She was in deep coma, with a large heart, tachycardia, pleural effusions, hepatomegaly and several other disorders including a blood sugar of 36 mmol/l (650 mg per cent). She died in a few hours, undiagnosed. Post-mortem examination showed the cause of death to be a large intracardiac tumour, previously symptomless. The hyperglycaemia can be attributed to 'some intracranial disaster' but is essentially unexplained.

Even an excess of ingested carbohydrate may cause glycosuria; for example, a bottle of Lucozade contains 150 g of carbohydrate, and a dehydrated child can drink that in an hour. There are, however, certain other causes of glycosuria which may give the paediatrician some trouble in diagnosis.

Salicylate poisoning

Salicylate poisoning can, in a few cases, give a very good imitation of diabetic pre-coma. The young child (and it is usually a toddler who has taken an overdose of aspirin) reaches a state of metabolic acidosis in three or four hours, and is hyperventilating at the time of admission. Both salicylate and acetone in the urine may give a positive ferric chloride test. A positive test after boiling the urine to get rid of acetone indicates the presence of salicylate, in therapeutic or toxic doses. In the early stages of salicylate poisoning there may be a transient polyuria. Finally, the child with salicylate poisoning may show hyperglycaemia. This seldom rises above the range of 11–17 mmol/l (200–300 mg per cent), but that is enough to take it to the top of the Dextrostix scale, which might confuse initial diagnosis. Further confusion could arise with euglycaemic ketotic diabetic coma (described on p. 181) which seems to be rare in childhood but which can occur in the teenager. Where there is doubt the important clue comes from the history, which is usually of five or six hours and seldom more than 24 hours in the child with salicylate poisoning, but not less than three days in the child with diabetes.

Hypernatraemic dehydration

Hypernatraemic dehydration in infancy is a common condition which may be associated with wide variations in blood sugar, including hyperglycaemia (Stevenson and Bowyer, 1970). Even the CSF figure for sugar may be well over 5.6 mmol/l (100 mg per cent). Here again the history is likely to be shorter than with diabetes, but that point is of little practical value in dealing with infants. The polyuria of the occasional infant with diabetes disappears into his nappy, and the thirst, which he is unable to slake himself, appears as irritability. The sodium level is a help, that of the diabetic when first seen rarely reaching that of hypernatraemic dehydration. Pretreatment sodium levels in 84 recent diabetics can be tabulated as shown in *Table 1.2*.

TABLE 1.2

Sodium levels in diabetics

mmol/l	Numbers
<120	1
120–129	15
130–139	65
140–149	11
150–159	0
>159	1

The overlap of diabetes and hypernatraemic dehydration is almost non-existent. The patient with the level 159 was a boy of three years who also had a blood sugar of 77 mmol/l (1400 mg per cent) and was in fact a case of non-ketotic hyperosmolar diabetic coma. There should be little cause for confusion about the diagnosis. Confusion usually arises because the baby with hypertonic dehydration has had a lumbar puncture because he was drowsy, and a high sugar level in the CSF is taken to mean diabetes. It should not do so.

Severe hyponatraemia has been described in association with hyperlipidaemia in ketoacidosis (Bell, Hilton and Walker, 1972).

Convulsions

Convulsions may produce hyperglycaemia. Spirer *et al.* (1974) describe 39 children with an average age of two and a half years. During or just after the fit the blood sugar was more than 8.3 mmol/l (150 mg per cent) in 13, and in six of these was more than 11 mmol/l (200 mg per cent). Two hours later, the range was 2.5–5.8 mmol/l (41–105 mg per cent). The hyperglycaemia appears to be mediated through catecholamines. In rats given electric shocks there is an increase in catecholamines (*see* p. 153) but after adrenalectomy there is hypoglycaemia.

Renal glycosuria

Renal glycosuria in childhood is less common than in adults, but may occur, particularly if there has been a heavy ingestion of carbohydrate (see the following section on the glucose tolerance test).

Acute pancreatitis

Acute pancreatitis may simulate diabetes. Chronic pancreatitis may in fact produce diabetes, as in cystic fibrosis, but that is not being discussed here. Acute pancreatitis presents with abdominal pain which may be in the left upper quadrant, and frequently with a raised blood sugar, thus resembling the abdominal manifestations of diabetic ketosis. Amylase and urinary diastase are raised. Malone (1974) discusses the possibility of pancreatitis and diabetic ketoacidosis occurring together. Amylase is not characteristically raised in diabetic ketoacidosis. It may be, but if a rise occurs it lasts less than four days. Malone reported four patients in their early teens who had raised amylase persisting for a week to a month. All had severe abdominal pain, and he suggested the syndrome could be due to concomitant pancreatitis.

Transient diabetic state

A transient diabetic state may occur in some ill children, and indeed in some who are not ill at all except that glycosuria has been found by chance and confirmed by the presence of hyperglycaemia. Such situations are discussed below.

THE GLUCOSE TOLERANCE TEST

If a child presents with a high blood sugar and the symptoms of diabetes a glucose tolerance test (GTT) is not necessary, and indeed if the child has to have insulin at once, as is often the case, a GTT is not practicable. The GTT is of value when glycosuria has been stumbled upon almost by accident.

It is important at this stage to define certain terms which are used in relation to diabetes.

(1) A potential diabetic is a child with a strong family history of diabetes.
(2) A latent diabetic is a child who has had a temporary diabetic state, either chemical or clinical, when under stress.
(3) A chemical diabetic has an abnormal glucose tolerance test, but no symptoms of diabetes.
(4) A clinical diabetic shows the symptoms and signs of diabetes.

A child may fall into two categories, for example he may be both a potential and a chemical diabetic. It should be noted that in Britain the term 'pre-diabetes' is only used retrospectively, and is applied only to the early clinical state of a child who has since developed diabetes, for example the pre-diabetic spurt in growth. This is a possible source of confusion, because in other countries 'pre-diabetic' may be used as a synonym for 'potential' in the sense used above. The above classification is simplified for the purposes of this book. It is given in more detailed form by Oakley (1968).

The test is done first thing in the morning with the child fasting. Glucose is given by mouth and subsequent fluctuations in the blood sugar are observed. Glucose gives a sharper and higher rise in blood sugar than a normal carbohydrate meal. The amount given varies with age, and from country to country. The standard amount in the UK is 50 g, in the USA 100 g, and surprisingly either dose gives very similar results.

Doses in children are: up to three years, 2.0 g/kg, or a shade more; from three to nine years, 1.75 g/kg; from ten years, the standard 50 g.

This assumes that the children are about normal weight for age. A small ten year old would be given 1.75 g/kg. Glucose is nauseating at times and is therefore best given in about 200 ml of water to which an unsweetened flavouring agent (for example fresh lemon juice) has been added. Lucozade is 16 per cent glucose.

It is standard practice in adults to test the blood sugar at zero, half, one, one and a half, two and three hours, but it is undesirable to prick children more often than strictly necessary and tests at zero, one and two hours are usually sufficient. The highest rise is usually seen at half an hour, and one can expect the blood sugar to have returned to near the fasting level by two hours. The test can be prolonged if reactive hypoglycaemia is suspected.

Standards vary in interpreting the test. The WHO suggest that a blood sugar of less than 6.7 mmol/l (120 mg per cent) at two hours is normal, over 7.8 (140) abnormal. Upper limits of normal in Australia are taken as 6.1 (110), 9.4 (170) and 6.7 (120) at zero, one and two hours. Equivalent figures quoted by Pyke (1968) are over 5.5 (100) when fasting, 10.0 (180) at half an hour, 8.9 (160) at one hour and 6.7 (120) at two hours. Capillary specimens may give readings about 10 mg higher than those quoted. The two hour specimen is probably the most reliable as a sharp initial rise is sometimes seen in a healthy person. One abnormal reading suggests that the test should be repeated, three such readings are usually taken as 'diagnostic'.

With the adult it is possible to obtain urine specimens to coincide with the blood specimens but in the child this is often impossible, so that diagnosis of renal glycosuria may be rather difficult. In the very young child it is worth including a sugar test-strip in the napkin.

Certain errors may affect the test results. If the preceding diet has been low in carbohydrate glucose tolerance may be unduly low and a peak of over 11.1 (200) may be obtained with a slow decline thereafter. Conversely, if the subject has been on a very high carbohydrate intake (for example 400 g daily) the blood sugar may show only a small maximal rise with several ups and downs during the test. For this reason it may be desirable to admit children to hospital for at least a day before the test to ensure an average carbohydrate uptake, but in practice the test can usually be done as an outpatient provided one is satisfied that the child is being fed normally. It is not good practice to hasten to do a GTT before a child has fully recovered from the systemic upset of an illness.

Apart from such errors that may arise within the test there are also potential difficulties in interpreting the results. The elderly have a higher normal range than the young. In addition, the figures of a GTT are not always reproducible. McDonald, Fisher and Burnham (1965) carried out repeated GTTs on 334 convicts. Nine per cent of the prisoners had at least one abnormal curve but none were abnormal at all times, suggesting that GTTs done in normal subjects will give an abnormal curve about once in 40 tests. Another study concentrated on the figure at two hours and found that if two GTTs were done 24 per cent of the subjects had results both above and below 6.1 mmol/l (110 mg per cent) which is near the border of diabetes.

In summary, it is not always easy to say 'This is an abnormal curve' and one certainly should not assume that such a statement can be construed as 'This is a diabetic curve'.

THE TRANSIENT DIABETIC STATE

It is known that some children may show a short phase of impaired glucose tolerance which can loosely be termed 'transient diabetes'. This is not a very good term as there are no diabetic symptoms or signs and the state is only one of *chemical diabetes*. Thirteen such cases were described by Court (1968) and most paediatricians will remember a few of their own. They are found to have glycosuria either in the course of an acute infection or at routine urine testing, for example at the time of admission for a minor surgical operation.

When glucose tolerance tests were done the children described by Court all had a peak sugar of 10.5 mmol/l (190 mg per cent) or over and two-hour levels of 7.7–13.3 mmol/l (140–240 mg per cent) in 12, the other having a level of 19.7 mmol/l (356 mg per cent). 'In most cases' the GTT was repeated a few days later and was similar. The follow-up was one to four years in 12, 10½ years in the other. None had developed symptoms of diabetes. GTTs were repeated after the follow-up period on ten patients, none of whom had a peak above 8.3 mmol/l and only one had a two-hour reading over 6.6 mmol/l (6.8 mmol/l (123 mg per cent)).

The follow-up period for most is rather short and Court does not suggest that none of these children will become diabetic in the future. In a series of 134 child diabetics Pond and Oakley (1968) included four, all with close relatives who were diabetic, who were found to be diabetic when routine tests were done because of 'slight or unrelated symptoms'.

John B, a boy of seven and a half years, became anorexic. The next day he was vomiting and febrile and two days later his family doctor found him dehydrated and with sugar in his urine. He was admitted the same day, and he said he had had thirst (drinking a bottle of Lucozade) and polyuria during the previous 24 hours. He was very dehydrated and flushed and his breath smelled strongly of acetone, but ketones were not detected in the urine. His Astrup and biochemistry, apart from a blood sugar of 23.2 mmol/l (417 mg per cent) and a blood urea of 10 mmol/l (60 mg per cent), were virtually normal. There was no family history of diabetes. He was put on a drip, first of saline then of half strength saline and 5 per cent dextrose, but insulin was not given. By the next morning he was sitting up reading a comic, well hydrated, with a blood sugar of 5.4 mmol/l (98 mg per cent). His blood sugar was normal thereafter and there was no glycosuria after the first specimen. A glucose tolerance test done six days later was flat. He was symptom-free for the next eight months, and was then discharged from follow-up. The most interesting and unusual thing in this history is the short burst of polyuria and polydipsia.

Transient diabetes after burns

After burns, as after many injuries, there may be an almost immediate rise in blood sugar, presumably due to adrenalin action. This is mild, symptomless and short-lived. It should not be confused with the very rare but serious complication known as 'burn-stress pseudo-diabetes' or 'adrenal cortical hyperglycaemia'. Rosenberg *et al.* (1965) collected six cases, two of whom had died. The onset was nine to 29 days after burning. Diabetic symptoms are present, and the condition is essentially one of hyperosmolar non-ketotic diabetic coma, and is treated as such. If the patient survives the diabetes disappears; but one patient followed up after a year had abnormal glucose tolerance, though symptomless.

Transient neonatal diabetes is discussed in Chapter 9.

Interpretation of GTT

When one happens upon a slightly abnormal GTT, what should one say to the parents and what sort of follow-up is indicated? I think one should explain the findings to the parents at the outset and add that this situation is quite common and rarely leads on to diabetes (which is not known to be true, but a half truth that spares years on tenterhooks is justified). The need for a further GTT in six months 'to be absolutely sure' is stressed, and the mother is asked to recite the main symptoms of diabetes (drinking too much, passing a lot of urine and wetting the bed, but excluding signs with protean causes, such as lethargy) so that she can bring the child back if anything suggestive of diabetes appears. Unless there is a family history of diabetes to suggest a longer follow-up, a normal GTT after six months should mark the end of surveillance. This is a personal opinion, but I believe that a cardinal duty of the paediatrician is to reduce anxiety when possible. if one takes a hopeful line one will be proved wrong at times but one has to accept that. To be able to say 'I was never wrong. I may have taken a little time to interpret the facts fully, and I may have given years of anxiety to mothers and to children in their formative years, but I was never wrong' is to talk of failure.

A case for consideration

Margaret McD was admitted at the age of one and three-quarter years suffering from codeine poisoning. She had pneumonia and had been given syrup of codeine phosphate for her cough. A routine urine test showed sugar. There was no history of diabetic symptoms so a GTT was done when she had recovered from her illness *(Table 1.3)*. The fasting figure was on the high side, with the rise thereafter being small and irregular, the kind of curve one might get from a patient who had previously been on a high carbohydrate intake, but she had been on ordinary ward diet. A single urine specimen was obtained at two hours and showed 2 per cent sugar. This suggested renal glycosuria as at no time in the two hours had the blood sugar been above 8.2 mmol/l (150 mg per cent). The mother stated that she had had GTTs performed since her pregnancy and had renal glycosuria, although she had also been put on a low carbohydrate diet. The maternal grandmother was on an oral agent for maturity onset diabetes. The test suggested that the child had both chemical diabetes and renal glycosuria.

TABLE 1.3

Date	Venous blood sugar in mg (hours after oral glucose)					
	0	½	1	1½	2	3
September, 1966	110	146	127	127	150	—
October, 1966	81	116	123	165	165	154
September, 1972	68	158	207	194	127	102
December, 1976	74	—	108	118	108	92

The test was repeated after a month. This time there was a bigger rise, but the peak figure was again late (one and a half to two hours) and again highly suggestive of diabetes. The delayed rise now indicated a preceding low sugar intake, but she had been readmitted to the ward before the test was done. Because of the suspicion of diabetes developing, and in an attempt to delay its onset, she was put on a carbohydrate intake appropriate to a diabetic. Her mother was quite happy about this as it paralleled her own diet and she had no qualms about her daughter's immediate future as she herself was getting on well. Follow up was therefore sustained.

The results of a third GTT done as an inpatient in 1972, when she was nearly eight, are shown in *Table 1.3*. The curve is different in shape. The peak figure is now at one hour and the two-hour figure has dropped well, though not into the normal range.

By 1975 she still showed no overt signs of diabetes. At her first admission her height and weight were both on the 25th centile, now they are above the 50th, possibly a sign of growth increase before overt diabetes appears, certainly evidence that she does not have diabetes of a degree to hold her back. During all this time her urine has been tested before breakfast and the evening meal on three days a week. If a positive is obtained, which happens about once in three or four months, the urine is tested four times a day for the next three days. The results are usually negative, but three times in eight years she has had two-day episodes of chemical diabetes associated with febrile infections. Because of the timing of the tests renal glycosuria is likely to have been often missed.

The last GTT in 1976 was normal. The two-hour blood was accompanied by a urine showing 2 per cent glycosuria.

There is no doubt that this girl has a low renal threshold and now has a normal GTT, but she had signs of chemical and latent diabetes in the past. Her future remains uncertain. If I were asked if I thought this child was going to develop diabetes I should spin a coin before replying. Were such a form of arbitration denied me, I should reply that I thought not. But I am of an optimistic turn of mind.

REFERENCES

Bell, J. A., Hilton, P. J. and Walker, G. (1972). Severe hyponatraemia in hyperlipaemic diabetic ketoacidosis. *Br.med.J.*, **4**, 709

British medical Journal (editorial) (1979). Diabetes and the gut. **1**, 1743

Court, J. M. (1968). The significance of abnormal glucose tolerance in childhood. *Austral. paed. J.*, **4**, 60

Fajans, S. S., Floyd, J. C., Pek, S. and Conn, J. W. (1969). The course of asymptomatic diabetes in young people, as determined by levels of blood glucose and plasma insulin. *Trans. Ass. Am. Physns*, **82**, 211

Feldman, J. M. and Lebovitz, Francine L. (1973). Tests for glucosuria: an analysis of factors that give misleading results. *Diabetes*, **22**, 115

Katz, L. A, and Spiro, H. M. (1966). Gastro-intestinal manifestations of diabetes. *New Engl. J. Med.* **275**, 1350

Kohn, B., Norma, M. E., Feldman, H., Thier, S. O. and Singer, I. (1976). Hysterical polydipsia (compulsive water drinking) in children. *Am. J. Dis. Child.*, **130**, 210

Lloyd, June K. (1964). Diabetes mellitus presenting as spontaneous hypoglycaemia in childhood. *Proc. R. Soc. Med.*, **57**, 1061

McDonald, G. W., Fisher, G. F. and Burnham, C. (1965). Reproducibility of the oral glucose tolerance test. *Diabetes*, **14**, 473

Malone, J. I. (1974). Juvenile diabetes and acute pancreatitis. *J. Pediat.*, **85**, 825

Oakley, W. G. (1968). *Clinical Diabetes and its Biochemical Basis*. Ed. W. G. Oakley, D. A. Pyke and K. W. Taylor, p. 253. Oxford; Blackwell

REFERENCES

Pildes, Rosita S. (1973). Adult-onset diabetes mellitus in childhood. *Metabolism*, **22**, 307
Pond, Helen M. (1971). Diabetes mellitus. In *Recent Advances in Paediatrics*. Ed. D. Gairdner and D. Hull, p. 317. London; J. and A. Churchill
Pond, Helen M. and Oakley, W. G. (1968). Diabetes in children. In *Clinical Diabetes and its Biochemical Basis*. Ed. W. G. Oakley, D. A. Pyke and K. W. Taylor, p. 590. Oxford; Blackwell
Pyke, D. A. (1968). Diagnostic tests. *ibid.* p. 284
Rosenberg, S. A., Brief, D. K., Kinney, J. M., Herrera, M. G., Wilson, R. E. and Moore, F. D. (1965). The syndrome of dehydration, coma and severe hypoglycaemia without ketosis in patients convalescing from burns. *New Eng. J. Med.* **272**, 931
Spirer, Z., Weisman, J., Yurman, S. and Bogair, N. (1974). Hyperglycaemia and convulsions in children. *Arch. Dis. Childh.*, **49**, 811
Stephenson, J. B. P. (1971). Uraemia as a determinant of convulsions in acute infantile hypernatraemia. *Arch. Dis. Childh.*, **46**, 676
Stevenson, R. E. and Bowyer, F. P. (1970). Hyperglycaemia with hyperosmolal dehydration in non-diabetic infants. *J. Pediat.*, **77**, 818
Tattersall, R. B. (1974). Mild familial diabetes with dominant inheritance. *Quart. J. Med.*, **43**, 339
Tattersall, R. B. and Fajans, S. S. (1975). A difference between the inheritance of classical juvenile onset and maturity onset type of diabetes of young people. *Diabetes*, **24**, 44
Valerio, D. (1976). Acute diabetic abdomen in childhood. *Lancet*, **I**, 66

CHAPTER 2

Strictness, Liberality and Control

> Prophecy is the most gratuitous form of error.
> George Eliot, *Middlemarch*.

> The dead hand pushes all of us into intellectual cages; there is in all of us a strange tendency to yield and have done.
> H. L. Mencken, Introduction to *In Defence of Women*.

Some years ago there appeared on television a middle-aged human male who was pleased to accept the description of 'typical football hooligan'. 'Yes', he said, 'that's right, you could call me a hooligan, yes.' When asked about the need for violence he explained, 'Well, this chap next to me says Smith is playing well and I say he's not, and if he says the same again, well, you can't go any further, you just put the boot in.' This is reminiscent of the attitude which was once discernible in the more rabid supporters of either strict or liberal regimes in the treatment of childhood diabetes. The two camps now seem to have gone some way towards settling their differences, and not before time. It seems appropriate to discuss the matter here, as obviously the writer's own position will be reflected throughout this book.

Advocates of a strict regime based their case largely on the importance of avoiding diabetic complications in later life. To bring this about they recommended a diet controlled in protein, fat and carbohydrate supplemented by frequent injections of short-acting insulin, often given on a sliding scale based on pre-prandial urine sugar results. The first priority was to prevent the blood sugar rising above normal, and if it did it was to be hammered down again instantly. It was natural that these ideas should hold sway in the years after the introduction of insulin. Here was a new drug, almost miraculous in its effect, which turned night into day. 'Who wants a vacation', asked Joslin in 1924, 'when he can watch mere ghosts of children start to grow, play and make a noise and see their mothers smile again?' Entrusted with insulin, it was a doctor's duty to use it to the full. When he did so, complications no longer appeared in childhood. We now forget that in the 1920s arteriosclerosis was common in diabetic *children*. It was not seen before then as diabetic children died within days of diagnosis. In 1932 Joslin wrote (in his foreword to Priscilla White's book *Diabetes in Childhood and Adolescence)* 'This small volume . . . brings hope to the diabetic adult by its story of the rise and fall of arteriosclerosis in the child. Today, hardening of the arteries, which caused concern in children five years ago, appears only in the neglected or inadequately treated boy or girl. Using the same methods ... can we not defer the premature appearance of this complication in adults?' Had we been doctors then we would all have shouted 'Yes!' and applied ourselves to the strict control of our diabetics. Now we are not so sure.

The history of diet for diabetic children is one of steadily diminishing restriction. In the pre-insulin era, Naunyn prescribed for all diabetics a carbohydrate-free diet, replacing the carbohydrate with fat. Allen recommended a period of complete starvation, followed by a diet designed to produce undernutrition. Joslin paid particular attention to the manner of lowering the calorie intake, cutting down first on fat to the point of elimination, then on protein and lastly on carbohydrate. Before insulin was discovered children were maintained for their short lives on a very low carbohydrate diet, and it is natural that this regime persisted into the insulin era, but children so treated did not grow properly. There was then a tendency to allow more carbohydrate, but protein and fat were also watched and a target of so many calories a day was set, involving a definite amount of the three main constituents and a balance of the ketogenic: antiketogenic ratio. Some older readers may remember how these principles were enshrined in the Lawrence Line diet, which was popular in Britain in the late 1940s.

I quote one example of the seriously over-treated diabetic child. This was a little American boy whose father was serving at the submarine depot ship in the Holy Loch, and 'little' is the operative word. He was half a head shorter than his younger brother and he looked pale, listless and miserable. He was having three injections of insulin daily if he was lucky, four if his evening urine showed sugar. The danger of such a regime is its tendency to produce subclinical hypoglycaemia with its attendant irritability and misery and a failure in growth. An adult who has been changed from a strict to a liberal regime may tell of the sudden upsurge in well-being. I therefore proposed to admit this lad at the end of the week, but he did not come. When I followed this up, his father said that he was going to Hawaii forthwith. I am used to my patients fleeing across the border to England, but this was going too far!

Diabetic dwarfism was common among children at one time, due to either a diet too restrictive to allow growth or so restrictive that the parents did not keep to it, so that the child had too much carbohydrate without adequate insulin cover. It should be remembered that diabetic dwarfism was commonest at a time when medium and long-acting insulins had not been introduced, so a change from a depot insulin to soluble insulin was not necessarily effective. Hamne (1962), who seasons a paper on growth with pleasing tales from the past, tells us that when Engels took over the diabetics of Falun in 1943 he was amazed by the number of diabetic dwarfs he found, all being theoretically on a very restricted diet, which they all seemed to be ignoring. Very restricted diets defeat their own ends.

It was children such as these who gave rise to the idea that a more liberal approach to control might be better. Supporters of the liberal regime drew attention to normal growth and normal psychological maturation as being just as important as, if not more important than, the amount of sugar passed in the urine.

Jackson and Guthrie (1972), writing from a clinic where control could be classed as strict, state that the major difference between their clinic and some others is that insulin is given as often as necessary to attain and maintain good control. This means that at least two doses of medium-acting insulin will be needed if the child is to eat as other children do. Here is an example of strictness in one respect (insulin injections) allowing liberality in another (diet), which emphasizes that the difference between strictness and liberality is not simply that between black and white. Another feature of the 'strict' clinic is frequent urine testing, done about four times daily. The liberal view is that this might encourage obsessionalism, and that two tests are adequate for most purposes.

Murthy and Jackson (1974) stress that their regime *permits* normal growth, which few would dispute, but their regime includes 'using high quality food, and intensive education of the parent and child', which would exclude a number of Glasgow cases, as there are variables to be considered. At some clinics the patients come mainly from the middle class and have cooperative parents, at others the socio-economic background is much poorer. Physicians at the first type of clinic are striving to convert 'fair' to 'good', at the second to convert 'bad' to 'fair', and this may to a certain extent give them a difference in outlook. This is not, however, a difference in principle, as both are aiming at as good control as is possible in the circumstances.

Another hindrance to final understanding is the difficulty in reporting on complications in relation to control. One can use a simple model, such as shown in *Figure 2.1*. The only debate is about how many of those with fair control develop complications. However, it can be argued that such debate is sterile, as the model is too simple and should really be more like that shown in *Figure 2.2*, where the broken lines represent areas of uncertainty. However, it would be very difficult to produce convincing results using the second model, so the debate is likely to continue, which is no bad thing. All can agree on the fundamental view, that all cases must be treated with enthusiasm and the desire to do one's best.

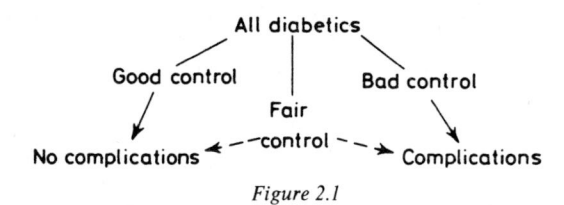

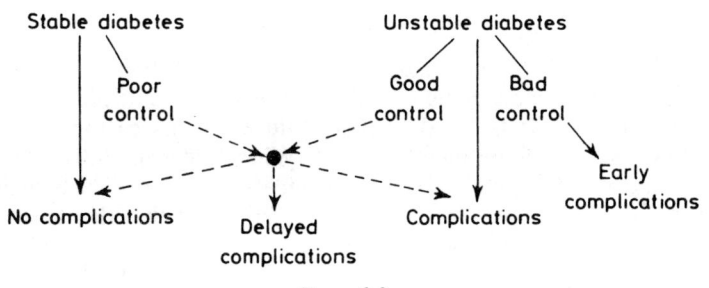

Figure 2.1

Figure 2.2

DIET

Limited carbohydrate is the diet most commonly used. The daily carbohydrate intake is measured according to the child's age, using the formula

100 or 110 + 10 × age in years = the daily requirement of carbohydrate in g.

Thus a three-year-old gets 130–140 g, a seven-year-old 170–180 g and so on, up to about 220–230 g per day. Protein and fat are allowed free, i.e. unmeasured. Exponents of the limited carbohydrate diet argue that the irregular and sometimes excessive intake of carbohydrate, often as sugar (which is allowed by the completely free diet) will at times involve a very sharp rise in blood sugar, will interfere with the utilization of the exogenous insulin and will thus cause instability of the diabetes and frequent ketosis, particularly in the insulin-dependent diabetes of childhood. The intake of carbohydrate, they say, should be moderate and evenly spread through the day as three main meals buffered by three snacks. The patient is, of course, allowed extra carbohydrate to cover unusual exercise.

The usual meaning of *free diet* is that not even carbohydrate need be measured, but that sugar, jam and sweets should not be taken and meals should still be given at regular times. Isaaksen is quoted by Hamne as finding that if he ordered diets of 150–180 g carbohydrate, what left the kitchen was 108–214 g and what was consumed was 50–195 g per day, which made nonsense of prescribing precise diets. Most of us have seen instances of a child being given an incorrect amount of carbohydrate* at a meal in hospital, but the conscientious parent may at times be more reliable than the hospital where a chain of many links is involved in getting a child's food from the kitchen to his table. Indeed, some children on a free diet may be more regular in their carbohydrate intake than others who are theoretically on limited carbohydrate. Might it not at least be more realistic to put children on a free diet? If the child is not restricted in his diet, might he not cooperate better with other restrictions necessary in his management, and might he not become independent sooner if he feels he is like other children in his eating habits? Opposition to such notions was brisk. When Söderling advocated a free diet (which he did in 1935) Tillgren, at a meeting of the Swedish Medical Association, exclaimed 'It is to be hoped that this business of free diet is only a case of an infant malady in the paediatricians themselves. There is then a chance that it will cure itself'. That is what is meant by 'putting the boot in'.

The *completely free diet* expects that regular meals will be taken, but allows the child sugar, jam, sweets, etc. The argument seems to be that if one is prepared to go as far as the free diet, why not go the whole hog and let the child be *really* like other children? This leads to consideration of the *high carbohydrate diet*. In the Indian subcontinent, for example, socio-economic and religious factors may dictate that an adequate calorie intake can only be obtained if the

---

* One patient recently told of a dramatic tug-of-war he had had over his plate with an auxiliary helper who was crying 'But you're a *diabetic*! You're not allowed to *eat*!' A less determined child might have given in and left his physicians wondering why he had been hypoglycaemic overnight.

carbohydrate intake is 300–400 g per day. In requirements of insulin or oral antidiabetic drugs these patients seem to differ little from Western diabetics. Is such a diet too low in bulk for Western intestines? But would vascular complications be less if the intake of protein and fat is low? These questions are still under debate (Bierman et al., 1971), and there has recently been a considerable swing in views on the diabetic diet. A much more detailed consideration of the diabetic diet will be found in Chapter 13.

It will be seen elsewhere (p. 59) that I am prepared to allow a free diet if I think it desirable, but this would not be given at the outset of treatment. The main indication for allowing a free diet seems to me that the child, though reasonably stable, appears to be almost obsessional about his diabetes; to be taking it too much to heart. Others allow free diet when social conditions are bad and the mother seems lacking in intelligence. This is reasonable enough (if they cannot manage limited carbohydrate, why prescribe it?) but I like to persevere with limited carbohydrate for these cases in the hope that I will, at least, get across the idea of regular meals. The same parent of limited intellect is apt to translate the suggestion of a free diet as 'The doctor said it did not matter what he ate or when, and I suppose it doesn't matter much about this insulin either'.

Insulin

Having a liberal attitude to the use of insulin means that one tries to give as few injections to children as possible. All, whether strict or liberal, would agree that insulin should be given often enough and in sufficient quantities to keep the blood sugar reasonably controlled; but argument would then develop on the meaning of the word 'reasonably'. This is a matter of opinion rather than fact, for which reason argument is likely to become all the more heated. The physician using one morning injection of Lente insulin (IZS) is prepared to accept that there will be post-prandial hyperglycaemia, but thinks this relatively unimportant if the daily urine sugar loss is less than 50 g. Agreement probably also exists on the general proposition that there are two main considerations in deciding on a regime for the diabetic child:

(1) his immediate welfare;
(2) his protection against long-term complications.

The physician with a liberal attitude argues that one should concentrate on the first point as there is no known way of ensuring that the second consideration can be met. All are agreed that the very badly controlled diabetic is heading for complications at an early age, and even the liberal physician does not countenance very bad control unless he thinks the child is virtually uncontrollable, due to unstable diabetes, mental inadequacy and/or a poor environment. Quite apart from its relation to future complications, very bad control detracts from the child's immediate welfare, the liberal's main concern.

A few years ago the liberals were walking very tall, sometimes jostling strict controllers off the sidewalk. It had been demonstrated (Siperstein, Unger and Madison, 1968) that significant thickening of the basement membrane of capillaries occurs in early diabetes and also in pre-diabetes (potential diabetes, in the British usage). If vascular changes had appeared before hyperglycaemia, surely these changes and the subsequent vascular degeneration must be independent of insulin lack, though perhaps genetically related to it? If so, why bother about strict control? The situation is, however, now more complicated than it was because some (Osterby-Hansen, 1970) have moved the direct negative and have said that the changes appear not before but after the onset of clinical diabetes; and others (Ireland, Patnaick and Duncan, 1967) have found similar changes in the type of secondary diabetes associated with haemochromatosis and chronic pancreatitis. The difference of opinion may arise from the technical difficulties involved in measuring minute structures which are not perfectly cylindrical. Such studies have not yet produced definite justification for either the strict or the liberal regime.

Control

I have written about 'good control' and have implied that it is not solely a matter of the level of sugar in the blood. In fact, it is now generally accepted that 'good control' is imaginary and we delude ourselves if we think control is ever better than barely adequate, a view which can be fitted in to the arguments on both sides of the strictness–liberality debate. Control is difficult to define and certainly cannot be classified by a single parameter, though this is sometimes done (for example by selecting the 24-hour urine sugar output) in seeking objectivity in a clinical study. My own definition of satisfactory control is that:

(1) the sugar in the urine is not constantly high;
(2) hypoglycaemia is infrequent;
(3) ketosis is absent;

(4) the child is happy at home and mixing well at school;
(5) the child is growing and maturing normally.

It is useful, however, to have in one's mind some figures. The standards used at the Joslin Clinic, as quoted by Priscilla White (1965), are given in *Table 2.1*.

TABLE 2.1

Standard of diabetic control in use in the Joslin Clinic (White, 1965)

Standard	Level of control			
	Perfect	Good	Fair	Poor
Hyperglycaemia, before meals	0	0	++	++++
Hyperglycaemia, after meals	0	+	++	++++
Urine glucose, g/24 hours	0	0–25	25–50	>100
Hypercholesterolaemia	0	0	0	++
Urine acetone	0	0	0—TR	++++
Growth	N	N	Satis	Retarded
Activity potential	N	N	Satis	Diminished

It would be pointless to go through the literature picking out variations from these standards. Some, for example, will accept a daily sugar loss as high as 60 g as satisfactory, but variations are really only a matter of terminology. All know that a loss of 25 g is better than a loss of 100 g. Differences simply depend on where one draws the lines to make the subdivisions, and what labels one puts on these subdivisions. Priscilla White (1965) puts the matter clearly and authoritatively when she says that today the only difference between strict and liberal control lies in whether we insist on 'good' as a level of control or whether we will also regard 'fair' as satisfactory; which is surely nothing to get red in the face about.

The trouble with my patients is that some of them never stay in one class of control for more than a day at a time. Author's licence is claimed for that statement, but it is certainly true that they have good spells and bad spells. Does one average this out and say they are moderately well controlled? This seems to me to be quite unjustified, because for all I know the very worst thing for a diabetic is to have good spells and bad spells*.

The difficulty in classifying control is reflected in our lack of precise knowledge of the relationship between control and complications. We know that the very bad are unduly prone to the early appearance of complications, but many believe that the results of fair control are as satisfactory as those of good control. This argues in favour of a liberal regime, but argument may persist for some time as it is ethically impossible to plan a properly controlled prospective study of the factors contributing to complications, and it is also difficult to carry out a retrospective study with an acceptable degree of accuracy. Those who wish to follow this debate further would do well to read the papers of Cahill, Etzwiler and Freinkel (1976) and Siperstein *et al.* (1977), together with the mediatory editorial by Ingelfinger (1977).

CONCLUSIONS

It will probably have been realized from the general trend of this discussion that, in the following pages, the scales will be tilted towards the liberal side. Basically, I use the limited carbohydrate diet but break the rules for some patients. I do not allow free sugar except in special circumstances. I doubt if it is as easy to get parents to adhere to a strict diet as it once was. Thirty years ago they could remember friends or relatives who had died because there was no such thing as insulin, and they were therefore ready to do what the doctor told them. Now the prognosis is recognized as relatively good and emphasis is (correctly) laid on the diabetic leading a normal life, so that parents may regard some laxity of control as excusable. I suspect it is easier to get them to cooperate if one's standards are not too strict. This is, of course, only theory, but I think it should be made clear as it has played some part in the evolution of my attitude towards childhood diabetes.

MONITORING CONTROL

In the past, the main standard of diabetic control has been the amount of sugar in the urine. Random blood sugars may have been done, but essentially the real regulator of insulin dosage was glycosuria. Now, with the introduction of meters for measuring blood

---

* An analogy might be that intermittent dieting producing a fluctuating weight is a bad thing for obese mice. They die sooner than if left fat.

sugar in the home, with glycosylated haemoglobin being recognised as a valuable index of long-term control and with the continuous monitoring in hospital of a wide field of biochemistry, it has become apparent that traditional methods are at best inadequate, at worst misleading (Malone et al., 1976). Blood sugars may swing violently from hour to hour, which invalidates the single random test, and urine sugar tests may swing from blue to orange with a rise of as little as 1.7 mmol/l (30 mg per cent) in the blood glucose. The traditional tests are useful but they must not be allowed to dominate completely our efforts to obtain optimal control. Apart from the more general parameters of control (growth, physical and mental well-being, freedom from severe hypoglycaemia and the symptoms of diabetes) there are now available more accurate estimates of glycaemia. These methods will now be discussed.

Glycosylated haemoglobin

Sugar in contact with haemoglobin produces a compound known as HbA_1, which is present in normal blood because normal blood contains glucose. This in turn has been subdivided into a-, b- and c-fractions, the ratio of the three remaining constant whatever the level of total HbA_1, and the c-fraction being much the largest. The papers by Gonen et al. (1977) and Williams and Savage (1979) are concerned with HbA_1, those of Tze, Thompson and Leichter (1978) and Heinze et al. (1979) with HbA_{1c}. The estimation of HbA_1 is the easier, and is coming into general use.

The high blood level of glucose in diabetes produces a high level of HbA_1. The particular value of estimating HbA_1 is that it gives a moderately long-term picture of control, indicating what has been happening over the previous two months, because glycosylated haemoglobin is stable and linked to the life-span of the red cell. It is independent of hour-to-hour and day-to-day variations in glycaemia, but correlates with a general impression of control, with growth and with glycosuria and glycaemia *provided they are measured over a long period.*

The bald statements of the preceding paragraph are not completely valid. Leslie et al. (1979) found some patients in whom the level of HbA_1 altered significantly in weeks rather than months and suggested that the test should be done repeatedly to be of real value. Svendsen et al. (1979) consider the test valid when used to compare groups, the difference between good and bad control being clear-cut; whereas it is not valid in the 'moderate control' group where the level of HbA_1 did not always correspond with the degree of control suggested by other measurements. This may fit with the suggestion of Leslie et al. that more than one estimate of HbA_1 is necessary. Figures for HbA_1 may vary slightly with the method used. The method commonly used in the UK (BioRad) gives a normal range of HbA_1 in non-diabetics of 5.5–9 per cent of the total haemoglobin. Levels under 10 per cent indicate good control, over 15 per cent bad control.

A boy of eight years attended the clinic regularly in the two months after diabetes was diagnosed. He was in partial remission, needing only 6 units of Retard in the day. He then defaulted and we did not get him back for 11 months despite letters to his mother and the family doctor and visits by social workers. When at last we did get him back he had heavy glycosuria and acetonuria, had gained only 2 cm in height and had *lost* 1 kg in weight. He was still on his 6 units of Retard. His HbA_1 was 21.4 per cent. The highest reading we have had in patients we have considered to be very badly controlled at the clinic is 15.6 per cent. This indicates that even when one is near despair about a patient (doctor and child both doing badly) one should not give up, as the clinic is giving them *something*.

Gale, Walford and Tattersall (1979) point out that HbA_1 may sometimes be misleading. A patient may be badly controlled because he is hyperglycaemic by day and hypoglycaemic by night, yet the two extremes combine to give an average 'satisfactory' figure for HbA_1.

The estimation of glycosylated haemoglobin appears to be a very promising way of indicating the general level of control over a period of weeks or months, but as yet we do not know enough to use this tool with absolute precision. Its limitation is that although it tells us that something is wrong it does not tell us *what* is wrong, which is where the home monitoring of blood sugar and the use of the 24-hour fractional urine test come in.

Monitoring blood sugar in the home

Various small machines are now available for estimating blood glucose, and they can be used in the home (Sönksen, Judd and Lowy, 1978; Walford *et al.*, 1978). Their accuracy has been discussed by Ross and Borthwick, (1979). The appearance of a figure for blood glucose as illuminated digits has a certain excitement about it; one could even run family sweepstakes on the results. If the user can be taught to correlate the results of several tests each day with insulin, meals and exercise there is a good hope of improved diabetic control, not so much because of the gadgetry *per se* but because of the patient's increased interest in his diabetes and the feeling that he is getting on top of it.

Unfortunately, the apparatus is difficult for children to use, as we have found by trial on the wards. The technique must be precise, particularly in timing. Children under 12 seldom understand much about diabetes (p. 85), and it is necessary for the child himself to understand the significance of the results to obtain full benefit from the method; being told what to do by a parent is not very likely to increase his interest. It appears that a new system less liable to operator-error and still quite cheap will soon be on the market, and when that happens a further effort to involve child diabetics can be made. For the present, profiles in hospital are employed as second-best.

The 24-hour fractional urine test

There is a difference of opinion about the value and relevance of estimating the amount of sugar passed in a 24-hour period. Some use the estimation as their main standard of control. Others, and until recently I was one of them, say that the collection imposes artificial conditions which make the answer unreal. Thus, if the collection is being made at home the child and his parents are on their best diabetic behaviour, whereas if he is in hospital the result is irrelevant to his diabetic state at home. However, Forman, Golstein and Genel (1974) reviewed the value of the 24-hour fractional quantitative urine glucose test (which had previously been described but had never found general acceptance) and concluded that it was a useful test. I have since used the test myself and now agree with Forman and his colleagues.

The urine is collected throughout a 24-hour period. It is divided into four fractions, urine passed from 0800 to 1200 hours, 1200 to 1600 hours, 1600 to 2000 hours and 2000 to 0800 hours. If the overnight urine is not passed until, say, 0815 hours it is included with the overnight specimen and not with the 0800 to 1200 hours collection. If a child's day begins, for example, at 0700 hours, all the quoted times should be brought forward an hour. The child should be asked to pass urine at the end of each collection period. The volume of each of the four specimens is measured, the percentage content of sugar is determined (preferably in the laboratory, but a rough estimate can be obtained in the side-room) and the total loss of sugar in g in each collection can be worked out. It is possible to carry out the test on a child at home. If this is done the mother is asked to bring a note of the volume of each urine collection, but she need only bring an aliquot of each specimen in four universal containers to each of which two drops of benzoic acid have been added.

The examples given by Forman, Golstein and Genel demonstrate clearly the value of the test, and are quoted here with permission.

Example 1

Time of specimen	Vol. (ml)	Total glucose (g)
0800–1200	113	4.0
1200–1600	135	0.0
1600–2000	240	1.3
2000–0800	480	6.2

Comment: A total daily loss of 11.5g is completely acceptable. There is no need to increase insulin. But both morning and evening sugar percentages would have been high, suggesting that an increase in insulin would be indicated. The family doctor had been increasing insulin inappropriately because of morning glycosuria and acetonuria, presumably a Somogyi effect (p. 115).

Example 2

Time of specimen	Vol. (ml)	Total glucose (g)
0800–1200	460	27.2
1200–1600	120	0.2
1600–2000	10	0
2000–0800	870	35.8

On NPH 40 units and soluble 5. Main point is that the volume of the third specimen is so small that very little sugar in it would have suggested the need to raise NPH. Family doctor had in fact reached NPH 120, Sol 10 before admission. This was not satisfactory. Patient could have another dose of soluble at night, or Lente or two doses of NPH. The high dose given at home was a response to afternoon glycosuria, which was probably also a manifestation of the Somogyi effect.

Example 3

Time of specimen	Vol. (ml)	Total glucose (g)
0800–1200	1020	108.0
1200–1600	960	101.0
1600–2000	420	39.8
2000–0800	720	65.5

Atrocious control. Child denied symptoms (could be due to large bladder). On Semilente-Ultralente mixture. SL to be increased more than UL (note gross loss of sugar between 0800 and 1600). All specimens show about 10 per cent sugar, which would not bring out the particular need for SL. This case was investigated because her denial of symptoms was belied by plateaux in height and weight.

Example 4

0800–1200	240	1.3	On Lente.
1200–1600	No spec.	0	Both pre-breakfast and pre-tea specimens would give sugar readings of over 2 per cent on simple testing. The need, however, is not for an increase of Lente alone but for the addition of Ultralente.
1600–2000	1800	55.8	
2000–0800	960	30.7	

A disadvantage of the test is that some diabetics show considerable day-to-day variation. Levinsky, Trompeter and Grant (1976) found good correlation between two collections from the same child, separated by a month or two. The apparent disagreement between these two statements may be due to the fact that I have used the test mainly on patients doing badly, rather than on those doing well.

A doubt may arise as to whether a full 24-hour specimen of urine has been obtained, and for this reason the daily output of creatinine should be measured at the same time as the sugar. It is accepted that the daily output of creatinine is at least 15 mg/kg body weight/day, and a figure less than this indicates that a full 24-hour specimen has not been obtained. In practice, I feel safer using a figure of 18 mg/kg/day.

Occasionally one has a pleasant surprise.

One boy seemed well but had consistently high urine sugars as shown by the five-drop test. He was admitted to investigate the possibility of renal glycosuria, but this proved to be unnecessary. His four urine collections showed 1.2, 1.6, 1.7 and 1.8 per cent sugar, which appeared as one reading of 1 per cent and three of 2 per cent, yet his total loss for the 24 hours was less than 20 g. If one stops to think that 2 per cent of a litre of urine is only 20 g one realises how unhelpful the five-drop test may be.

The 24-hour fractional test may show *when* control is worst and insulin can be adjusted accordingly, but a consistently high output during the day raises the possibility of overtreatment and/or emotional factors being involved.

Infusion pumps and hospital monitoring

A pump may be used to control the constant infusion of insulin, with added boluses to cover meals, and good results have been obtained from the subcutaneous route (Pickup *et al.*, 1979; Tamborlane *et al.*, 1979a and b) as well as the intravenous. At present this can only be regarded as a research project to be carried out in hospitals with sophisticated laboratories. A spin-off of interest to all clinicians, however, is the way this method can demonstrate control of lipid and amino acid as well as carbohydrate metabolism. For example, Alberti, Dornhorst and Rowe (1975) have suggested that diurnal levels of growth hormone and the alanine/pyruvate ratio may be better indicators of diabetic control than the blood sugar. Such observations have no practical application at present, but indicate clearly that in the days when we claimed to control diabetes by observing only meals, exercise and urine sugar we were groping in the fog: however I still do my share of groping!

Hepatomegaly

The clinical and x-ray assessment of liver size may be taken as an indicator of overall diabetic control during a period rather longer than that indicated by HbA_1 estimations. Serial readings are of most value. The significance of hepatomegaly is discussed later in the chapter on complications.

ENVOI

I should like to end this chapter with a plea for better understanding. It may be true that the man who expects strict control drives the difficult cases away from his clinic (while some of the others are diet-breaking on the sly), and it may be true that those of us who accept moderate glycosuria are idly allowing our patients to drift into mortal danger, but both sides should accept that they are trying to work towards the same end, a healthy adult. Let us look for similarities as well as differences for each has something to learn from the other.

REFERENCES

Alberti, K. G. M. M., Dornhorst, A. and Rowe, A. S. (1975). Metabolic rhythms in normal and diabetic man. In *Contemporary topics in the study of diabetes and metabolic endocrinology*. Ed. Shafrir, E. New York and London; Academic Press
Bierman, E. L. (1971) on behalf of a committee. Principles of nutrition and dietary recommendations for patients with diabetes mellitus. *Diabetes*, **20**, 633

REFERENCES 35

Cahill, G. F., Etzwiler, D. D. and Freinkel, N. (1976). Control and diabetes. *New Engl. J. Med.*, **294**, 1004

Forman, B. H., Golstein, P. S. and Genel, M. (1974). Management of juvenile diabetes mellitus: usefulness of 24-hour fractional quantitative urine glucose. *Pediatrics*, **53**, 257

Gale, E. A. M., Walford, S. and Tattersall, R. B. (1979). Nocturnal hypoglycaemia and Haemoglobin A_1. *Lancet*, **II**, 1240

Gonen, B., Rubenstein, A. H., Rochman, H., Tanega, S. P. and Horwitz, D. L. (1977). Hemoglobin A_1: an indicator of the metabolic control of diabetic patients. *Lancet*, **II**, 734

Hamne, B., (1962). Growth in a series of diabetic children on identical treatment with 'free diet' and insulin, 1944–60. *Acta paediat.*, **51**, Suppl. 135, 72

Heinze, E., Kohne, E., Meissner, C., Beischer, W., Teller, W. M. and Kleihauer, E. (1979). Hemoglobin A_{1c} in children with long standing and newly diagnosed diabetes mellitus. *Acta paediat. scand.*, **68**, 609

Ingelfinger, F. J. (1977). Debates on Diabetes. *New Engl. J. Med.*, **296**, 1228

Ireland, J. T., Patnaik, B. K. and Duncan, L. J. P. (1967). Glomerular ultrastructure in secondary diabetics and normal subjects. *Diabetes*, **16**, 628

Jackson, R. L. and Guthrie, R. A. (1972). The child with diabetes. *Missouri Medicine*, **69**, 351

Joos, T. H. and Johnston, J. A. (1957). A long-term evaluation of the juvenile diabetic. *J. Pediat.*, **50**, 133

Joslin, E. P. (1924). *The Treatment of Diabetes Mellitus*, 3rd ed. p. vi. London; Henry Kimpton

Leslie, R. D. G., Pyke, D. A., John, P. N. and White, J. M. (1979). Fast glycosylation of haemoglobin. *Lancet*, **I**, 773.

Leslie, R. D. G., Pyke, D. A., John, P. N. and White, J. M. (1979). 'How quickly can HbA_1 increase?' *Br. med. J.*, **II**, 19

Levinsky, R. J., Trompeter, R. S. and Grant, D. B. (1976). 24-hour urinary glucose excretion in assessment of control in juvenile diabetes mellitus. *Arch. Dis. Childh.*, **51**, 463

Malone, J. I., Hellrung, J. M., Malphus, E. W., Rosenbloom, A. L., Grgic, A. and Weber, F. T. (1976). Good diabetic control—a study in mass delusion. *J. Pediat.*, **88**, 943

Murthy, D. Y. N. and Jackson, R. L. (1974). Growth in diabetic children. *Lancet*, **I**, 736

Osterby-Hansen, R. O. (1970). Electron microscopic study of glomeruli from young patients with short duration of diabetes; the mesangial region. *Diabetologia*, **6**, 59

Pickup, J. C., Keen, H., Parsons, J. A., Alberti, K. G. M. M. and Rowe, A. S. (1979). Continuous subcutaneous insulin infusion: improved blood glucose and intermediary-metabolic control in diabetics. *Lancet*, **I**, 1255

Ross, I. S. and Borthwick, J. L. (1979). Performance of home blood-glucose meters. *Lancet*, **II**, 257. (refers to previous correspondence)

Siperstein, M. D., Foster, D. W., Knowles, H. C., Levine, R., Madison, L. L. and Roth, J. (1977). Control of blood glucose and diabetic vascular disease. *New Engl. J. Med.*, **296**, 1060

Siperstein, M. D., Unger, R. H. and Madison, L. L. (1968). Studies of muscle capillary basement membranes in normal subjects, diabetic and prediabetic patients. *J. clin. Invest.*, **47**, 1973

Sönksen, P. H., Judd, S. L. and Lowy, C. (1978) Home monitoring of blood-glucose. *Lancet*, **I**, 730

Svendsen, P. A., Christiansen, J. S., Andersen, A. R., Welinder, B. and Nerup, J. (1979). Fast glycosylation of haemoglobin. *Lancet*, **I**, 1143

Tamborlane, W. V., Sherwin, R. S., Genel, M. and Felig, P. (1979a). Reduction to normal of plasma glucose in juvenile diabetes by subcutaneous administration of insulin with a portable infusion pump. *New Engl. J. Med.*, **300,** 573

Tamborlane, W. V., Sherwin, R. S., Genel, M. and Felig, P. (1979b). Restoration of normal lipid and amino acid metabolism in diabetic patients treated with a portable infusion pump. *Lancet*, **I,** 1258

Tze, W. J., Thompson, K. H. and Leichter, J. (1978). HbA_{1c}: an indicator of diabetic control. *J. Pediat.*, **93,** 13

Walford, S., Gale, E. A. M., Allison, S. P. and Tattersall, R. B. (1978). Self-monitoring of blood-glucose. *Lancet*, **I,** 732

White, Priscilla (1965). The child with diabetes. *Med. Clin. North Am.*, **49,** 1069

Williams, M. L. and Savage, D. C. L. (1979). Glycosylated haemoglobin levels in children with diabetes mellitus. *Arch. Dis. Childh.*, **54,** 295

CHAPTER 3

The First Admission

In this chapter the management of a diabetic child who is not acutely ill will be considered up to the time he is discharged from the ward. The management of ketoacidosis will be considered in a separate chapter. It will be assumed that the patient has been diagnosed early, that his blood sugar is around 17–28 mmol/l (300–500 mg per cent), that his urine shows only one or two pluses of acetone, that no weight loss is apparent to a new observer and that he has walked into the ward. There is time to take stock.

The first day

Assuming he has not been admitted in the evening there is no reason to put the mild diabetic to bed. His surroundings will more quickly become familiar and his apprehension will be more quickly stilled if he is allowed to wander round the ward. He can have the normal ward diet. It is better to withhold insulin so that an untreated fasting urine and blood sugar can be obtained the following morning. During the first day all urine specimens are tested for sugar and ketones. Although it may not be strictly necessary in the mild diabetic, blood should be taken for electrolytes and gases as well as for the blood sugar level. Haemoglobin estimation will be done as a routine, so the PCV can be done as well. These investigations are all essential in the moderately ill diabetic and should be done in the mild case, largely to give a base-line for the study of more serious cases.

Communication with child and parents begins on this first day. This subject is so important that it is given a chapter to itself (Chapter 5).

The initial insulin

Insulin is begun on the morning of the second day, after a fasting blood sugar has been done and before breakfast. It is customary to begin treatment with a short-acting insulin, Actrapid MC or Leo Neutral RI. Schoolchildren can be begun on 10 units subcutaneously three times a day and pre-school children on 6 units three times a day. The physician must be prepared for a rapid modification of this schedule as many children with slight ketosis are very sensitive to insulin. The urine may be clear of sugar by the time the second dose (before the mid-day meal) is due, and that dose could be reduced or omitted altogether. If the urine is still clear by the time of the evening meal, 8 units could then be given instead of 10. It may, however, take two or three days before the dosage can be reduced to two injections a day. Around that time an odd little phenomenon may occur. It might be assumed that if a child's urine has been cleared by 24 units in 24 hours it should stay clear on a smaller dose, perhaps 18 units, but this does not always occur. Indeed, there may be a tendency for insulin requirements to rise in the first few days, and fall slowly thereafter. There appears to be a transient period of resistance to insulin, but why this occurs is uncertain.

While the child is still on soluble insulin the question of deliberately giving him a hypoglycaemic attack has to be considered. The idea is that if a mother has seen a hypo attack being successfully treated she will feel more confident about recognizing and treating such an attack at home. There is no doubt that the fear which dominates home management at first is the fear of hypo attacks, and the mother who has seen a hypo attack being treated in hospital is glad of it, but she prefers the attack to happen by mistake. If she is given the option she is likely to reply, 'Well, I would like to see it, but I don't think I would like you to do it to him.' That is the majority opinion in our Parents' Group. However, the mother may not be the best judge of this situation and it may be unfair to ask her. I myself do not induce hypo attacks, as the day-time attack is usually easily dealt with, but those who induce a hypo attack as a routine are certainly convinced of its value. However, I doubt if even they would give the child a convulsion in the middle of the night, which is what really worries the parents. If a hypo attack is to be induced the usual dose of morning insulin is given and food withheld until the hypo occurs.

An attempt to change to a depot insulin may be made in all except the prepubertal children, who will almost certainly need two injections a day. The timing of the change varies. Acetone should be absent from the urine and the total daily need for soluble insulin should be fairly constant. If the case has gone smoothly, and has not shown an unexpected rise in insulin requirements on the second day of insulin, the change can be made on the third day, but irregularly fluctuating urine sugars would make it advisable to delay a day or two longer. The choice of a depot insulin will be discussed later in this chapter.

Diet

While the patient's initial insulin dosage is being stabilized he is being fed, and it is therefore appropriate to discuss here just how he should be fed. It will be remembered that here we are discussing the child who has walked into the ward, not the ketoacidotic child. The diabetic diet and its rationale are discussed fully in Chapter 13. What is given here is just enough to start the patient on solid food.

I begin on the basis of limited carbohydrate, and ask the dietitian as soon as possible to make an assessment of the child's average daily intake. If the formula (p. 23) says he should have 160 g of carbohydrate daily but he is taking 180 g, then I would give him 180 g unless he were obese. It will often be found that, if sweets (candies) are deleted from his previous intake, the residual carbohydrate will be surprisingly close to what the formula suggests.

Assuming one is prescribing a limited carbohydrate diet, one then has to decide how to divide it up during the day. A diet of 170 g might be divided 30, 20, 40, 20, 40, 20, though some would prescribe more at the main meals and less at the snacks. (If one does so, one is more likely to get a pre-prandial negative reading from the urine.) One principle is to keep breakfast relatively small, because normal children under the age of eight seldom take 'a good breakfast'. However, the scatter of carbohydrate will depend on the type of insulin used. If the child is on two injections of a rapid-acting insulin (which I do not recommend) he may need a bigger breakfast, if on a long-acting insulin he may need relatively more in the evening. Even on soluble insulin I would start our hypothetical mild case on a distribution such as that suggested above, on the grounds that adjustments can be made for hunger if it appears. One other suggestion can be made. Milk (lactose) and some fruit (fructose) or a sweet biscuit may have too short an overnight effect on the blood sugar and increase the risk of hypoglycaemia before breakfast. I like the last snack to be starchy, possibly with a little protein and fat. An egg sandwich would fulfil the requirements, and most children can digest it.

Stabilization

After a few days the diabetic comes under a fair degree of control. The patient cannot, of course, be stabilized until he goes home and leads his normal life. The request 'Please admit for stabilization' should be re-phrased 'Please admit to eradicate gross imbalance'. If one is trying to impress on a diabetic that he is not so very different from others, the shorter the time he is in the hospital the better. The 'I'm going to get this right' brigade, who keep children in for months, are in danger of putting themselves before their patients. One week is ideal, two weeks or more are necessary in most cases. There was a time when it was thought that deliberate overtreatment in hospital for the first few weeks improved the long-term prognosis. I doubt if many hold this view now, and I like to discharge patients as soon as possible, i.e. as soon as the child is stable and the parents understand the management.

LONG-TERM THERAPY AND THE CHOICE OF INSULIN

One can hardly blink these days without another new insulin appearing on the market. In an attempt to guide the reader towards making a choice I shall

(1) consider the length of action of insulin;
(2) discuss short-, medium- and long-acting insulins without differentiating between the old and the new; and
(3) compare the old and new insulins.

Length of action

We may talk of a 'short-acting insulin', but we must remember that there are a number of variables which affect the onset and duration of its action.

The *site of injection* is important. It is well known that injecting into an area of fat hypertrophy can cause irregular absorption of insulin, but so may changing from one apparently undamaged old site to a new one. The paper by Henry *et al.* (1978) stresses how very important this factor may be. In this one patient the half-life of elimination of soluble (regular) insulin from a much-used site was 8.9 hours, from a completely new site 0.9 hours. This is doubtless an extreme example. One cannot even say that use of an old site may convert a short-acting insulin to a medium-acting insulin. In this case it virtually immobilized the insulin altogether.

Exercise may act on the blood sugar in two ways, by increasing the level of insulin and possibly by delaying the emptying of the stomach (Zinman *et al.*, 1978). Furthermore, exercise of a specific part may hasten insulin absorption; for example injecting into a leg and riding a bicycle will give quicker absorption than injecting into a leg and reading a book (Dandona, Hooke and Bell, 1978).

Individual variation may also play a part. Dixon, Exon and Malins (1975) propounded the attractive hypothesis that whereas a lot of insulin antibodies in the blood caused insulin resistance, a few antibodies would cause only 'buffering' which would prolong the action of insulin. Unfortunately (for those who like a good hypothesis) Ortved Andersen (1975) has failed to reproduce the results on which the hypothesis was based. However, it does seem to be an observable fact that the length of action of any one insulin may vary from patient to patient.

Groups of insulins

The insulins in common use in the UK are summarized in *Table 3.1*.

Short-acting insulins are used in the treatment of diabetic ketoacidosis and as routine therapy in combination with a medium-acting insulin. I think that short-acting insulins used two or three times a day as continuing therapy are too likely to cause rapid swings in blood glucose, which can predispose to the Somogyi phenomenon (p. 115). Mauriac's syndrome (dwarfism, hepatomegaly and some Cushingoid features) was common in the early days of insulin, becoming much rarer when the first long-acting insulin (PZI) was introduced. If a child goes out of control on one injection of a depot insulin the answer, as far as I am concerned, is not to put him on two injections of short-acting insulin but to change to two injections of medium-acting insulin, possibly introducing a little short-acting insulin later, either as an addition to the medium-acting insulin or as a substitute for part of it. There are exceptions. I remember one girl who did better on two small injections of soluble insulin than on two larger injections of Rapitard (which I used more often then than now), but it is better to start with the rule rather than the exception.

Semilente and Semitard are neither short- nor medium-acting, the duration of action falling between the two. Semilente was frequently given mixed with Lente, and indeed several of my patients who have been diabetic for many years are still on that mixture. Even those are being changed to the newer insulins if they become

TABLE 3.1
A list of the insulins in common use in the UK, to which a list of synonyms is appended

Action	Duration in hours (Peak)	Type Old	New
Short	1–8 (3–6)	Soluble Nuso	Actrapid MC Leo Neutral RI
Short-medium	1½–15 (5–9)	Semilente	Semitard MC
Medium	2–24 (4–12)	Lente Isophane Rapitard	Lentard MC Monotard MC Retard RI
Long	4–32 (7–28)	Ultralente PZI	Ultratard MC

Synonyms
Soluble: insulin injection BP, regular, standard
Semilente: insulin zinc suspension (amorphous) BP, prompt IZS, IZSA
Rapitard: biphasic insulin injection BP
Isophane: Isophane insulin NPH BP, NPH (neutral protamine Hagedorn)
Retard and Monotard: pork isophane
Lente: insulin zinc suspension BP, IZS
Ultralente: insulin zinc suspension (crystalline) BP, extended IZS, IZSC
PZI: protamine zinc insulin injection BP.

Note (1) MC and RI insulins are pork, British insulins are beef.
Note (2) Lente is a mixture of 30% Semilente and 70% Ultralente

Lentard is a mixture of 30% Semitard and 70% Ultratard
Two other mixtures are available:
Mixtard is 30% Leo Neutral and 70% Retard
Initard is 50% Leo Neutral and 50% Retard.

Very new insulins
Short
  Hypurine Neutral
  Neusulin
Medium
  Hypurine Isophane
  Neuphane
  Neulente
Long
  Hypurine Protamine Zinc.
All are highly purified beef insulins.

unstable or as they approach their teens. Some use Semilente in combination with a short-acting insulin, usually twice daily, but I have never done so myself. One came my way recently. He had had a severe hypoglycaemic attack at 3 pm and he had a three-finger liver, which surprised me not at all. It is possible that one morning injection of Semitard may control a very young child for a short time during the early stages of his disease. In the pre-school and early school years diabetes is relatively stable, the pancreas retaining the ability to secrete some endogenous insulin and, as the young child does not eat overnight, there may be little or no tendency to hyperglycaemia during the night hours. Even in this group, however, I find that one injection of a medium-acting insulin is likely to give better control.

The *medium-acting insulins* are the rocks on which insulin

therapy is based. One morning injection may suffice during the remission ('honeymoon') period. This may last for months or years, but then insulin requirements will rise and two injections a day are indicated. The level of insulin dose when the change should be made is about 1 unit/kg body weight/day, but this is a rule of thumb which I have myself broken at times. When going to two injections, it is customary to lower the daily total by 10–20 per cent, giving two-thirds in the morning and one-third in the evening, but this is only the starting-point and subsequent changes will be indicated by the urine sugars. As puberty approaches it will almost certainly be necessary to give twice-daily injections of a mixture of short- and medium-acting insulins. The paediatric custom is to begin with another 2:1 ratio, two-thirds of each injection being medium-acting and one-third short-acting. In saying this I am aware that some adult physicians give more of the short- and less of the medium-acting. What has been said applies to the child who becomes diabetic in his early years. Should the onset be at ten or 11 it is probably best to begin right away with two injections.

When one is using *mixed insulins* twice daily, it is necessary, at least for a time, to test the urine four times a day. The short-acting morning insulin is adjusted to the mid-day urine, the medium-acting morning insulin to the late afternoon urine, the short-acting evening insulin to the bed-time urine and the medium-acting evening insulin to the morning urine. It may be possible to drop out one insulin, for example, the evening short-acting if the bed-time urine is consistently free from sugar. Testing four times a day is easy enough in hospital but may be more difficult when the child is back at school, though the mid-day urine can be tested with Diastix.

With intelligent, cooperative and interested parents *and children* it is possible to maintain the four daily tests but usually I try to lessen the burden. This can be done by testing only in the morning and late afternoon, asking the parent to keep the short-acting insulin constant and to adjust the medium-acting one only. They can test four times on occasional days, and the short-acting insulin can be altered at the clinic. This works quite well as long as the diabetes remains under control. The regime may seem too strict and so it may prove with a hostile child, but in practice it may give a compensatory freedom particularly to the teenager whose life varies from day to day and even more from night to night. If he wants to eat more than usual in the early part of the evening and then stay out till 1 am, he can take a little more of his short-acting insulin that evening and rather less of the medium-acting one (Farquhar, 1976).

I doubt if anyone who runs a diabetic clinic is ever very keen to lay down rules on the giving of insulin, there are so many exceptions.

When skimming through the records of the last 200 patients to be discharged from the clinic at the age of 13 years I found that three of them had left us (some years ago) on one morning injection of Semilente. Their morning urine sugars had been satisfactory, so there seemed no real reason to change. Again, I have sometimes found that after changing to twice daily injections the evening injection is gradually cut out again because of consistently clear morning urines, so that the patient goes back to one injection a day, on a lower dose than before and better controlled. Presumably a minor form of second remission has been induced. One simply has to consider each patient as an individual.

Old or new insulin

In making the choice between the older and newer insulins four points may be considered.

(1) Should we use pig or beef insulin, or does it not matter?
(2) What harm is done by the impurities in 'impure' insulin?
(3) Is there any immediate benefit to be seen from one or the other?
(4) Is there any long-term benefit to be hoped for from one or the other?

(1) Many studies have shown that when a change is made from beef to pork insulin the requirement of insulin drops. This is explicable on the grounds that pork insulin is less likely to be immunogenic because pork insulin differs from human insulin in one amino acid, whereas beef differs in three*. Åkerblom and Mäkelä (1978) have shown that children produce antibodies more readily than adults, but that purified insulins produce less than conventional insulins. It is possible, however, for a child to be relatively well controlled with a low level of free insulin in the blood, as the rate of dis-

---

* Guinea-pig insulin differs from human insulin in 15 amino acids. It is believed that guinea pigs never sleep for more than 10 minutes at a time because if they did so in the wild predators would get them. At least they would be safe from insulin manufacturers. Bewick (1829) treated 'The Guinea-Pig or Restless Cavy' with remarkable intolerance.

'Great numbers are kept in a domestic state, but for what purpose can hardly be determined. They have neither beauty nor utility to recommend them; their skins are of little value; and their flesh, though eatable, is far from being good. Their habits and dispositions are equally unpleasant and disgusting: void of attachment even to their own offspring, they suffer them to be devoured the moment they are brought forth. ... They pass their whole lives in sleeping, eating, and in the propagation of their species. They are by nature gentle and tame; they do no mischief, but seem to be equally incapable of good.'

sociation of the antibody–insulin complex and the rate at which cell-receptors take up insulin are other variables.

(2) Proinsulin and desamido-insulins are recognized impurities in conventional insulins, and Bloom *et al.* (1979) have drawn attention to the presence of other pancreatic hormones (glucagon, pancreatic polypeptide, vasoactive intestinal peptide and somatostatin) in these insulins, but not in the new highly purified insulins. These impurities are capable of producing antibodies, an alarming thought when one considers the wide distribution of VIP and somatostatin in the body. There is no evidence that antibodies have yet produced a disaster and some think the risk is over-rated (Pyke, 1978). Proinsulin is also immunogenic. The evidence is academic rather than clinical, but it is enough to turn me against the older insulins.

(3) The established benefits of the purified insulins are that they do not produce lipoatrophy (though they may cause local hypertrophy) and they are less likely to produce local allergy. They are of great value in severe insulin resistance, which is rare.

(4) The long-term benefits of the newer insulins are not established, as indeed they cannot be until they have been used for many more years. They may even have long-term disadvantages, but on a theoretical balance they might be helpful. Nobody likes flies in his soup, and one regards circulating antibodies with similar distaste. Specifically, it has been suggested that insulin antibodies may play a part in producing diabetic microangiopathy.

Another factor that must be considered is cost. The cost factor is to a certain extent offset by the lower doses needed of purified insulin. Our own figures for the relative insulin requirements are given in *Table 3.2*. One caveat must be issued about these figures. The children on the older insulins were treated before those on the newer, and recently we have been paying closer attention to the possibility of over-treatment (p. 117), but it is unlikely that this is a significant factor during the first few months at least. The difference in requirements between the two age-groups, whether on older or newer insulin, stresses the insulin resistance of the prepubertal and pubertal years, and any study on children should be closely controlled for age.

There is a strong majority opinion that children should be treated with the new purified insulins. At our clinic we use Leo Neutral RI and Retard RI and occasionally Semitard MC. Actrapid MC and Monotard MC are doubtless just as good as the first two, but using a

TABLE 3.2

A comparison of the old and the purified insulins in terms of the dose needed

Insulin	Age at onset (years)	Daily dosage in units/kg body weight at various times after diagnosis (numbers)			
		3 months	6 months	1 year	2 years
Older types	Under 9	0.70 (49)	0.86 (47)	0.97 (47)	1.03 (44)
MC or RI	Under 9	0.41 (26)	0.63 (21)	0.76 (11)	0.75 (2)
Older types	9 or over	0.73 (27)	0.98 (29)	1.33 (24)	1.42 (17)
MC or RI	9 or over	0.54 (18)	0.68 (14)	0.84 (10)	1.10 (5)

(Note: Griffin, Smith and Baum (1979) report similar findings, but they are set out differently)

limited number of insulins makes management easier in hospital and clinic.

Insulin for the infant

This subject is dealt with in Chapter 9, after considering neonatal diabetes.

Summary of the insulins

(1) One injection a day of a medium-acting insulin should suffice in the remission period.
(2) One injection of a medium-acting insulin to which a small amount of a short-acting insulin is added may be enough for a time thereafter.
(3) The older child will probably need two injections daily.
(4) Approaching puberty he is likely to need two injections of short- and medium-acting insulins combined. This over-rides (1)–(3) above.

(5) When *beginning* to use medium- and short-acting insulins in combination, give twice as much medium- as short-acting.
(6) When using two injections a day, *begin* with twice as much insulin in the morning as in the evening.
(7) Consideration of the needs of the individual over-rides these suggestions (Werther and Baum, 1978).
(8) Urine-testing twice daily is usually enough, but short spells of testing four times a day are often helpful.

Further discussion of possible adjustments to insulin dosage appears in Chapter 6, The Outpatient Clinic.

'Oral agents'

Three possible benefits have been attributed to oral antidiabetic agents in the management of juvenile diabetes mellitus.

(1) They might delay the onset of clinical symptoms in chemical diabetes, or in children at special risk. This is discussed on p. 226. It remains a matter for academic study, but the results so far are not very promising.
(2) They have been used to attempt to prolong the remission phase (p. 199) but the results are difficult to assess and there is certainly no striking benefit.
(3) There is an impression among postgraduate students that somebody somewhere once said that they were a useful adjunct to insulin in stabilizing unstable diabetes. This is probably a reference to Krall, White and Bradley (1958). Seventy-two juvenile diabetics were treated for periods of one to 16 months. Sixty-four showed improvement in blood sugars but 34 of these gave up the oral agents because of gastro-intestinal side-effects. The remaining 30 cases were kept on treatment for an average of seven months, with the conclusion that 'long-term' cases did better than expected in respect to insulin requirements. Nobody is likely to start a crusade on such results, and the oral agents are not now in general use as an aid to control.

I once put a girl with mild diabetes on oral agents, largely to see what happened. She responded well, and when our paths crossed at a meeting some 12 years later she was still well controlled, and still on oral agents. Since then I have not come across a child diabetic sufficiently mild in the initial stages to merit a further trial of oral agents, and it seems best to accept the rule that the oral agents have no part to play in the management of juvenile diabetes mellitus.

Mixing insulins

There are various ways of mixing insulin but I shall describe only that which is now used in our clinic, as it seems to be the easiest. The short-acting insulin is taken up first. Air is injected in the same amount as the insulin which is to be withdrawn. If this is not done a vacuum will eventually form in the vial making withdrawal difficult and the insulin frothy. There will always be a bubble in this insulin, representing the dead space of air in the needle and nozzle of the syringe. It is removed by working the plunger while the needle is still in the insulin. A second needle is inserted in the vial of medium-acting insulin to allow air to run into the vial. This means that insulin can be withdrawn from the second vial without injecting air through the syringe. The 'clear' insulin is withdrawn first. It matters little if a little clear insulin gets into the cloudy insulin by mistake as it is converted into cloudy and conforms to the labelling on the vial, but if cloudy gets into clear some clear will be converted to cloudy and the contents of the vial will no longer strictly conform to the labelling. With good technique this should not happen, but it is safest to allow for slight errors. The mother who complains she is always getting bubbles in the syringe is probably tugging at the plunger instead of withdrawing slowly.

It will be seen that when we draw up, say, 6 units of clear insulin we are in fact drawing up 6 units plus the amount necessary to fill the dead space in the needle and nozzle of the syringe, and this additional insulin will be carried into the barrel of the syringe when the cloudy insulin is drawn up. Academically, this causes inaccuracy in measuring the insulin; but clinically it mattes very little as long as the technique is the same from day to day.

The care of equipment

It seems odd that the best way of keeping diabetic equipment is still being discussed but recent work suggests that we may have been over-careful. There are now doubts about the best needles to use, the best syringes and the best way of keeping both of these.

A special insulin syringe must be used. These syringes all have the marking 'BS 1619' and though they may vary slightly in shape and may be of 1 ml or 2 ml in volume the marking BS 1619 guarantees that they are graduated at 20 units/ml. Patients coming from overseas may have syringes marked at 40 or 100 units/ml. There is much talk of introducing the 100 unit/ml syringe as standard in the UK but at the time of writing it is still talk. Needles should be 25 gauge, ½ to ⅝ inch long.

The older system of boiling syringes has now been discarded. Syringe and needles are now kept in a plastic case which is half filled with industrial methylated spirit (obtained on prescription from a chemist). Surgical spirit sounds more scientific but is to be avoided as it tends to be greasy. The needle may be left on the syringe while it is in the case. The methylated spirit should be changed weekly. The needle fits into a spring at the bottom of the carrying case, this protects the tip of the needle. For everyday use any well-covered vessel is satisfactory.

Before the injection is given care must be taken that the syringe is free from methylated spirit, which is done by working the plunger up and down ten or 12 times. After the injection has been given a little industrial spirit should be taken into the syringe to rinse out any last trace of insulin, and then discarded. Parents note that after injection a little insulin may run back from the needle into the syringe and fear that the child has not been given the correct amount of insulin, but they can be reassured that the 'dead space' in the needle is allowed for in the markings on the syringe.

Needles should be handled with care and should not be banged against the walls of the container. Some parents find a needle is blunt after using it once or twice, others use the same needle for weeks. This is usually blamed on the very tough skin of the child or the incompetence of the manufacturer but is more likely to be due to rough handling.

Many parents like to use disposable syringes and disposable needles. The disposable needle is always sharp (and indeed may be used three or four times if kept in spirit) and the parents were probably trained with disposables in hospital and are apprehensive of a change. It is now possible for hospitals to issue disposable needles to children, which is the practice at our clinic.

Greenough, Cockcroft and Bloom (1979) have recorded observations which indicate that many of the standard recommendations are unreal, unnecessary and uneconomic. Forty per cent of their patients kept their syringes dry and only 18 per cent boiled them daily. They seemed none the worse for it. It was shown that the average life of a glass syringe costing £2.16 was three months. The life of a disposable syringe costing 5.9p (with needle) is about two weeks, so it is much cheaper to use disposables. After initial use they are returned to the packet with needle attached and kept in the fridge. They are not kept in methylated spirit as this would remove the markings, but as no spirit has to be cleared from the syringe the time taken over injection is shorter and sterility appears to be perfectly satisfactory. In a letter of comment Oli (1979) agreed with Greenough's findings, stressed the great economic advantage in a country like Nigeria where diabetics pay for their treatment and added that, as few Nigerians had fridges, he had found it completely effective if syringe and needle were put back in the packet, which was then put in a well-covered pot, which was in turn put in a hole in the ground 'dug as deep as the hand can reach'. He had had no case of infection in his five years of running a diabetes clinic. I have dwelt on this subject at some length not because it is 'fun medicine' (which in a way it is, for I have been grinning to myself all the time I have been typing this), but to show that today's accepted ideas may be unacceptable tomorrow.

Ancillary aids to injection are the Palmer Injector ('the gun')* and the Hypoguard*. Neither of these is the complete answer to problems of injection. One very conscientious girl, mentioned elsewhere, was determined to give her own injections but sat for an hour with the point of the needle indenting her skin. Given 'the gun', she sat for an hour with her finger on the trigger. Neither device actually injects the insulin, added thumb-power being necessary. It is true that many children are helped by these aids but some are not and they should not be advised to get one as a routine. Needless expense to the parents might be spared if the hospital outpatient clinic held a gun which could be lent for a trial period to prospective buyers. Messrs. Hypoguard have recently offered one of my patients a trial of the Hypoguard injector on approval.

Publicity has recently been given to an instrument which injects insulin by compressed gas, without the use of a needle. It is not always painless—insulins cannot be mixed—a supply of compressed gas must be available and it is very expensive. The British Diabetic Association is strongly opposed to its use.

Insulin should be stored at a temperature of 4–10 °C, although it may withstand 15 °C, i.e. in a cool place or a refrigerator, but not the freezing compartment. It should not be frozen, nor should it be left at a window on a sunny day or on a shelf above a fire, but in general it is easy to keep. Insulin may be accidently frozen during air travel if it is in the luggage compartment, so it should always be carried in the hand luggage.

* 'The gun' may be obtained from Messrs. Palmer Injectors Ltd., 166 Buchanan Street, Glasgow G1 2LN, Scotland.

A comprehensive postal service, including various plastic cases and disposable needles and syringes, is organized by Messrs. Hypoguard Ltd., 49 Grimston Lane, Trimley, Ipswich IP10 0SA.

Disposable syringes and 25G × ⅝ in needles may also be obtained from Messrs. Steriseal Ltd., Redditch, Worcs., England.

The injection

Several *sites* are available. These are the antero-lateral quadrants of the thighs, the lower abdomen and the tops of the upper arms. Patients would have considerable difficulty in injecting themselves in the buttock, so that site should not be used in hospital. The best site for children is the thighs. The injections have to be spread out, and I usually suggest using the left thigh on Mondays, Wednesdays and Fridays and the right on Tuesday, Thursdays and Saturdays, working down the thigh as the week progresses. On Sundays the mother can give the injection into the top of the upper arm, over the deltoid, which keeps her in practice if the child is giving his own injections on other days. The trouble with injecting children is that there is very little room. It is difficult to keep the injections well spaced out and as soon as they begin to cluster there is risk of fat hypertrophy occurring. The above scheme allows for each upper arm being used only once a fortnight, which minimizes the chance of fatty tumours forming. Unfortunately, very few children will tolerate injections in the abdominal wall and only five out of the 120 or so attending my clinic do so. 'It is frightening before you start and it seems to hurt more at first, but you get used to it', I was told by an adult diabetic of many years standing who now uses the abdominal wall as a routine. It is not surprising that most children balk at the idea.

A fold of subcutaneous tissue is pinched up and the needle is inserted as nearly as possible at a right angle into the skin, certainly not less than at an angle of 45 degrees. The plunger is withdrawn to make sure the point of the needle is not in a vein and the injection is then given. It is important that it is given into the subcutaneous tissue. At too low an angle it may be given into the deeper layers of the skin, and this seems more likely to happen when the gun is being used in the hands of children.

Testing the urine

Sugar in the urine

Certain fallacies in readings given by Clinitest, Clinistix and Ketodiastix have been mentioned in Chapter 7. They will not be repeated here as it is now assumed that a diagnosis of diabetes has been definitely made.

The parents and the child, if he is old enough, are usually instructed in urine-testing by a senior nurse or sister, but the physician should check the technique from time to time.

A check list, copies of which could be given to the parents if the physician so desired, is:

(1) Test-tube and dropper should be dry.
(2) Only the dropper supplied with the set should be used.
(3) The dropper should be held vertically over the tube while the drops are released. Resting the little finger of the right hand on the index finger of the left makes this easy.
(4) After measuring two drops of urine into the test-tube the dropper should be rinsed before finally taking up the water.
(5) The test-tube should be washed out as soon as the test is complete, and turned upside down to drain.

Belmonte *et al.* (1967) advised that the 'two-drop' test should be used as a routine. They used two drops of urine plus ten drops of water, which gives a scale of urine sugar up to 5 per cent, and it is only at that level that the 'orange flash' (known as the 'pass through' in the USA) begins to occur. In other words, there will be no mistake at a 3 per cent sugar level, for example, whereas there could be with the five-drop method. Furthermore, laboratory checks suggested that the two-drop method was slightly more accurate (Dorchy and Loeb, 1977). The two-drop test is now being much more widely used in diabetes clinics. A 5 per cent reading with two drops can be repeated with one drop, to see if it is nearer 10 per cent.

It is obvious that the five-drop test is only roughly accurate. If the true sugar reading is 1.5 per cent, the test could be reported as either 1 per cent or 2 per cent, a considerable range of error. A reading of 2 per cent means 2 per cent *or over*, which can be anything up to 10 per cent. In the presence of constant 2 per cent readings it is advisable to determine just how much sugar is really being lost in the urine.

Other tests for sugar

Clinistix offers a semiquantitative estimate of urine sugar. It reacts to glucose only, and not to other reducing substances (in contrast with Clinitest). It is of little value as a routine test as its upper limit extends only to 0.5 per cent sugar in the urine, but it is of value as a screening test and also in some special circumstances, for example the child who is not yet out of nappies, or the enuretic child in whom one wants an idea of the overnight sugar loss. Clinistix can be incorporated in the nappy, in the bed, or inside the pyjamas.

Diastix is a test quantified up to the usual 2 per cent. It exists in combination with Ketostix as Ketodiastix *(see below)*. The colour range of Diastix is from blue to brown. The disadvantage of Diastix is that it involves measuring a precise period of time, the same applying to Clinistix, Acetest and Ketostix. The time may be incorrectly measured, particularly if the tester is trying to make up his mind between two shades, and it also means that he must own a watch with a sweep second hand. However, if a child has to test his urine at school or is away for the day or on holiday, Diastix may be valuable as they are not bulky and can be used in the school latrines or behind a bush. They are no cheaper than Clinitest, and Clinitest has a fixed end-point so that it matters little if there is slight delay in reading the test.

Tes-Tape is used more in the USA than it is at present in the UK. It is specific for glucose. The colour range is from yellow to blue-grey. Like Diastix it is easily portable. A possible disadvantage is that it is read at 1 minute, but if the reading at that time is 0.5 per cent or more the final reading is made at 2 minutes. This feature could lead to the tape being mis-read by a slapdash parent.

Colour-blindness (Thompson *et al.* 1979) should be considered if a child seems to become confused in reading his urine tests. Yellow-blue colour-blindness may appear in some children and make reading Tes-Tape difficult, while red-green will do the same with Clinitest. A change in the method of testing should get around this problem.

Testing for ketones

The popular phrase 'testing for acetone' is misleading. One is testing for acetone and acetoacetic acid, and there is usually more of the latter than the former.

The older tests, Rothera's nitroprusside test and Gerhardt's ferric chloride test, are now seldom used as the modern tests are more easily performed. The ferric chloride test is the least sensitive test for ketones and may be negative when Acetest scores +++.

An *Acetest* tablet, which reacts in a manner similar to Rothera's test, is placed on a white surface and a drop of urine is put on the tablet. If ketones are present a purple colour appears, the intensity of the colour being compared to a printed colour scale after exactly 30 seconds. One problem is that the inexperienced user may score + for the slight alteration in the shade of the tablet produced by simply wetting it, on the grounds that 'there must be *some* acetone there'. He should be warned of this beforehand.

Ketostix strips act on the same chemical principles as Acetest but are slightly less sensitive. If the ketone is acetone alone, a weak positive first appears at a level three times higher than that needed to produce a similar result with Acetest.

Ketodiastix has two test areas, one for ketones and the other for sugar, and is simply a combination of Ketostix and Diastix, which have already been discussed.

Testing the blood for sugar

The most reliable method of measuring blood sugar is to measure the true glucose. 'Blood sugar' includes other reducing substances. The percentage difference between the two figures is small when the blood sugar is high. There is also a slight difference between capillary and venous blood, clinically unimportant except possibly in a doubtful glucose tolerance test.

Dextrostix uses a peroxidase–chromogen system similar to Clinistix. Technically, it is more difficult to use in children than in adults. The finger is pricked and a drop of blood quickly and evenly applied to the test area. This is washed off after exactly 60 seconds, for which purpose a plastic bottle which emits a narrow jet of water on pressure is useful. The test area is compared with a standard colour chart. In children one prefers to prick the back of the thumb rather than the pulp as this is less painful, but it does mean that the spreading of the drop on the test area is more difficult. Add to this the fact that washing off the blood is by no means instantaneous and 'exactly 60 seconds' becomes an impossible goal. However, allowing for a degree of inaccuracy, Dextrostix has its uses. It is useful to know at once when a high blood sugar had been reduced into the Dextrostix scale (upper level 14 mmol/l, 250 mg per cent), and useful to know if it disappears off the bottom of the scale, presaging hypoglycaemia.

The reflectance meter uses Dextrostix, as described above, but the strip is then inserted in the meter, a contact is made and a reading is obtained photoelectrically on a wide scale (up to 55 mmol/l, 1000 mg per cent). The meter is standardized before each session by means of a standard strip. It has the built-in disadvantage of Dextrostix and tends to under-estimate high values, but I find it useful in certain circumstances, for example, in giving instant bedside readings when following the progress of a very ill patient, or in doing spot checks on outpatients when one wants to know immediately if the blood sugar is 2.7, 13.8 or 27.7 mmol/l (50, 250 or 500 mg per cent). More recent devices for measuring blood sugar are described in Chapter 2.

Testing the blood for ketones

It is possible to test for ketones in the blood using either Acetest or Ketostix, and either plasma or serum. One method is to spin down heparinized blood and dip a Ketostix in the supernatant. If the reaction is definitely positive it can be repeated on plasma diluted two, four and eight times. One can then follow serially at the bedside the progress of ketosis, although in practice this seldom seems necessary.

Urine testing at home

When should urine be tested, and for what? In hospital the urine is usually tested 4-hourly, but one cannot expect the patient to test the urine more often than four times a day at home—before breakfast, before the mid-day meal, before the main evening meal and at bed-time. I think it desirable to test four times a day from the first discharge from hospital to the first or second outpatient attendance, but thereafter twice a day (before breakfast and the main evening meal) is probably enough *as a routine* in most cases. If a child is showing signs of poor control a further spell on 'four times a day' is indicated. One patient has as parents a doctor and a nurse who feel happiest testing every urine specimen two days a week and omitting all urine testing on the other days, unless the child has signs of polyuria or thirst, or of an infection, however mild. This system seems to work well with them and I see little point in arguing.

The first urine specimen passed in the morning may contain sugar which entered the bladder some 10 or 12 hours before, while the blood sugar may be low at the time the urine is voided. This may lead the parent to wonder how the child can be hypoglycaemic when there is sugar in the urine. Double-voiding in the morning helps to get round this difficulty. The child passes urine on rising and again 20 or 30 minutes later. The first specimen gives an indication of what has been happening during the night, the second of the state of affairs on getting up in the morning. It is customary to chart the second specimen, but I like to see both of them charted as they are two different sources of information. Double-voiding can, of course, be done at any time of day. It is often difficult to get cooperation from the younger children, who cannot see the point of micturating when they do not feel the need, but it can be done successfully with some very young children so it is always worth a trial.

There is no need to test for ketones as a routine, but it should be done if the urine shows 3 per cent or more of sugar, and also throughout illness. The presence of ketones in a sugar-free morning urine is not uncommon in small children, and is indicative only of overnight carbohydrate starvation. The same may be seen in the non-diabetic child, particularly if he has been vomiting.

On adjusting the insulin

Various schemes are in use for the adjustment of insulin dosage at home. These are described in Chapter 6. At the first discharge from hospital the insulin is lowered to allow for increased activity at home, a drop in the region of 10–20 per cent being suitable for most cases. One assumes that the child is being seen again in about a week. Will his requirements fall during that week as he enters into a remission period (p. 197) or will they rise due to some untimely infection or to anxiety in the home? Considering these possibilities one may feel inclined to instruct the mother on adjusting the insulin to cover such variations, and indeed the situation should be explained to her, but I think it rather unkind to saddle her with the personal responsibility of changing the insulin during her first few days at home. On the other hand, I do not want to saddle her with hypoglycaemic attacks or the effects of a febrile cold contracted in hospital just before discharge, so I compromise by asking her to telephone if the urine is either free from sugar or showing a steady 3 per cent or more for 36 to 48 hours.

At the time of discharge

The need to communicate with the parents throughout the child's stay in hospital is discussed at some length in Chapter 5. An adequate interview shortly before discharge takes the best part of an hour. The following matters should be covered:

(1) Equipment is checked.
(2) Interplay of diet, insulin, exercise and blood sugar is discussed.
(3) Hypo attacks: most likely time of occurrence, manifestations, treatment.
(4) Chart keeping.
(5) Indications for altering insulin dose: possibility of infection, or marked fall in insulin needs even before first clinic visit.
(6) The possibility of behaviour problems on first going home.
(7) When best to 'phone for advice, and how to get in touch with the Outpatient Clinic. In addition to the hospital numbers I give the

new diabetics my home number, saying that they will almost always find me home between 6 and 6.30 pm.
(8) What should be brought to the Outpatient Clinic, i.e. the morning urine specimen and the urine charts and, at the first visit, the insulin and syringe for checking.

REFERENCES

Åkerbloom, H. K. and Mäkelä, A-L (1978). Insulin antibodies in the serum of diabetic children treated from the diagnosis of the disease with highly purified insulins. *Acta paediat. scand.,* Suppl. 270, 69

Belmonte, Mimi M., Sarkosy, Eva, and Harpur, Eleanor R. (1967). Urine sugar determination by the two-drop Clinitest method. *Diabetes,* **16,** 557

Bewick, T. (1820). *A General History of Quadripeds,* p. 377. Newcastle-upon-Tyne; Longman, Hurst, Rees, Orme and Brown

Bloom, S. R., Adrian, T. E., Barnes, A. J. and Polak, J. M. (1979). Autoimmunity in diabetes produced by hormonal contaminants of insulin. *Lancet,* **1,** 14

Chance, G. W., Albutt, E. C. and Edkins, S. M. (1969). Serum lipids and lipoproteins in untreated diabetic children. *Lancet,* **I,** 1126

Dandona, P., Hooke, D. and Bell, J. (1978). Exercise and insulin absorption from subcutaneous tissue. *Br. med. J.,* **1,** 479

Dixon, K., Exon, P. D. and Malins, J. M. (1975). Insulin antibodies and the control of diabetes. *Quart. J. Med.,* **44,** 543

Dorchy, H. and Loeb, H. (1977). Comparative value of semi-quantitative tests for glucosuria in juvenile diabetes. *Pediat. adolesc. Endocr.,* **2,** 42 Karger; Basel

Editorial, *Br. med. J.,* (1976) **I,** 484

Farquhar, J. W. (1976). Diabetic Adolescence. *International Diabetes Federation Bulletin,* **21,** (no. 3) 6

Greenough, A., Cockcroft, P. M. and Bloom, A. (1979). Disposable syringes for insulin injection. *Br. med. J.,* **1,** 1467

Griffin, N. K., Smith, M. A. and Baum, J. D. (1979). Reduction of insulin dose on changing diabetic children from standard to monocomponent insulins. *Arch. dis. Childh.,* **54,** 123

Henry, D. A., Lowe, J. M., Citrin, D. and Manderson, W. G. (1978). Defective absorption of injected insulin. *Lancet,* **2,** 741

Krall, L. P., White, Priscilla and Bradley, R. F. (1958). Clinical use of the biguanides and their role in stabilising juvenile-type diabetes. *Diabetes,* **7,** 468

Oli, J. M. (1979). Disposable syringes for insulin injection. *Br. med. J.,* **2,** 273

Ortved Andersen, O. (1975). In *Immunological aspects of diabetes mellitus,* (ed. Ortved Andersen, Deckert and Nerup), *Acta endocr.* (Copenhagen), Suppl. 205, 240

Pyke, D. A. (1978). In *Insulin: proceedings of the Nordisk symposium* (ed. Hulst), p. 77. Utrecht; Bunge Scientific Publications

Thompson, D. G. Howarth, F., Taylor, H., Levy, I. S. and Birch, J. (1979). Defective colour vision in diabetes: a hazard to management. *Br. med. J.,* **1,** 859

Werther, G. A. and Baum, J. D. (1978). Once- versus twice-daily insulin for diabetic children. *Br. med. J.,* **2,** 52

Zinman, B., Vranic, M., Albisser, A. M., Hanna, A. K., Minuk, H. L. and Marliss, E. B. (1978). Exercise and insulin absorption. *New Engl. J. Med.,* **298,** 1202

CHAPTER 4

Behaviour

It is now appreciated that there is an important interplay between the behaviour of a diabetic child and his diabetic state. The old attitude was that if a patient was poorly controlled he was making mistakes with his insulin or his diet and if he said he was not he was lying. Though this was understandable when insulin was new and wonderful, such an attitude can now be regarded only as an unwarranted assault on the patient's integrity.

The management of the young diabetic is of necessity full of danger to his emotional development. He receives painful injections, often from those who should be most loving to him. The need to adhere strictly to a timetable, even during the holidays, comes into his life too soon. He cannot eat what he likes when he feels like eating it, nor dare he choose to miss a meal when he is enjoying himself at play. He is regularly put to the test, or at least his urine is. However hard his parents try it is difficult for them to prevent a glimmer of pleasure at a negative test or a slight frown at a strongly positive one; so he finds himself facing constant praise or blame, which is bad for any child and particularly bad for a child who feels he cannot really be held responsible for what is happening. Above him hangs a cloud of over-protection, from which rain down the words 'I don't think you had better' and 'No, you can't'.

The average child will wriggle and yell when he is first given his injections at home. He feels resentment. He notes that his mother, now on her own, is anxious. He may have to succumb to superior force over his injections, but he can show her who is in the driver's seat when it comes to taking his measured carbohydrate. He will tend to negativism which may well spill out of the home and into the school. He may try to cling to his own personality by bizarre behaviour, and less specific signs of behaviour disorder may appear.

A boy of seven developed diabetes. His mother, herself a diabetic, was very competent. Despite this, the boy at once gave trouble at meal times. His school work deteriorated badly and he developed encopresis. Previously one of the family, he began to dissociate himself from family affairs, or if he did accompany anyone he insisted on going on roller skates. There were constant rows. When changed from a limited carbohydrate diet to a free diet he was back to his old self in a fortnight, his encopresis gone, his school teacher delighted. His mother's experience of diabetes enabled her to say that his daily carbohydrate intake was never more than 20 g away from that originally prescribed.

This history is quoted as an extreme but essentially normal reaction to the onset of diabetes. He resented his diabetes and reacted briskly against it, which is a healthy reaction in a young child. It is not surprising that a child reacts in this way. What is surprising is that the reaction is mild in most, and that children get over it quickly, except for those who already have some deep-seated disturbance.

Over-protection

The next history concerns a boy who showed a mild form of the initial reaction, but who drifted on into a reaction that can be regarded as abnormal. Children with a passive disposition may welcome over-protection. They do not go out much and may even accept diabetes as a sign of distinction. They submit to their regime with pleasant resignation, except possibly for some amiable diet-breaking.

A boy developed diabetes at the age of three. Apart from transient screaming at injections and a passing jealousy of others at table, his first two years were uneventful. He was on a Lawrence Line diet (which measures protein and fat as well as carbohydrate) but tended to become obese. Thereafter he had four readmissions in four years because of ketoacidosis. His mother was uncertain of his management in many ways. He was kept indoors to be safe, a situation with which he readily complied. By the age of four he was 11 lb (5 kg) overweight for his height. Despite prolonged efforts at education, his mother consistently underscored his urine sugars and he showed fairly frequent acetone as an outpatient. He mixed very poorly at home, but found the ward regime suited him well and at the age of nine said he would be glad to come back into hospital at any time. Even in hospital he succeeded in diet-breaking in the ward kitchen. He was then sent to a diabetic hostel where he did very well, playing in the school football team and taking only an occasional extra chocolate biscuit; this did not upset his urine sugars, which were now good. He was changed from Lawrence Lines to a limited carbohydrate diet. He came home after nine months, apparently well-controlled but now 20 lb (9 kg) overweight for height. He soon returned to his indolent ways and took very little exercise. He would slouch into the clinic with an ingratiating leer and settle down with his comic while others got on with matters of no great concern to him. He was eventually persuaded, at the age of 11, to join the local athletic club, but gave it up soon after as 'I got blamed for pulling the lassies' hair', perhaps the most one could hope for in the way of athletic prowess from this lad. He then mooned off to attend at an adult hospital, 14½ lb overweight for his height, which was that of a boy one and a half years older.

Were it not that one knows never to become emotionally involved with a patient, certain flutterings in the spirit of this boy's physician could easily have been mistaken for an urge to shake and belabour. There seems little doubt, however, that his mother's uncertainty played into the boy's hands.

The essential of the boy's attitude seems to have been a failure to come to grips with his diabetes. He hardly reacted to it at all. A downright refusal to have anything to do with his diabetes was beyond his emotional compass. There are, however, some children who show the 'adolescent reaction' and who seem set on denying the existence of their diabetes.

The adolescent denial

The adolescent reaction is normal. A boy in his early teens realizes that he must soon stand on his own two feet. Further learning he will accept if he can see its usefulness; but if he can see no future in learning his wish to be himself will take over. He realizes he must leave his family. He sees that the opinions held in his family have not always been right and he will feel bound to tell the family so, yet if he has had a happy childhood he may again take his long-forgotten teddy to bed with him. He will get the glimmer of an idea that the whole system of school, family and his individual life works under some over-riding national law. But, if he has been unhappy, he may reject the school, the family and the law. Diabetes can scarcely make a child happy, and so the young diabetic, long before adolescence, may slip into this adolescent denial of any authority, even the authority of fate. In the pre-adolescent years the child is already beginning to break from the family. His behaviour tends to be that of his peers modified by the family attitude. If he comes from an average background the child of five years does not cheat at school. At the age of ten he knows it is priggish to withhold knowledge from a friend who is suffering during a school examination. He has moved from home morality to peer morality, and the diabetic child, like any other child, wants acceptance from his peers, so there is a tendency for the diabetic child to deny the essential difference that lies in his diabetic state and join his group. It is only a tendency. How clearly it will be seen will depend on the happiness of his family background.

A girl developed diabetes at the age of nine. She rebelled strongly against her regime, and would rush screaming into the middle of the road at meal times. After a few months she was readmitted to hospital and put on a free diet, but this did not have the good effect seen in the case first described in this chapter. Indeed, all it did was to undermine the mother's confidence rather more, and she was having to carry the burden herself. Her husband, outwardly a pleasant enough fellow, held certain unfortunate dogmatic opinions. He quite liked his own children, of which he had five, but he did not like any other children. He was fond of his wife and appreciated her difficulties but felt that the direct care of his children was none of his business. Nothing would shake him in those deep beliefs.

Matters became worse. The child did at least take her injections and has continued to do so but she refused to produce urine specimens for testing. The mother then gave up, apart from doing the injecting. The child was admitted to a diabetic hostel and eventually settled quite well, giving her own injections and testing her own urine. As soon as she went home she resumed her old ways. Further scenes culminated in an attack on her mother with a kitchen knife when it had been suggested that she might accompany her father to the laundrette. On psychiatric advice she was readmitted to the hostel, and the cycle repeated itself. She has been in the hands of the police, who considered her the ringleader of a gang of teenage housebreakers, but the householder dropped charges when he heard that the girl was a diabetic. She has just graduated to an adult hospital. She intends to be married by the time she is 16. Through all this she has remained remarkably stable on whatever dose of insulin she was on when discharged from hospital or hostel. She had only one unplanned admission in four years, for hypoglycaemia.

Symptoms of disordered behaviour

These histories have been quoted to show how some children reacted to their diabetes. They are vivid and serve as an introduction to a more scientific study of behaviour in diabetes. Such a study, long and valuable, has been made by Koski (1969) under the appealing title of 'The coping processes in childhood diabetes'.

It is difficult to assess a child's reaction on his first admission to hospital. Is his anxiety caused by his diabetes or simply by being in hospital? On one thing, however, Koski is definite; the severity of the psychological reaction in hospital does not relate to future diabetic control. Indeed it may be that the more placid the child in hospital the worse will be the control. If one accepts this as possibly true it is not difficult to see why. Nobody is caring enough, perhaps not even the doctors. The troublesome patients get the attention while nobody notices that the drifters have started quietly drifting.

Koski gives a long list of symptomatic reactions and compares their appearance in groups which were classified as good to fair (GF) or poor (P) as regards their diabetic control. There were 30 in each group. After discharge from hospital behavioural differences became clear. Disturbances in social behaviour are much more common in the poorly controlled group. Such disturbances appeared 24 times in the P group, three times in the GF group, the most common symptom in the P group being passive resistance (nine), with withdrawal or autistic behaviour second (five) and aggressive behaviour third (three). The GF group showed rather more anxiety (12:10) but whereas free-floating anxiety was much commoner in the GF group (9:1) as were specific fears (5:1), frank anxiety attacks were more common in the P group (5:3). A little anxiety seems to be good for you. Stealing and lying were not common in this Finnish series, contrary to my own impression in Glasgow, but enuresis was (GF five, P eight). After considering these and other factors, Koski evolved psychiatric diagnostic categories, as in *Table 4.1*.

TABLE 4.1

Diagnosis	GF	P	Total
Normal adjustment	11	4	15
Mild adjustment disorder	8	8	16
Psychoneurosis	8	4	12
Personality trait disorder	3	14	17

The behaviour of a psychoneurotic child has ups and downs with good spells. The behaviour of a child with a personality disorder is always somewhat warped.

The children in the GF group had better school records. In those with above average school performance the ratio was 2:1 in favour of the GF group, in the below average group the ratio was reversed. Six children in the P group had had to repeat a class twice, there were none in the GF group. This scarcely seems to be a matter of intelligence. The average IQ (Terman–Merrill, Form L) in the GF group was 102, in the P group 99. This implies a failure of achievement rather than intelligence.

That a hen-or-egg situation exists must now be clear. Which comes first, the behaviour disorder or the poor diabetic control? It is what Sir Walter Scott might have called 'a guid gangin' plea'.

I have ane *(a law affair)* myself—a gangin plea that my father left me, and his father afore left to him. It's about our back-yard—ye'll maybe ha'e heard of it in the Parliament House, Hutchinson against Mackitchinson—it's a well-kenn'd plea—it's been four times afore the fifteen, and de'il onything the wisest o' them could make o't, but just to send it out again to the Outer House. Oh, it's a beautiful thing to see how lang and how carefully justice is considered in this country! *The Antiquary*

Behaviour disorder against diabetic control is a gangin plea, but one which is not yet ready for discussion. The behaviour of a diabetic child is one factor; the natural stability of his diabetes and the attitude of his parents are others. It is time to consider the part played by the parents.

The family reaction to diabetes

It has been my custom recently, when a child has been diabetic for a month or two, to ask the parents to put in writing their feelings until the present. I ask them to tell me what they have felt about diabetes, and also about what help, or lack of it, they have so far received. This is in no sense a scientific enquiry. They receive no questionnaire. If I think the parents are not used to putting things on paper I do not ask them to do so. The following letter, quoted *verbatim* and *in toto* (the influence of Scott lingers on) should be regarded only as a text.

'Your son has diabetes and is going to require insulin for the rest of his life.' At the time, these were the most shattering words we had heard, and we received them in a state of dull shock. We knew there were diabetics, but in a different sort of world from ours, and now we were suddenly expelled into that world.

We didn't exactly doubt the doctors, accepting that our son was diabetic, but were quite sure that early treatment would cure him. When it dawned on us, our first thoughts were of his life, having continuous injections—how would it change him? Schooling, careerwise—how would he suffer in that field? But our main thoughts centred on getting him home as quickly as possible, and into the family again, to be cared for.

We are more enlightened now on the subject and accept his condition, finding assistance in reading and talking about it, though occasionally a feeling of resentment occurs.

The emotional and dramatic use of the word 'expelled' will have been noted. For the rest, I have chosen this letter partly because it is very clear and partly because it covers the main points in a small space.

The points brought out in the letter illustrate a normal family reaction to the first diagnosis of diabetes. There are bewilderment and shock, wishful thinking ('we ... were quite sure that early treatment would cure him'), anxiety for his future, and resentment. Some regard the 'Why did it happen to us?' reaction as a sign of guilt, and it may be so. These feelings are most common in the group who go on to good control. If the parents do not feel shock and anxiety and do not try to wish themselves out of this situation they do not care very much. Another feature in concerned parents is insomnia, which may go on for months. Talking about it can bring great relief. 'Thank God!' a mother said recently. 'I thought I was going mad: there are others like me, then?' She would have passed through that phase if nothing had been said, but anything that increases a parent's confidence in the doctor at an early stage is of value.

The good family will also frequently, without urging, adjust their diet to that of the diabetic child. They tend towards a diet a little lower in carbohydrate and fat and higher in protein, and sugar and jam no longer appear at table. This is most easily done in small families and depends on the readiness of other children to make small sacrifices, which in turn depends on the age and understanding of the non-diabetic children, but much can be done with tact. *The more members of the family involved the better will be the diabetic control.* Eleven families had modified their diet in Koski's GF group, none in the P group. In the good families all the older members will have some knowledge of diabetes, and will be able to supervise injections if the need arises. One tends to think of the problems of the diabetic child and to forget the considerable problems of a mother who is left to cope with diabetes on her own. Shared responsibility is good for the whole family. One must also remember that the parents who ask the most questions, often apparently trivial to the physician, are probably the most concerned. They can be helped to incorporate their anxieties into the care of the child, and it is well worth trying to give that help. The patient who appears at a general medical clinic with a written list of questions or bodily complaints is well known and will be diagnosed almost certainly as 'psychosomatic' but such a list at the diabetic clinic has to be gone through painstakingly. The listmakers are the ones who care most and the fact that they are vivid in their imagination and anxieties is just a part of their ability to care.

Failure to cope

The poor family has such problems that it cannot care effectively for the diabetic child. The main problem may occasionally be lack of intelligence, but is more likely to be an unwillingness to take arms against a sea of troubles. A built-in rejection of all authority, including doctors, may often be the main stumbling block, and such parents may have to deny their own incompetence by omnipotent thinking ('I'm with him 24 hours a day, the doctors can't tell *me* anything about diabetes'). The omnipotent thinker is also a danger to others as he is apt to sound off with bad advice to others less experienced whom he has cornered at the clinic or in the ward.

> A girl became diabetic at the age of eight. Her control was poor. It soon emerged that *all* the family were well known to the school authorities because of their frequent absences. The mother simply failed to send them and had twice been taken to court. The father took his weekly pay packet straight to the greyhound track, which determined the family fortunes for the week. The mother became a bingo addict and was often out of the house when her children needed her. One accepted lack of adherence to diet with resignation, but one worried about her insulin—not so much about whether she was getting the correct dose as whether on some days she was getting any insulin at all. Despite periods of institutional care she eventually developed Mauriac's syndrome (p. 256).

It seems that rejection of authority may include rejection of one's own authority, i.e. irresponsibility.

Low intelligence

The parent who is slow to understand may still care about his child and it is worth persevering with such a parent. He may have the added difficulty that his child is more intelligent than he is, and the child may be going out of his way to confuse the parent further. Frequent clinic visits are necessary, but the pleasure of these parents at getting something right at last can be touching and rewarding.

The interplay of persons

It is not being argued that stability or instability of a child diabetic is controlled solely by his emotional state, although it is influenced by it. Indeed, it was pointed out in a case quoted previously in this chapter that one girl's diabetes remained surprisingly stable during a hectic emotional career. But it probably remains true that some diabetics are inherently more stable than others and that some are only apparently unstable because of ill-advised treatment. Yet there can be no doubt that the interplay of personalities, emotions and social background can affect diabetic stability. These are fine words, worth a place in any textbook, but what do they mean?

A relatively simple approach to diabetics as persons rather than diseased objects has been provided by Farquhar (1976) in an outstanding paper which suggests that diabetics may be divided into *cans, can'ts, won'ts* and *would-if-they-had-been-told-hows*. (One cannot help thinking that if the results of the therapy of diabetes had been published under these four headings instead of *en masse* we would, by now, have a better understanding of what therapy can do; but that is by the way.) Farquhar's types seem particularly relevant to adolescents who are taking over their own diabetic care.

The subject can be looked at a little more closely. How do average children respond to different types of parent? Tattersall and Jackson (1980) give a succinct analysis of this problem and I have borrowed freely from them. Certain types of parent will tend to produce certain types of children, and I have the gall to think that this can be expressed fairly simply, as in the following table.

TABLE 4.2

Parent	Child
(1) Over-anxious	Over-dependent, may go so far as to *demand* attention from others
(2) Self-pitying	Attention-seeking, even resorting to diabetic trickery
(3) Rejecting	Rebellious
(4) Obsessional	Anxious
(5) Feckless, anti-establishment	Feckless, anti-establishment

This table refers to 'the average child'. 'The average child' is as rare as 'the textbook case'. Some children develop definite personalities very early in life, and may even be born with them. A child with a strongly self-assertive personality will show rebellion more often than the table indicates, a very passive child is likely to remain passive whatever type of parent he may have. Nevertheless, I believe *Table 4.2* has value in providing a starting-point from which to consider the parent–child relationship and its bearing on diabetic control.

How does one recognize the different types of parent?

(1) The *over-anxious* parent is all too ready to do the right thing in order to avert disaster. The mother may sleep in the child's room and accompany him to school.

> A diabetic of two years' standing came into my care recently. His mother was still weighing all his food. 'So you won't be able to eat in restaurants?' said I. 'Oh, yes, we do,' she replied. 'We take the scales with us.' I told the boy himself that he did not need to test his urine before, during and after a game of football (which he was doing), indeed he only needed to test it twice a day. His look of radiant delight came as a revelation to me.

Over-anxious parents are ready, almost without thinking, to do anything the doctor says.

(2) A *self-pitying* mother will use clinic time to talk of her difficulties and how she has courageously surmounted them. She sits as near as she can to the doctor with the child squeezed out, and at the end of the interview one realizes that the child has hardly been mentioned. Urine charts may have been discussed, but not the child.

(3) The *rejecting* mother goes further than the self-pitying mother. She too tends to monopolize the interview and sits close to the doctor, but adds a few steely looks flashed at the child from time to time. The child has let the family down by developing diabetes. I have heard a mother say 'Trust him to get diabetes! It's just the kind of thing he would do, and he's the only one in the family who would have done it!' Such statements are never made in jest, even when accompanied by a smile.

(4) *Obsessional* parents are described in some detail on p. 124. There is a superficial resemblance to both over-anxious and rejecting parents, but obsessional parents are made of sterner stuff. Over-anxious parents may seem quite ready to be trampled on; obsessional parents are prepared to do the trampling. Rejecting parents wish they could see the back of their diabetic

child; obsessional parents will always strive to get him to toe the line.

(5) *Feckless* parents have just been described under the heading of 'Failure to cope'. Their children, like other children, learn from them by example. Diabetes gets the same treatment as other problems—pretend it is not there and it will go away. Ideally, such children should be sent quickly to a diabetic hostel but their parents will not let them go because they think that this is the establishment having another go at their rights and abilities as parents. The children may pick up this turn of mind and may cheat with their diabetes simply for cheating's sake, so that no doctor is in a position to tell them what to do. These are Farquhar's 'can'ts'. They need infinite patience. The diabetic regime must be simple to the verge of laxity. There is only one rule, and that is 'Do not lose them'.

Psychiatric help is seldom needed, even with the difficult cases. The great majority of cases are best managed without *formal* referral to a psychiatrist. On the other hand, an informal chat with a psychiatrist over hospital lunch can be of great value. One can discuss how this family might react to the appearance of an experienced psychiatric social worker trying to assess the family background. If psychiatry is practised at all it is probably best practised at a superficial level (*see* p. 178). Many of the problems of the diabetic child are real problems of management (injections, diet, time-schedules) and it is the duty of the self-respecting physician rather than the psychiatrist to modify these problems as best he can.

I have been trying to foresee difficulties. I hope I have not suggested that all diabetic children are heading for behaviour disorders. It should now be pointed out that more than one study (for example Sterky, 1963) has shown that there is no difference in the incidence of emotional disturbance between diabetic and non-diabetic children if one excludes the immediate reaction to diabetes and the adolescent denial reaction, the latter being particularly common in girls. This may be true, but if it is, Koski's finding that 17 of her 60 diabetics were incapable of even marginally healthy living implies a very high rate of personality disorder in the general population. My own clinical impression is that Koski is right. However, the matter is largely academic. The doctor can only deal with one patient at a time and if he has an emotional problem one tries to help, whether he is diabetic or not.

A point which is often stressed in the literature (though it has never to my knowledge been scientifically investigated) is that if a child shows disturbed behaviour when he develops diabetes there were disturbed family relationships in the family before the diabetes appeared (Belmonte, 1963). This is certainly my own clinical impression. I do not believe that the appearance of diabetes in a child can be blamed for a breakdown in relationships within the family. It is more likely to weld a divided family together, though it does not always do so. The power-shifts which may occur in a family when a child becomes diabetic are described by Wishner and O'Brien (1978), the mother and the diabetic child rising in the pecking order.

In looking at the family background of diabetes we are really looking at associations rather than cause and effect. The diabetic who does well comes from a stable background and the whole family has a positive attitude to the disease. They realize that, with knowledge and continuing observation, good control can be obtained and that an outwardly normal life can be lived. Ludvigsson (1977) covers this ground and mentions that regular exercise is a favourable sign, perhaps not for itself alone, but as an indicator of a well-balanced family life.

Despite the importance of the family, it should be remembered that the brunt of caring for the diabetic child falls on the mother. Studies have demonstrated the appearance of anxiety symptoms in the mothers of diabetic children, but the fathers are relatively unaffected.

Emotion and blood sugar

So far, emphasis has been laid on the effect of his disease and his environment on the diabetic child. We have considered factors which might affect his social adjustment and have discussed the chances of his long-term control being good or bad. There remains to be discussed the possible influence of emotional stress on diabetic control at any given moment.

That adrenalin raises the blood sugar is well known. Some parents may spontaneously relate transient hyperglycaemia to definite events, for example, school examinations, and it seems reasonable to think them right and to accept adrenalin as the mediator. Other mechanisms exist. The level of growth hormone, an insulin antagonist, may fluctuate with socio-emotional influences. Hyperthyroidism may lead to high blood sugars and concomitant hyperthyroidism makes diabetes more difficult to control. Removal of the cerebral cortex in animals causes hyperglycaemia, which is attributed to overaction of the sympathetic system; this makes it theoretically possible for a relative imbalance between cortical and sympathetic action to affect diabetic control. The important role of emotional factors in producing recurrent ketoacidosis has been established by the work of Baker and his group and is referred to on p. 179.

Does the emotional upset seen in some diabetic children result from poor diabetic control producing despondency, loss of self-confidence and lack of interest, or is poor diabetic control the result, in some instances, of emotional disharmony? It is likely that both suppositions are true and that sometimes a vicious circle may be set up. This problem is still being discussed. From the practical point of view one can say that poor diabetic control, behaviour disorder in children, and social and emotional problems in parents tend to go together. One should try to modify all three aspects in the hope that improvement in one field will show some associated improvement in another.

In the face of uncertainty and conflicting evidence one is justified in having a working hypothesis. Any diabetic child will show an initial adverse behaviour response which can usually be made transient by adequate management of the child, his diabetes and his parents. If there are adverse social and psychological factors in the child or his background before the diabetes appears then it will take longer to obtain control of his diabetes, which may in fact never be properly controlled at all. These comments assume secondary importance if the child's inherent diabetic state is unusually stable or unusually unstable.

I have tried to set out the problems of behaviour in some sort of order, but it may give some encouragement to others if I admit that I still make wrong judgements. Let me conclude this chapter with a cautionary tale.

One girl was a problem from about the age of ten. She was known in the clinic as 'The Wee Soul', because her mother always referred to her as such. She was a nocturnal diet-breaker ('She was down in the night and had five French cakes, but you can't really blame her, the wee soul'). Her urine charts were very poor. Having had a hypo attack which alarmed her mother she proceeded to have several more, although circumstances suggested that these were not genuine attacks. 'The wee soul, she's always hypo when I go to get her from school. I just have to walk her up and down till she gets better.' During several explanations of why walking up and down was not the accepted treatment of a hypo attack the mother would gaze at me with the blank stare of one saying to herself 'The poor fool, can't he see I'm talking about *her* hypo attacks?' Unfortunately, the wee soul was moved to a classroom beside which ran the public street, with the result that her mother could peer in the window at will. When she did so, her daughter toppled from her seat on to the floor. Unable to bear this any longer, the mother at last irrupted into the classroom, picked up the prostrate form in her arms and cried to the world 'How would you like it if your child was suffering from an incurable disease?'

Eventually she left us at the age of 13. I saw her again a year later, during the Christmas season, when I found her doing a holiday job in a baker's shop. We were separated by a huge pile of French cakes. I transcended good taste so far as to wink at her, to which she responded with a maidenly blush.

At the same time we had another girl of the same age. Her mother had severe rheumatoid arthritis, both parents were elderly and neither was very bright. They tried very hard, but their daughter went her own way. Her urine usually showed ketosis and she had no interest in her illness. She was re-admitted 'for education' but was surly and uncooperative. A psychiatrist failed to make worthwhile contact with her. She turned her back, literally, on attempts to educate her. We staggered along till she left us at the age of 13. One day, some years later, I made a routine visit to a maternity hospital to exchange views with the babies. I was greeted by a despairing obstetrician, 'Will you please talk to one of the mothers? She's 18, her baby's illegitimate and she's completely blind, and I know it's very sad and I should be more understanding, but she's completely impossible and I can do nothing with her, and I'm only asking you because you knew her earlier, she is a diabetic.' Sure enough, it was our patient. The nurse who was leading her carefully by the hand was The Wee Soul.

I had written them both off in my mind as hopeless cases. One was, the other was anything but. Once The Wee Soul no longer had to manipulate her mother, she blossomed. The matron described her as 'a very promising young nurse, reliable, conscientious'. One should not stick to a first judgement; one keeps it constantly under review.

REFERENCES

Belmonte, M. M. (1963). The future of the diabetic child. *Can. med. Ass. J.*, **88**, 1112

Farquhar, J. W. (1976). Diabetic adolescence. *International Diabetes Federation Bulletin*, **21**, (No. 3), 6

Koski, Maijo-Liisa (1969). The coping process in childhood diabetes. *Acta paediat. Scand.*, **58** Suppl. 198. (This long paper quotes 149 references on behaviour)

Ludvigsson, J. (1977). Socio-psychological factors and metabolic control in juvenile diabetes. *Acta paediat. Scand.*, **66**, 431

Sterky, G. (1963). Family background and state of mental health in a group of diabetic schoolchildren. *Acta paediat.*, **52**, 377

Tattersall, R. B. and Jackson, J. G. L. (1980). Social and emotional complications. In *Complications of Diabetes*, ed. Keen, H. and Jarrett, J. Second edition. London: Edward Arnold

Wishner, W. J. and O'Brien, M. D. (1978). Diabetes and the family. *Med Clin. N. Am.*, **62**, 735

CHAPTER 5

Communication and Education

The need for communication between the diabetic child, his parents and the medical staff is so much taken for granted that there may be some who have not seriously considered how best to set about communicating. It is unrealistic simply to pour out a flood of learning in the expectation of a parent absorbing it all, like a sponge. The release of information must be carefully timed and suited to the understanding and temperament of the parent and the child.

Talking to the child

The pre-school diabetic child can learn little from formal teaching but he can learn a fair amount from example and imitation. An occasional four-year-old may seem anxious to inject himself and may indeed be able to do so, but he cannot be expected to begin to understand the basis of diabetic management. He can be shown foods he can take in unlimited quantity and others which he should leave alone, but his interest may not extend beyond scepticism. His education comes largely through the education of his mother. If his actions show that he has found no reason why diabetics should behave like this the only answer may be to say 'You remember how ill you felt before you came into hospital? You don't want to feel as ill as that again, do you?' Even to the older rule-breaker one cannot say 'If you carry on like this you'll be blind by the time you're 20, if you live that long.' Communcation with the pre-school child can only be at a superficial level as regards his diabetes, but one can try to boost his self-respect for the future by praising all that is going well.

An attempt can be made to instruct the schoolchild in a very simplified physiology of diabetes. He can be told that his symptoms when he was first admitted were due to the sugar in his blood being too high; that stuff called insulin brings the blood sugar down to what it should be and that as he lacks insulin he has to be given it by injection; and that sugar in his urine is about the same as it is in the blood and that a lot of high tests mean that he needs more insulin. He is also taught how to test his urine by a nurse, a sister or a doctor, or all three at various times (p. 52).

There is little hope of successfully instructing the younger child about hypoglycaemic attacks. His reaction to hypoglycaemia is likely to be irritability and confusion so that he does not take his sugar. His mother should ensure that anybody he spends much time with (for example grandmother, school teacher) knows the signs of a hypo attack and knows to give him two dessert spoons (20 g) of sugar, possibly as Lucozade or Dextrosol. The older child, in whom hypoglycaemia shows as faintness, pallor and sweating, has a better chance of aborting his attack by giving himself sugar and should be told what a hypo attack is and why it is most likely to occur before meals and after exercise. This seldom works out in practice. I use a simple multiple choice questionnaire (*see later in this chapter*) with the older children, and the one question they invariably get right is how to treat a hypo attack. When thinking clearly they know what to do about hypoglycaemia, but they almost always forget when befuddled by hypoglycaemia.

Attempts at further instruction in physiology and anatomy are probably futile, possibly dangerous. Kaufman and Hersher (1971) describe the beliefs of five teenagers, aged between 13 and 19 years. They were patients at a teaching children's hospital linked to a university. All were well educated and had received 'programmed instruction on a teaching machine'. The children were able to accept the relationship between sugar and insulin, but beyond that their notions became bizarre. One, who had eaten a great deal since her diabetic mother died, knew that her stomach would be bigger than the normal stomach due to over-eating. She thought her pancreas was normal but suspected that her stomach would eventually fill her whole body. Another was convinced that when insulin was cut off by the clogging or severance of tubes coming from the pancreas the pancreas would then fill up with a kind of dirt that spread throughout the body. Vomiting was due to sugar building up around the stomach in a bulky layer, compressing the stomach and squeezing the food back out the mouth.

The information received by a diabetic child will be limited by his understanding and distorted by his psychological make-up. It might be argued that if a diabetic child is not instructed in elementary physiology and anatomy he will still worry about his diabetic insides and it would be better to give him facts as a basis for his fantasy rather than leave him completely in the dark. It appears more likely that his mind can be adequately occupied in coping with simple rules of thumb covering the diet-sugar-insulin-exercise relationship. We hope that further instruction will do good. We should be aware that it might do harm. Undue introspection begets confusion, confusion begets loss of confidence and loss of confidence slows the maturation of a child's personality.

How much one tells a child depends on one's assessment of the child within his family and perhaps teaching machines are not very good at this. However, many hospitals have booklets which can be issued to the parents and the older children. Those booklets have a value less as manuals of instruction than as reference books to which the mother can turn to see if she has remembered correctly what the doctor has told her. The basis of instruction is free-ranging conversation and its first aim is to produce trust. The mastery of diabetes will come in time.

Talking to the mother

Nurses, ward sisters, dietitians, house-officers and more senior doctors all have a part to play in instructing the diabetic child and his parents. It is therefore very desirable that the mother should be able to live in hospital during the child's first admission. It helps her to get to grips with diabetes more quickly. If she is living out she will be given little set pieces of instruction, but if she is living in she can also ask sudden questions as they come into her head. She is managing the child herself before she goes home, which helps to bridge the gap when she leaves hospital. Above all, she will have the opportunity to get to know those who will be looking after her child in future and she has a chance to appreciate the medical resources that are behind her.

The *nurse* sees much of the child as she gives his injections, supervises his urine testing, brings his meals, changes his bed and so forth. The mother will also probably see more of the nurse than she sees of any one other person in hospital, and some mothers find it easier to talk to a nurse than a doctor. Because of this the nurse must beware of being tempted into assuming the role of the doctor. She should confine her medical comments strictly to the matter in hand, for example injections or urine testing, if she possibly can. If she is cornered she should say as little as possible, 'We don't need to worry about that now, you can ask the dietitian in the morning'. She should

COMMUNICATION AND EDUCATION

never lie to the child, for example 'It's only for a day or two' or he will lose confidence in the long run. She should not indulge in prognostics; a breezy account of lipoatrophy is out of place, even if she has just seen a striking case. What has been said suggests that the role of the nurse is essentially negative: that all she has to do is keep her nose clean. It is not so. A passing comment from the mother ('We are all very fond of ice-cream') may be more important than a studied reply given to a dietitian. She may learn that Granny is a compulsive eater whom the patient often visits, or that father sees no reason to be sober at weekends. She may learn that 'just a normal boy' means that he accepts the family belief that each day should be ordered according to the phases of the moon and that football is forbidden by the Great Pyramid. All this information is of great value to the medical staff, and the nurse may be in a unique position to get hold of it.

The role of the *ward sister* overlaps those of the nurse and the hospital officer. She is the Wise Woman, and the shorter her skirts, the worse! If injections are going badly it is she who will have to take over. She, more than anyone, is in a position to impress on the parents that there are many different people trying to help. She can stress the continuity of care in such phrases as 'You'll bring him back to the ward to see us when you're visiting the clinic, won't you?' She, with her experience, can say 'You're worried, aren't you? You're bound to be' and cheer the mother up, whereas a junior nurse saying the same thing might only cause depression. She alone can say 'You'll like Dr X, he's a kind man' or 'You'll like Dr X, he's a hard man', and get away with either. The sister must know her consultant, and the consultant must know his ward sister. If she plays her cards right, the patient's mother will ask her to tea, and if the question is raised, the consultant should encourage her to go.

The *house-officer* or *registrar* is likely to be the first of the medical staff to make contact with the patient as he checks him in and carries out the first medical examination. Here again he must be careful not to say too much. An example of saying too much to an excited parent has been quoted by Richard Asher ... 'The doctor looked down his throat and told me the ear drum had grown right into the throat and was hanging down like a sausage. He cut it off and said if he'd been five minutes later the child would have been dead'. By restricting one's comments one is not trying to keep the patient in the dark, one is trying to avoid confusion at the outset of a life-long illness. It is best to start off with 'This appears to be diabetes, but there are one or two other tests to be done. Whether it is or not, the treatment is clear'. One has in mind the occasional ill child, usually young and free from polyuria and polydipsia, who may have marked hyperglycaemia in the course of a febrile illness yet be normal in a day or two and show no signs of diabetes years later. The house officer will later explain the need to give fluids and salts, the need for insulin and the undesirable presence of acetone. One must accept as natural the possibility that the parent is poised to blame ulterior forces for his disaster, and nothing that in any way might be regarded as criticism should pass between medical and nursing staff in the presence of a parent. The house officer, newly qualified, should consult with the ward sister on the best line to take, remembering that whatever the diagnosis it is better to be friendly than authoritarian. As the days pass the house officer must never forget to ask the mother how *she* is feeling. It is easy for a house officer to drop into a chair for a moment and have a casual chat with the mother. It is more difficult for the consultant, inhibited by the presence of his entourage. The mother is the lynch-pin in managing diabetes and she should feel she is at least on equal terms with the others, not just a useful middle-woman between the very important doctor and the very important patient. If one approaches the bedside and asks 'How is Johnny today, Mrs McTaggart?' the sensitive, anxious mother may take this to mean 'I suppose you're making a hash of things, eh?' Mrs McTaggart is probably a lot more worried than Johnny. 'How are things doing today, Mrs McTaggart, did you sleep all right last night?' is a better form of approach. Mrs McTaggart knows that the doctor is going to care about Johnny. She gets a boost from knowing that the doctor cares about *her*.

The role of the *dietitian* is of great importance, because she may be trying to introduce the parent to abstract thought. It falls to the dietitian to explain the mysteries of carbohydrates, proteins and fats and almost inevitably she is also involved in explaining the connection between insulin and carbohydrate metabolism. She has to talk about blood sugar when discussing carbohydrate, she can hardly discuss blood sugar without discussing the effects of insulin. The nurse can say 'Now put five drops of urine in this test-tube, see what I'm telling you love, what a shame you've put in six. ... Wash it out and try again ... no, not that test-tube, a dry one, ten drops of water, that's it, and pop in the tablet ... yes, I know it's got blue spots dear, they all have ... and *up* it goes in a lovely fizz, you weren't watching, no it doesn't matter that you've dropped it on the floor, let's try again' and the mother can see it all happening with her own eyes. But the dietitian cannot say 'Oh, see this great lump of starch *slowly* turning into sugar ... now, it is positively *oozing* into the blood ... ah, my goodness, this is our lucky day, here comes a molecule of insulin ...' She is trying to teach theory to one who may not have a theoretical turn of mind. The dietitian needs to be patient, learned, intelligent and kind, which is a lot to expect from the salary she is paid.

The *consultant* is relatively unimportant in the first few days. He should be sure that he is well informed about his patient before he approaches the bedside. The mother may have saved up her questions for him alone. There are some mothers who speak easily to nurses, others who feel that consultants are the only worthy recipients of their thoughts (possibly because the father thinks so, and one must be sure to talk to the father in such circumstances), but always one is looking for those who have mastered the simple mechanisms of diabetes, those who feel they have won some small victory. Then one can ask the father to be present as well as the mother, recapitulate what little has been learned and make plans for the future. It is of great importance that the father should be brought in at this stage, if not before, and if it means that the consultation will have to take place on a Saturday then the consultant will just have to bite on the bullet.

Subjects discussed at the Saturday interview might well be:

(1) The effect of insulin lack on the blood sugar, and how this may well lead to polyuria, polydipsia and acetonuria.
(2) The interaction of the food, insulin and exercise on the blood sugar.
(3) The causes, timing and treatment of hypoglycaemic attacks, remembering that at this time the parents will be more fearful of hypoglycaemic attacks than of anything. The parent does not worry about the theory of a hypo attack, he is worried in case his child is going to die.
(4) Injection sites and the care of syringes, insulin, etc.
(5) Occasions for lowering or raising insulin.
(6) The action to be taken if a child develops an infection.

The consultant must attempt to allay natural anxiety before it arises. The sudden appearance of struggling in a previously cooperative child is a commonplace. So is the added worry whenever the child is out of the parents' sight. This can be marked when the child is at school, gross during the hours of darkness. It is worth repeating that the parents do not care a tuppenny hoot whether their child has a hypo or not, they are worried about his chances of dying. This is the great fear. This must be hammered out.

The parents must not be allowed to feel that at discharge a lifeline is being cut. They should be told that, although given an appointment, they can in fact attend the clinic at any time, and they should also be assured that a telephone call will not be regarded as the silly panic of inadequacy but as a sensible use of the experience of others.

Communication at the time of discharge

The *family doctor* will, of course, receive a discharge letter from the hospital. This letter should be sent immediately as the doctor is being asked to be the first line of defence in a continuing disease. It is a good practice to send him a copy of the booklet used at the clinic because diabetes in childhood is relatively rare and he may not have had to deal with a child diabetic before, and also because the booklet should ensure that the family doctor and the clinic take the same line. There are certain points of legitimate disagreement in the management of diabetes, for example in the diet or the type of insulin used, but these minor differences may seem major to the parent. Even slight differences in phrasing or emphasis may be taken by the parent to imply disagreement between doctors. It is easier for doctors to fit in with the central regime of the clinic than for the clinic to fit in with the different ideas of different doctors. At the same time the family doctor should not feel that he is being cut out. I think it a pity that although I receive many phone calls from patients I get relatively few from doctors.

The *school medical service* should also be kept informed. In a large city it may be possible to attain the ideal of a school medical officer sitting in at the diabetic clinic for a few sessions to find out how that clinic deals with its problems. This medical officer is then in a very good position to see that the child is well integrated into the school. The welcome given to a diabetic child varies from school to school and from teacher to teacher. The effect of a mild hypo is unpredictable. The reaction of one teacher may be 'get that child out of here! Special School for *him*!', whereas another teacher may become very interested in the problems of the diabetic and may indeed become quite expert in telling a genuine hypo from a slight touch of hysteria or an attempted confidence trick. The school medical officer is best placed to settle such problems that arise in school and it is a pity that the liaison between the clinic and the school medical service is sometimes not as good as it might be.

If that is the case, there is a short pamphlet published by the British Diabetic Association (BDA) called *The Diabetic at School* which may prove useful. The doctor can give two copies to the mother, one for the head teacher and one for the class teacher. It is obtainable from the British Diabetic Association, 10 Queen Anne Street, London, W1M 0BD.

The *school teacher* wants to know
(1) A little about the nature of the disease.
(2) The recognition and treatment of hypo attacks.
(3) The how and where of urgent medical help.
(4) What punishments are suitable for the diabetic child (for example, he should not be 'kept in' beyond a meal-time).

Ideally, this information should be passed on by the school medical officer.

Home visiting is another ideal probably attainable only in the larger centres. Some hospitals have a nursing sister whose task is to follow a patient with a long-term illness (for example, coeliac disease, diabetes, cystic fibrosis, certain orthopaedic problems) into his home immediately after discharge. In the case of the diabetic the sister might well appear on the morning after discharge just after the injection should have been given, to find out if all is going smoothly and to give advice if it is not. No doubt she would also accept a cup of tea if it were offered and two-way communication can thrive in such a relaxed atmosphere. The mother can pick up a few nursing details particularly suited to her circumstances and the sister can report back to the hospital on the atmosphere in the home.

Until now the appointment of such a nurse to work in the community has depended on the chance coincidence of a nurse, ready and capable of doing such a job and of such a job existing where a nurse wants to do it. Recently, however, a training course has been provided specifically to produce nurses with the necessary skills. In the USA such schemes have been extended to regions (Giordano *et al.*, 1977).

A hospital social worker can enlist the aid of a local social worker in visiting the home or the district nurse can be asked to supervise injections, but such solutions are probably second best unless the district nurse knows the family already. The nursing sister has a chance to know the patient before his discharge and her extra medical knowledge, particularly concerning childhood diabetes, can be an advantage.

The outpatient clinic

Little will be said here about the workings of the clinic, which has a chapter to itself. It is at the clinic that the parents' diabetic horizons are widened. They learn, without indignation if they are gently led, that the management of diabetes is not as simple as was first made out. The paediatrician in his turn learns more about the home and mutual understanding increases.

All would agree that the aim in managing childhood diabetes includes outward normality. A mother who is tentatively injecting oranges and viewing her first exchange list should not be bothered with such notions unless they occur to her. There cannot be even outward normality until the parents are themselves coping with diabetes. In the early months at the clinic one can begin to push gently the expectation of normality in the end. The British Diabetic Association, particularly through the journal *Balance*, can help in this respect. It is a sane journal, different from the hectically sad journals of societies for fatal diseases, and all parents should be urged to join the BDA. Indeed, membership of the BDA might be considered as prescribable under the National Health Service. The time for pushing the idea of normality is the first few months after discharge from hospital, but otherwise that is a period of consolidation.

FURTHER EDUCATION

There are many more diabetic adults than diabetic children, so it is natural and indeed right that the meetings of the British Diabetic Association tend to concentrate on the adult diabetics. There is therefore a case for forming a special group for the parents of diabetic children.

The parents' group

The parents' group should serve an area, not a hospital, as judicious out-breeding will improve the stock. The group should be formed under the wing of the BDA, as this may make it possible to use premises outside a hospital. Meetings should not take place in hospital if an alternative can be arranged, partly because parents might come to regard other hospitals as 'inferior' and partly because parents talk more freely in a non-clinical atmosphere.

Any paediatrician starting such a group should first consult his colleagues in the area to make sure he has their goodwill as some might suspect the impending propagation of heresy, and such physicians should be particularly urged to attend an early meeting. These early meetings will of necessity be arranged by the physicians, but the parents should be encouraged to form their own committee as soon as possible, and refer back to the BDA for guidance in running their own affairs. As I see it, the principle behind these meetings is that doctors and parents should meet as experts in their own fields, medical experts and Our-Jeannie experts. It is not only the parents who will learn from these meetings. Doctors can benefit too, particularly if the meetings are kept informal. A long talk from a doctor followed by a few questions from the floor will not do. A short talk followed by a rambling discussion is much better. The doctor should be asking questions as well as answering them. 'How many are still wetting the bed?' followed by 'How many of you think it is due to diabetes?' gives useful information to everybody quickly.

The presence of one doctor is essential, but two doctors taking different sides in a discussion is better and three doctors having an argument is splendid—as long as they can agree on a final opinion. Obviously there should be no clash on major issues, but doctors can discuss the pros and cons of giving insulin during the remission period, or take slightly divergent views on the significance of a behaviour pattern described by a parent. Such episodes help a parent to think, instead of always being on the receiving end of instructions. The doctor can always talk at a certain parent while gazing steadfastly in another direction, a procedure which would only give offence in the outpatient clinic.

A dietitian is almost essential, and social workers should be encouraged to attend. It is useful to have up one's sleeve a list of sensible teenagers who can describe their days as diabetic children, and a visit from a school teacher can be arranged.

It is true that the parents with the poorest knowledge of diabetes are the ones least likely to attend, but trying to help the good parents is still well worth while. I have learned, for example, that it is difficult even for good parents to see what is involved in balancing dependence and independence in the child. 'How can we make a child independent without encouraging him to be irresponsible?' leads to a good deal of confused muttering. It is at least a help to realize that the confusion is there.

Teach-ins

A 'teach-in' for diabetic children and their parents carries the 'parents' group' one step further. One I attended recently was held over a weekend during the summer holidays at a residential college so that the children, the parents and at least some of the medical team could live in. All expenses were paid by the BDA and members of the BDA acted as child-watchers when necessary. Short talks were given on diet, holiday camps and various aspects of diabetes, and long discussions followed. Films were shown, short ones about diabetes and long ones about cowboys. Everybody ate together. In the intervals, worried fathers took on new life as agile goalkeepers and physicians were rebuked by their patients for smoking too much. Those who were silent on the first day were talking freely by the second. The parents appeared to benefit from it and the children were not too bored. At the end, one mother made a salutary comment, 'It's not so much what I learned, doctor, it was finding how many people were trying to help John and me'.

The trouble with such a meeting is that it is too expensive to run frequently. It requires organizing and many helpers have to give up a lot of time.

Holiday camps

The holiday camp allows the diabetic child to communicate with his peers, in deed if not in word. It is doubtful if there is a diabetician in the UK who does not approve of diabetic camps. The diabetic child learns how much he can really do without disaster supervening. He sees others giving their own injections and dealing with problems like his own. His independence is encouraged. He can become a member of a different, rather elitist group of his own, a thought which may sustain him if his nasty little school-fellows tease him about being a diabetic. His whole outlook on his diabetes can be altered. He may, for example, see and help a friend who is becoming hypoglycaemic, a great boost to his pride and self-confidence.

This leads to the observation that a diabetic at camp will learn in a new way, by observation of what his fellows are doing. True, there will still be instruction from above but some older children rather resent that type of instruction and do better by following their peers. The rebellious child may best be treated as part of a group to prevent him feeling 'picked on' *again*. The physician caring for a diabetic camp should consider the personalities of his charges and avoid appearing as just another physician laying down the law.

Nobody doubts the value of the camp, but unfortunately the literature on the subject is somewhat dowdy. Psychological tests have been employed in an attempt to demonstrate the improvement which occurred at camp, but without any real success.

This raises a principle in medical practice. If something cannot be proved, can it be ignored? The scientist, with reservations, might answer 'yes', the artist 'no', while the physician probably tries to keep an open mind, which lets bias in. It does seem, however, that children are happier when they come back from camp. The Craig Test for Jollity has not yet been devised so this remains a subjective opinion.

The only worry about the camps is that the children one most wants to see there, the over-protected and the self-content, elect to stay at home. Were they to go, the psychological improvement might be demonstrable.

What about the physician, particularly in relation to medical ethics? He must certainly be allowed to correct major errors of technique (on the grounds that it is the child rather than the home clinic which has gone wrong), and he must be allowed to change the dose of insulin; but should he be encouraged to change the *type* of insulin and the number of doses, except in an emergency? I realize that I disagree with many when I suggest that he should not; but my objection is pragmatic as well as ethical. A change may not be accepted by the parent who changes back to the old insulin as soon as the child is home. This makes it difficult for the home clinic who may have been considering just such a change after camp and who now fear that if they do make the change the mother will think they have no minds of their own. I think the authority of the physician with long-term care of the child should not be undermined, even unintentionally and with the best of motives. If I am at a camp and think a change should be made I write a personal letter to the home doctor suggesting that such a change might be indicated.

Any physician with a chance to attend a diabetic camp should go. It will be very good for his medical education. At the ordinary diabetic clinic there is not time to check on every point in management at each visit and some amazing errors can arise unknown to the physician. They come to light at camp and sometimes elsewhere and nobody should pride himself on his ability to manage diabetes until he knows what can happen. I shall give some examples.

(1) I came across one boy who had three vials of soluble and three vials of isophane floating around in a container of methylated spirit. The 'soluble' was no longer a clear solution. His technique was to take up the isophane first, insert the needle in the soluble and then pump the plunger of the syringe up and down three or four times, finally fetching up with the correct total dose—but in what balance between soluble and isophane, goodness only knows.

(2) The daily insulin requirements of another boy dropped from 148 to 40 units during two weeks at camp and even at the low dose he was having frequent hypo attacks. This raises the suspicion that there may be some days at home when he does not take any insulin at all. Such a suspicion is very difficult to verify, but there is a true

tale to be told. A physician, himself a diabetic, had charge of a diabetic camp and took his non-diabetic son along with him to help out. One day the physician went to one of the cabins to give the occupants a short talk on one aspect of diabetes. He was met at the door by his son, who asked 'Dad, how long can you go without your insulin?' 'I don't know', replied his father, 'I have never tried'. 'Well', said his son, 'This chap says he can go for four days, and this one says *he* can go for *six* days. ...'

(3) At a one-day seminar in another part of Scotland a father came up to me (quietly, I am glad to say) and asked me why his son got boils at his injection sites. I tried to persuade him that his son did *not* get boils at his injection sites, this being a very rare thing to happen, even once, but eventually he convinced me. It transpired that he kept the syringe and needles in uncovered, unboiled, unchanged water.

(4) I am certain that in all these cases the child had deviated from the instructions originally given, which leaves me asking 'What is going on in *my* clinic?' I shall tell you. A boy of seven years had been diabetic for eight months and had given no trouble during the remission period. It transpired that his insulin requirements had recently been rising and that he had begun to have hypo attacks.

Myself: When do they happen?
Mother: When he goes to his Granny's.
Myself: When is that?
Mother: Just after getting off the bus, walking up to her house, about half-past eleven.
Myself: Has he had his snack all right?
Mother: No, it's a long journey and I don't like him eating on the bus, it's not nice.
Myself: He must have his snack. How does he respond to his Dextrosol?
Mother: I don't give him Dextrosol. Oh, I know what you said, but a woman told me you can't give a diabetic sugar. I've tried him on snuff.
Myself: Snuff?
Mother: It's no good. This (*and she dumped a bottle of smelling-salts on the desk*) is much better. Livens him up at once.

After some discussion I suggested altering his insulin and introducing a little soluble. She did not like the idea. After a pause for thought she slapped down a packet of disposable needles bearing the legend 'Sterilised by Gamma Radiation'. 'Does this mean', she asked, 'that if I have him circumcised we won't have to change the insulin?'

It is perhaps just as well that the physician does not know all that is going on in his clinic or he might succumb to that dreaded affliction, brain-rot.

TOWARDS SELF-CARE

Self-care in diabetes, by which one means the ability to adjust one's insulin and diet to urinary findings and to expected stress, and to give one's injections, is the ultimate aim of education in diabetes. The journey really begins in the cradle. If little problems of eating, sleeping and voiding are not adequately dealt with there will be a rift in confidence between mother and child. If this wound does not heal, the onset of diabetes will open it further. The intelligence, personality and environment of the child are as much determinants of his fitness to look after himself as is his age, though age is very important. When should we encourage a child to stand on his own?

It may well be helpful here to consider the findings of Etzwiler (1962). By means of a questionnaire (*Figure 5.1*) he deduced that children did not have a reasonable knowledge of diabetes before the age of 12 or 13 years. He reached the important conclusion that to ask a child to care for himself before then could only lead to feelings of inadequacy and thus exaggerate the adolescent rebellion.

The only modification one would offer is that Etzwiler's work does not allow (and he never suggested that it did) for individual variations. Attending my clinic now is the only child of elderly parents, an intelligent somewhat obese lad of 11 who has no trouble with the questionnaire but who seems quite prepared to let his parents look after him indefinitely, so personality is important. There is also a boy of ten who got off to too good a start. He was giving his own injections at the age of four, which seemed to encourage his parents to leave him on his own. More often than not he attends the clinic without his urine charts, and almost always without his mother. A spell of sustained ketosis led to his readmission for stabilization. Minor faults of technique were ironed out and the mother was urged in a long interview to supervise the boy closely. When she returned to the ward immediately after that interview, her son, fascinated by his refurbished skills, asked her to come and watch him testing his urine. 'I can't be bothered', she replied. That boy's future is worrying. It has been shown (Collier and Etzwiler, 1971) that a child's knowledge of diabetes coincides closely with his parents' knowledge of the disease. In fact, knowledge of the disease is held in common in the family. If a family is irresponsible a child will need constant instruction, however good he may seem to be at

1   Have you ever read or has anyone ever read to you any books or articles about diabetes?
    (A) Yes
    (B) No
    (C) Don't know

2   In uncontrolled diabetes the blood sugar is
    (A) Increased
    (B) Decreased
    (C) Neither A nor B
    (D) Don't know

3   Insulin causes the blood sugar to
    (A) Rise
    (B) Fall
    (C) Neither A nor B
    (D) Don't know

4   *Soluble insulin acts
    (A) Fast, and for a short time
    (B) Slowly and for a long time
    (C) Neither A nor B
    (D) Don't know

5   *Lente acts
    (A) Fast, and for a short time
    (B) Slowly and for a long time
    (C) Neither A nor B
    (D) Don't know

6   When urine is tested with Clinitest tablets a red-orange colour means
    (A) Lots of sugar in the urine
    (B) Little or no sugar in the urine
    (C) Neither A nor B
    (D) Don't know

7   When urine tests with Clinitest constantly show a red-orange colour, do you need
    (A) More insulin
    (B) Less insulin
    (C) Same amount of insulin
    (D) Don't know

8   Is acetone in your urine
    (A) Good
    (B) Bad
    (C) Don't know

9   If acetone is in your urine, do you need
    (A) More insulin
    (B) Less insulin
    (C) Same amount of insulin
    (D) Don't know

10 If you feel shaky and dizzy you should
    (A) Take more insulin
    (B) Eat sugar
    (C) Lie down and go to sleep
    (D) Don't know

Figure 5.1. A questionnaire designed to test a child's knowledge of his diabetes. (By permission of Dr Donnell Etzwiler)

* These questions are phrased according to the insulins of which the child has experience.

managing himself. When we talk of gradually training a child for self-care we use words like 'communication' and 'education' both of which carry an intellectual connotation. We should realize that self-care will come when the child feels a need for it, and a need is emotional.

It has often been said that diabetics should be told they can lead a completely normal life. I think this is a mistake, particularly with children. The diabetic child knows perfectly well he is not leading a normal life. Since when were injections, urine-testing, diet and strict time-keeping 'normal' for a child? If the doctor goes on talking about a normal life the child may come to regard him as a fool, quite out of touch with reality. Even worse, the child may believe him and fail to realize that his disease must be taken seriously, which would be a horrible failure in communication. It is better to say to the older child precisely what one means, something along the lines of 'We all know diabetes is a terrible nuisance and it's bad luck that you have to put up with all this caper, but think of all you can still do. You can play all your old games, and when you are older and looking after your own diabetes nobody outside the family need ever know you are diabetic. You can take a job and get married in the normal way.' The last sentence contains two half-truths—not all jobs are available to diabetics and a few diabetic boys may be impotent as adults (Ellenberg, 1971)—but at this stage the half-truths seem justified.

Johansson, Larsson and Ludvigsson (1979) stress the need for educating the older child as well as the parents. When they interviewed child diabetics who had become young adults they found that more than half considered that the information they had been given about diabetes was 'highly inadequate'. The patients felt that their parents had been instructed but that they themselves had been largely ignored, even when they were old enough to understand. The dangerous time is in the early teens, when many leave a children's hospital and change to an adult hospital. The paediatrician may think that the adult physician will give information about the future diabetic life and the adult physician may assume that the paediatrician has already done so. In addition, about half the patients thought diabetic clinics were poorly run and that diabetic associations were of little help, which probably indicates no more than a negative attitude to society in some young adult diabetics. However, the medical profession has not been at its best in dealing with this problem.

REFERENCES

Collier, B. N. and Etzwiler, D. D. (1971). A comparative study of diabetic knowledge among juvenile diabetics and their parents. *Diabetes*, **20,** 51

Ellenberg, M. (1971). Impotence in diabetes: the neurologic factor. *Ann. intern. Med.*, **75,** 213

Etzwiler, D. D. (1962). What the juvenile diabetic knows about this disease. *Pediatrics*, **29,** 135

Giordano, B., Rosenbloom, A. L., Heller, D., Weber, F. T., Gonzalez, R. and Grgic, A. (1977). Regional services for children and youth with diabetes. *Pediatrics*, **60,** 492

Johansson, E., Larsson, Y. and Ludvigsson, J. (1979). Social adaptation in juvenile diabetes. *Acta paediat. Scand.*, Suppl. 275, 85

Kaufman, R. V. and Hersher, Betty (1971). Body image changes in teenage diabetics. *Pediatrics*, **48,** 123

Two books are also recommended

Peter and Mary are Diabetics. Produced by Novo Industri and distributed by Martindale Pharmaceuticals Ltd., Chesham House, Chesham Close, Romford RM1 4JX, Essex. A small booklet, useful in the early school years. Peter, a carefree little fellow, is kept up to the mark by Mary, who knows it all. The format allows certain dangers to be stressed in an impersonal and non-punitive way.

Notes for the Guidance of Parents of Diabetic Children by J. W. Farquhar, 2nd edition. Edinburgh, Churchill Livingstone, pp. 45. Price 95p. My personal feeling is that the instructions and explanations given are rather full for the parents of a child who has just become diabetic, but I recommend it after the parents have had a few months' experience of diabetes.

Appendix

New patients are discharged from the Royal Hospital for Sick Children, Glasgow (RHSC) with a printed booklet containing notes on management. These notes are meant to act as reminders of the initial instruction which has been given and are not meant to be a complete guide to the outpatient management of diabetic children. After parents have had some months of experience they are advised to buy the booklet by Farquhar, mentioned above.

Certain points should be made about the RHSC booklet.

(1) A blank space is left for individual instructions, telephone data, etc.
(2) Parents are asked to test the urine four times a day till first seen at the outpatient clinic.
(3) Parents are asked not to alter the insulin dosage before the first clinic attendance without first consulting one of the clinic doctors by telephone.
(4) The booklet also contains notes on diet. These are given in Chapter 13.

The introductory text of the booklet is given below. I have found that these bare bones suffice as an introduction.

DIABETES

Diabetes occurs when there is a lack of insulin in the blood. Insulin is produced by the pancreas, and normally helps us to use the sugar in our blood. If there is a lack of insulin, the sugar in the blood rises. The sugar in the urine depends on the sugar in the blood, and the urine sugar is easier to test. It is our aim in diabetes to keep the blood sugar near a normal level by the use of insulin. Factors which lower the blood sugar are insulin, exercise, and too little food. Conversely, lack of insulin, lack of exercise and too much food will raise the blood sugar, and so may most of the simple infections.

Injections of insulin are usually given into the outer part of the front of the thigh but the front of the abdomen can also be used. We seldom advise injecting into the buttocks in case the sciatic nerve is affected.

If you keep injecting in the same place, hard patches may form under the skin. Your child may ask you to inject into this place, as it is less painful in a hard patch. However, insulin is not regularly absorbed from a hard patch, so you must not give way to your child's wishes.

Syringe and needles. Your syringe bears the number BS1619, and any syringe that does so is satisfactory. In replacing needles, try to obtain size 25G.

Syringe and needles should be kept in methylated spirit. Surgical spirit should not be used. Before use, the plunger should be worked up and down in the syringe to dry out excess spirit, and then the needle is put on the syringe to dry out the needle. The methylated spirit should be changed weekly.

To avoid getting bubbles when you draw up the insulin into the syringe, inject from the syringe into the insulin bottle a volume of air equal to the amount of insulin you are going to withdraw.

Testing the urine. The urine should be tested ten minutes before breakfast and before the main evening meal.

(1) *Sugar.* Follow the instructions issued with your Clinitest tablets.
It is possible to have sugar in the urine when the blood sugar is normal or low, particularly before breakfast. Morning urine may, for example, be urine which has collected in the bladder between 10 pm and 8 am. The urine passed between 10 pm and midnight may contain much sugar, that between 6 am and 8 am, none, but both these urines mix in the bladder, so that you may find a positive result at 8 am even though the sugar in the blood may be lower than normal at the time. One can always check on this by testing an extra specimen of urine at 7 am, but the doctor will keep you right.

(2) *Acetone.* The urine need not be tested for acetone as a routine. The presence of acetone often means that there is a good deal

more than 5% sugar in the urine. The doctor will tell you when to test for acetone.

Hypoglycaemic attacks are usually called 'hypos'. They happen when the blood sugar is low. This is most likely to occur before a meal, particularly if a meal is late or has been missed, and it may happen on waking in the morning. An unusual amount of exercise, or a late night, may produce low blood sugar.

In a hypo attack the child is usually pale, clammy, drowsy and irritable. Any very odd behaviour, particularly before a meal, should make one think of a hypo attack.

The treatment is to give two pudding-spoonsful of sugar or glucose, washed down with a little water. Six Dextrosol tablets or half a tumbler of Lucozade are alternatives. Repeat in 5 minutes if the child is not improving. If you find it difficult to give the sugar, tell the doctor, because it is often possible to use an injection to help you. If you are not sure if it is a hypo attack or not, treat it as a hypo attack.

Diabetic pre-coma. The opposite of hypoglycaemia is a return towards the diabetic state your child was in before he was admitted to hospital. If the urine sugar is high for a long time you may notice that he is passing a lot of water and having to get up at night to pass water. This is a sign of the need for an increase in insulin, because if the signs are neglected your child may gradually drift towards diabetic coma. Hypoglycaemic attacks come suddenly. It usually takes several days for a child to develop diabetic coma.

Changing the insulin. The insulin is adjusted to the amount of sugar in the urine. If you find three or four readings of 3% or 5% *in succession*, and the reading is still high, raise the insulin by two units (one mark on your syringe). If you find three or four clear readings in succession, lower the insulin by one mark. If there is a hypo attack for which the reason is not obvious (such as being late with a meal), drop the insulin one mark. If your child is not on a single injection the doctor will give you special instructions.

Illness of any kind may lead to more sugar appearing in the urine, in which case you will probably have to raise the dose of insulin.

If your child is off his food because of illness, try to ensure that he gets all his carbohydrate ration, even in the form of sugar if all else fails. You will find a list of foods you can use in the 'emergency' in your diet sheet.

If your child's intake of food is low due to illness you may feel you should reduce the insulin. In fact, you may have to raise it. The rule is, *follow the urine* results, and if there is a lot of sugar in the urine raise the insulin. On the other hand if the urine is clear of sugar, which may happen if the child is vomiting and has no fever, the insulin should be reduced. Usually, if a child is feverish and not eating well he will still produce sugar from his own body tissues, and this sugar needs insulin to cover it as much as carbohydrate taken by mouth. Remember, adjust the insulin according to the urine results, not according to the food intake.

Exercise. It is often difficult to tell how much exercise a young child is going to take. If you know he is going to take more than usual, for example during a night at the Cubs, you can give him an extra 10 g of carbohydrate beforehand. If you realize afterwards that he has already taken much more exercise, give him an extra 10 g of carbohydrate.

CHAPTER 6

The Outpatient Clinic

> Sigh out a lamentable tale of things
> Done long ago, and ill done ...
> John Ford (1586–1640)

GENERAL CONSIDERATIONS

There are some who regard an outpatient clinic as an irritating interruption in the serious busines of ward medicine. I have never felt it so. The charm of the outpatient clinic is that one never knows what is going to happen next. Certain conversations which could only have taken place in a general paediatric outpatient clinic stand out in the memory. I once asked a mother about the family history, and got the reply 'Well, my husband's a transvestist, of course'. It was the 'of course' which gave the comment its air of mystery. The simple opening question 'Now, what is concerning you most about her?' has produced two memorable replies: 'A man on the bus said it was her glands, doctor' and 'To tell you the truth, he has never been himself all his days'. Life in the outpatient clinic is as real as a Thurber drawing.

It may be that the diabetic clinic at the Royal Hospital for Sick Children, Glasgow (RHSC) is not entirely typical of the clinics in Britain. The clinic must respond to the patients who attend it and in Glasgow we have more than our share of the underprivileged.

The social background of British children is described in *Born to Fail?* (1973), an account of 10 504 children born in one week in March, 1958 (The National Child Development Study). They had been followed up at seven years (1965) and 11 years (1969). Using standards of family composition (a large number of children, or a one-parent family, low income and poor housing), one child in 16 was at a social disadvantage in Britain. There were wide regional differences. In Southern England the figure was one in 47, in Wales and Northern Ireland one in 12 and in Scotland one in 10. Glasgow is socially the worst part of Scotland. According to the 1956 Census, only 2 per cent of houses in Birmingham consisted of one or two rooms, at which time the figure for Glasgow was 48 per cent. If overcrowding be taken as more than 1.5 members of the family per room then 18 per cent of British children were overcrowded either at seven or 11 years. The Glasgow figure for 1956 was 66 per cent. Admittedly, the Glasgow figures predate the national figures and Glasgow housing has improved in recent years, but the mothers of today spent their childhood in these very poor conditions and Glasgow now supports a legacy from the past and a burden in the present.

Many mothers with such a background are against 'the establishment', against clinics and against doctors. Talking to some of them is very difficult. Statements like 'Advice to parents regarding the exercise of a benign discipline is usually all that is required' are well-rounded and worthy but hollow. They sound as if they had come out of a computer, tonelessly*. It would be better to treat the parents to a couple of verses of *Afton Water* which might attract their interest and induce a cooperative frame of mind.

It is well established that one of the main features in maintaining good diabetic control is a good social background. The difficulties caused by overcrowding, poverty and inadequate control by adults are obvious in the care of the diabetic. In addition, parents in poor surroundings tend to resent medical clinics. In *Born to Fail?* it is stated that two-thirds of the mothers from good homes attended child welfare clinics regularly, but only one third of the mothers from poor homes did so, even though they were in need of supervision. It is another feature of the anti-establishment mentality. The poorest attenders are those who most need to attend. It may appear in this chapter and elsewhere that the writer runs into more trouble with his diabetics than others do; but it is hoped in the light of what is written above, that this will be accepted as reasonable by the charitable reader. If one concentrates on the difficult cases there should be little trouble in dealing with the easy ones.

Secular changes in the outlook of the country cannot be ignored. I took over this diabetic clinic 25 years ago and it seems to me that during that time the attitude of parents, particularly the good ones, towards the diabetes of their children has altered for the worse.

* After 1 Corinthians XIII, v. 1.

Perhaps the optimism of my youth has given way to the disillusionment of age. In fact, I know it has, but I do not think it has swayed my judgement in this case. Parents and children are now more anxious than they were. I do not say that diabetes is worse controlled than it used to be, but I think control is more difficult to maintain than it was. It is for the social philosopher to evaluate the causes of any increased anxiety in the population as a whole, but anxiety over medical matters seems to have been fostered by the press and television, writing or talking just a shade above the heads of the majority. This gives parents the feeling that they will never understand all there is to be known about these things while the very fact that they have been harangued makes them feel they *should* understand. This undermines their confidence in themselves without in any way increasing their trust in doctors. So much the worse for diabetic control.

CONSTITUTION OF THE CLINIC

The patients

It is now necessary to consider the setting up of a diabetic clinic for children. Who should attend? In Glasgow, children come to the RHSC until their thirteenth birthday and are then referred to an adult hospital, one of five hospitals depending on the district in which they live. In Edinburgh, which has the same rule about not admitting after the thirteenth birthday, patients attend the children's diabetic clinic until their sixteenth birthday, but are admitted to one adult hospital if inpatient treatment is needed between the thirteenth and sixteenth birthdays. This has the advantage for the paediatrician of allowing him to have a continuing say in management through the stormy years of adolescence, but it calls for cooperation between the two hospitals. The large paediatric unit in a general hospital has at least one advantage over a sick children's hospital: it is much easier for the paediatrician to follow the progress of his former patients. On the other hand, one should consider whether it is best for the patient to make a double change at 16, from one hospital to another and from school to adult life. I favour making the change at 13.

It is for the physician to decide for himself whether it is worth holding a special clinic for diabetic children. A tentative opinion is that if 20 diabetic children attend under one roof it is worth instituting a special clinic for them.

The clinic staff

The doctors

The advantage of having a diabetic clinic attached to a children's hospital is that the clinic will be big enough to be worth while but not so big that the personal touch is lost, which can happen at the clinics of some of the large adult hospitals. If only one or two physicians are running a clinic, the patient and his doctors come to know each other well, so that the patients and their parents come to believe that they are at least getting continuity of care. It is also easy for two physicians to consult together about any problem that is arising.

The dietitian

Should the dietitian have a room of her own or not? If the clinic is not too cumbersome, i.e. if it is held in one or two rooms, it seems preferable for the dietitian to sit in with the doctors. There can then be a prompt interchange of question and answer between parent, dietitian and doctor about any small point which arises. It is also desirable, however, that the dietitian should have another room available for lengthy discussions with an occasional parent. A few parents have difficulty in understanding the principles of diet at first and all of them should have a thorough check of the day's intake every year or so. Quite often, one finds that a 'well-trained' parent has quietly slipped into error. The doctor needs only a summary from the dietitian. A long dietetic discussion at the doctor's desk wastes clinic time.

Nurse-technician

The roles of the *nurse* and the laboratory *technician* have to be considered together. If a number of clinics are running together the hospital may supply a biochemistry laboratory technician to do the routine side-room work, including the testing of diabetic urines. If this is so, the nursing duties in the clinic may be carried out by an auxiliary nurse who may not be experienced in testing urines though well able to take the height and weight and fetch and carry in general. The alternative is to have a state-registered nurse who will measure the height and weight and also test the urine. The best system is probably that which gives the nearest approach to permanency. Junior laboratory technicians are under training and may return 1 per cent on a urine which the patient has scored as 2 per cent, in which case the patient is probably right. The nurse who has been with the clinic for years is trained in the ways of the clinic and can be trusted.

Social work

A *social worker* should be available. It is probable that the majority of patients have no serious social problems and a social worker giving her full attention for the time to the diabetic clinic may be a luxury, yet parent and doctor can learn much from a social worker. The contented mother need only stick her head round the social worker's door, but others welcome a good long chat about nothing much. There are some things which mothers will discuss more freely with social workers than with doctors or nurses, little things about their private lives which they feel ashamed to tell the doctor.

> Jean was a girl of eight whose diabetes unexpectedly went out of control. Questions were answered truthfully. Yes, she was taking her carbohydrate accurately. Yes, the urine testing and insulin injections were carefully supervised. No, she did not seem ill, she was still normally active. It was the social worker who finally supplied the full answer. Jean's elder brother had just become an abattoir attendant and with rather too much enthusiasm, persisted in showing Jean his how-to-do-it picture books on the slaughtering, skinning and evisceration of animals. Jean had gone off all animal food and dairy products, living mostly on bread and tea. Her nights were disturbed by dreams. Yet Jean's mother had been too embarrassed by this family upheaval to mention it to the doctor, and he in his turn (as can be imagined) had not thought to ask the vital question 'Has your son become an abattoir attendant and is he pestering your daughter with nasty pictures?'

This episode stresses that it is not enough for the doctor to tell the mother what should be done; the mother also has a duty to tell the doctor what is happening at home, and it is the business of the social worker to help her in doing so by supplying a sisterly shoulder for her to weep on.

'The trusties'

It may be that, in a smaller hospital or in a developing country, it will not be possible to have a dietitian at the clinic or a social worker on call. It should be possible, however, to enlist the help of one or two reliable mothers, a system which was begun at the Royal Hospital for Sick Children in Edinburgh. These mothers take it in turns to run a small stall at the diabetic clinic where disposable needles are issued and syringes are sold at bulk rates*, where meetings and diabetic camps are advertised and where the various publications and products of the British Diabetic Association are available. There is thus the opportunity for the mother of a new diabetic to discuss problems of management with a mother who has had considerable experience of the subject. This gets round the attitude 'What do they know about it? They have never had a diabetic child of their own', but the experienced mothers must not say anything which can be construed as different from the advice given by the doctor or dietitian. They should comment not on the amount of carbohydrate to be given, but on the form in which their own child found it most palatable. They should not be drawn into discussions on which is 'the best' insulin or how much should be given, but they can talk of how their own difficulties were resolved or disappeared. This introduces another parameter of care for the diabetic child, that of shared experience. One cannot measure the power of shared experience but I believe it to be great. It seems to be the instrument for tapping some primordial strength. A doctor may be second best in not having a diabetic child of his own but by seeing a mother and child for many years, he can develop an empathy which is close to shared experience. This is the justification of continuity of care.

It is true that meetings of the British Diabetic Association bring some (not very many) parents together, but such meetings are less intimate, less personal and therefore less real. Meetings for the parents of diabetic children can be arranged. The big meetings tend to pass on knowledge, the personal chats bring hope. The mother who is to become a counsellor should not be too shy or too uncertain to give advice, but equally she must be free from the urge to impress or domineer. The selection of suitable mothers can be made less invidious if their nominal function is to issue disposable needles.

Backing for the clinic

This will come from other specialties. Most important in childhood diabetes are the psychiatrist, the dentist and the ophthalmologist. The importance of maintaining close contact with these specialists will be discussed later.

---

* A physician cannot do this, it is indulging in trade.

A MORNING IN THE DIABETIC CLINIC

'If anything happens to that boy, you've got me to reckon with. I'm older than you are, but I'm kinda sneaky.'

Buck, in *High Chaparral*

'I do not kick against my fate,
I think that life is swell.
Contentedly I sit and wait
For the world to go to hell'.
Don Marquis

The mood of the doctor on entering the diabetic clinic may be one of brisk militancy or passive resignation. He is well advised to slip into emotional neutral before seeing his first patient. Mrs Smith may be intensely irritating. I have found, however, that I do not become so easily irritated since realizing that irritation usually resulted from a feeling that I was not doing a good job, either because I could not assess the situation clearly or because insurmountable social or intellectual defects seemed to be impeding the chosen line of treatment. One must also remember that to be as irritating as she is, Mrs Smith must have great problems of her own. Mrs Jones is not very clever, so she needs more help rather than less. Neither of them can be very happy, and care should be taken to avoid making them feel miserable or inept. The doctor should try to be considerate rather than kind, for kindness may slip into condescension. Even if it does not do so, there are times when he may want to be rather firm and if he has seemed very kind in the past, his sudden firmness may come to the patient as a slap in the face; but being considerate is consistent with being firm. It is foolish to hope to describe an attitude of mind, but craven not to try.

There, then, the doctor sits, a moral paragon with a skilled analytical brain. The first patient enters, bearing a slip of paper on which are written his height and weight and the urinary findings. His mother also enters, bearing urine charts. 'How many calories to a pomegranate?' she demands. The doctor considers the data on the slip of paper, the dietitian flicks through the pages of her reference books and the clinic has begun.

Height

The figures for height are mainly of long-term value. They should be entered on a *growth chart,* such as those constructed by Tanner and Whitehouse for British children (*Figures 6.1* to *6.4*), or by Nellhaus

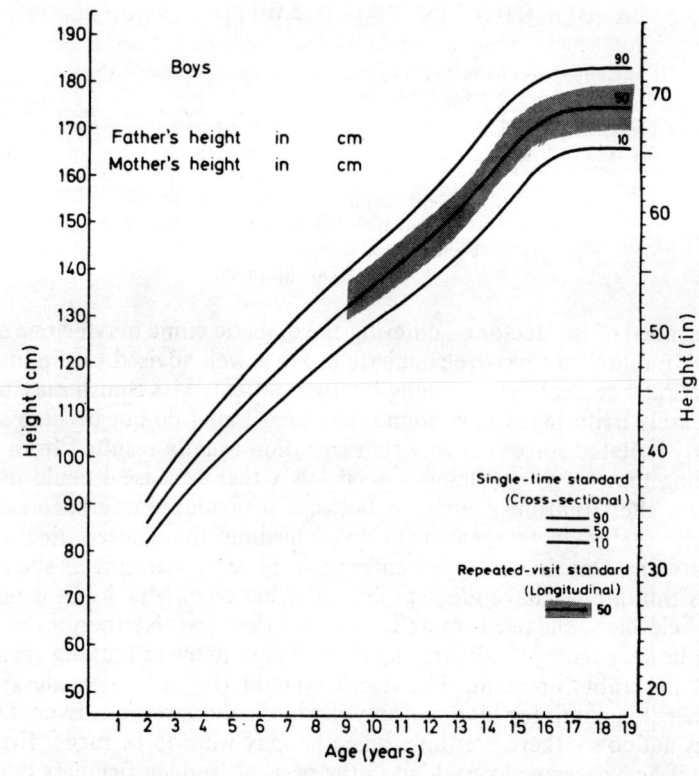

Figure 6.1. Growth chart: Height of boys. (This and the next seven figures are redrawn in simplified form from the charts prepared by J. M. Tanner and R. H. Whitehouse and are reproduced by permission. The more detailed originals are strongly recommended for clinic use. They may be obtained from Messrs. Creaseys, Printers, Bull Plain, Hertford)

for American children. The scale of the charts is small, and an entry about once in six months is enough to tell what is to be told. If a child's readings have for some time been on the 50th centile but then begin to fall below it, one can say that he is falling below his isodevelopmental pathway, which really means his expected rate of growth. Unfortunately, individual children often do not stick to the same centile throughout the growth period, even during that relatively smooth period of growth in the early childhood years. The prepubertal growth spurt is preceded by a period of a year or two in which growth slows down. In the majority, this slowing down is so slight as not to be noticed, but in some it is exaggerated and can be clearly seen. Even in families a common growth pattern may be seen, all the children slowing down at the age of six for example and

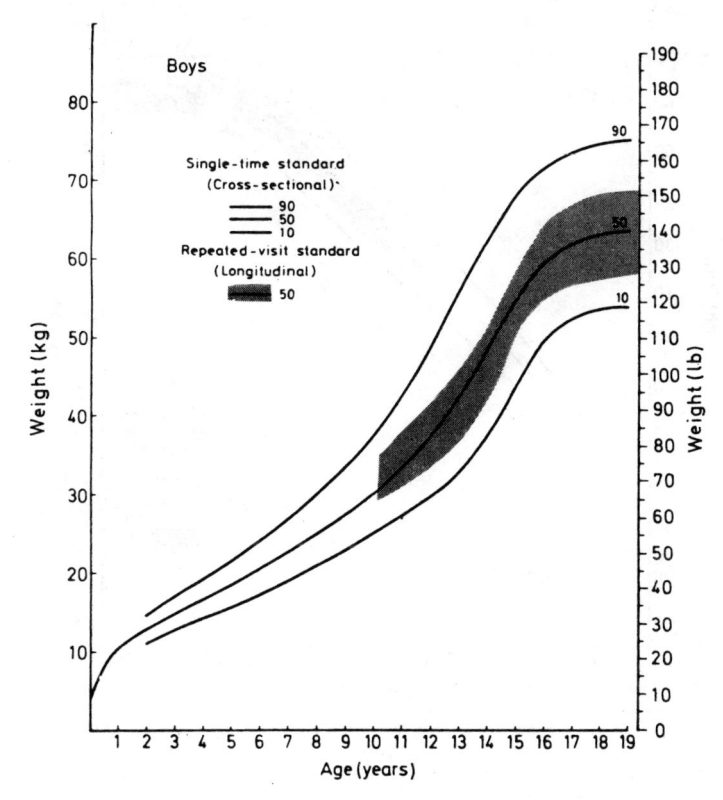

Figure 6.2. Growth chart: Weight of boys

speeding up again at the age of eight. I have been told by a kindly mother 'Not to *worry*, doctor, *all* my children do that at that age'. It is known that bad diabetic control may result in dwarfing. If we wait for dwarfing to warn us of poor diabetic control we will have lost a year or two in which the occurrence of dwarfing might have been prevented. Recording height is therefore of little immediate practical value, but two examples can be given in which height recording may be of use.

(1) A sudden increase (which would have to be double checked) over a period of three months is suggestive of a prepubertal growth spurt, and the mother can be warned and reassured in advance of

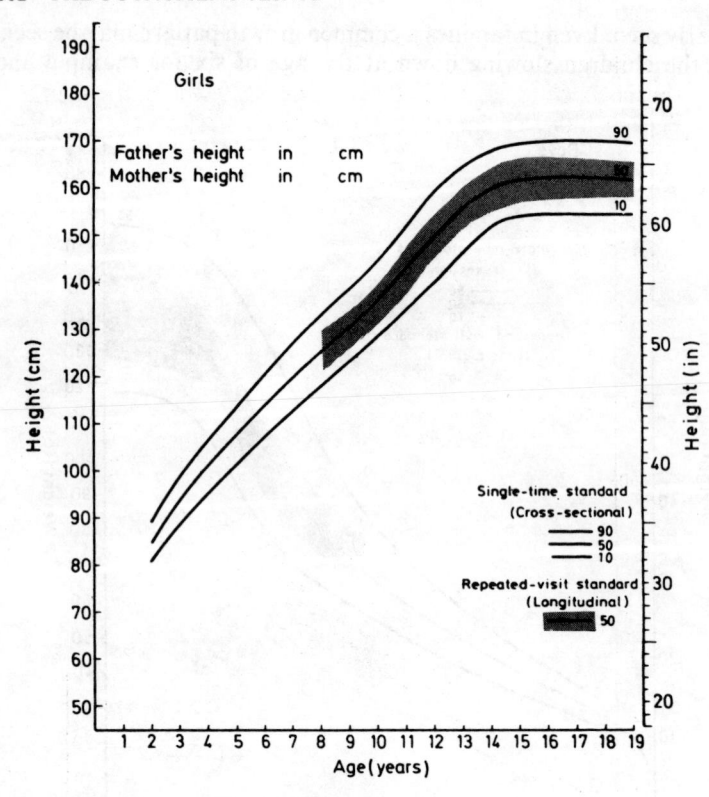

Figure 6.3. Growth chart: Height of girls

an impending increase in insulin or a possible change to a different type of insulin.

(2) An occasional child may show, quite consistently, an apparent tendency to shrink and expand. At successive visits he is up a centimetre, down half a centimetre, up a centimetre, down half a centimetre and so on. He is not really shrinking and expanding, except perhaps emotionally. We have probably all met this type of child in the general paediatric clinic, the 'leaner'. Many small children are asked to stand by the doctor's desk while the chest is auscultated in case they are frightened at the outset by being asked to lie down. An occasional child takes the opportunity to put a hand on the doctor's desk and sink gently sideways as if glad of the rest, even though he was sitting down five seconds previously. If one removes the light pressure of a stethoscope too

suddenly from the front of his chest he may topple forwards. These are the leaners, and I suspect them of being passive, unenthusiastic children. I think those who show fluctuations in height at each diabetic clinic visit fall into the same category.

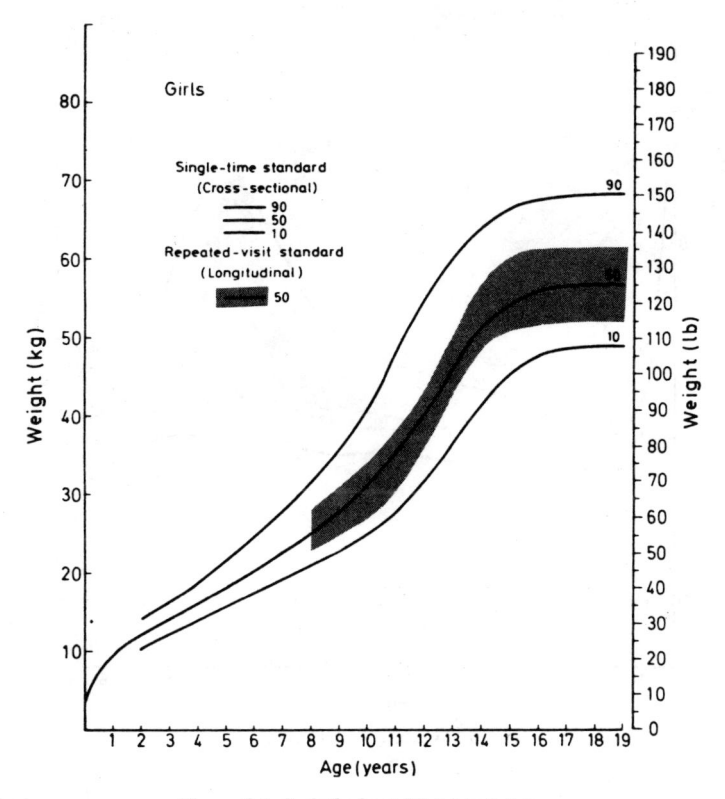

Figure 6.4. Growth chart: Weight of girls

The *bone-age* is a valuable investigation to have up one's sleeve. Serial readings are important here also, because maturation, like height, may proceed by fits and starts. Further, although height and maturation may proceed roughly in parallel, one may be fitting while the other is starting. If the height lags by the same amount as the bone-age this may simply be due to an individual variation in the child's growth pattern and may be consistent with adequate diabetic control.

The *velocity chart (Figures 6.5 to 6.8)* is particularly suited to demonstrating alterations in the rate of growth over relatively short

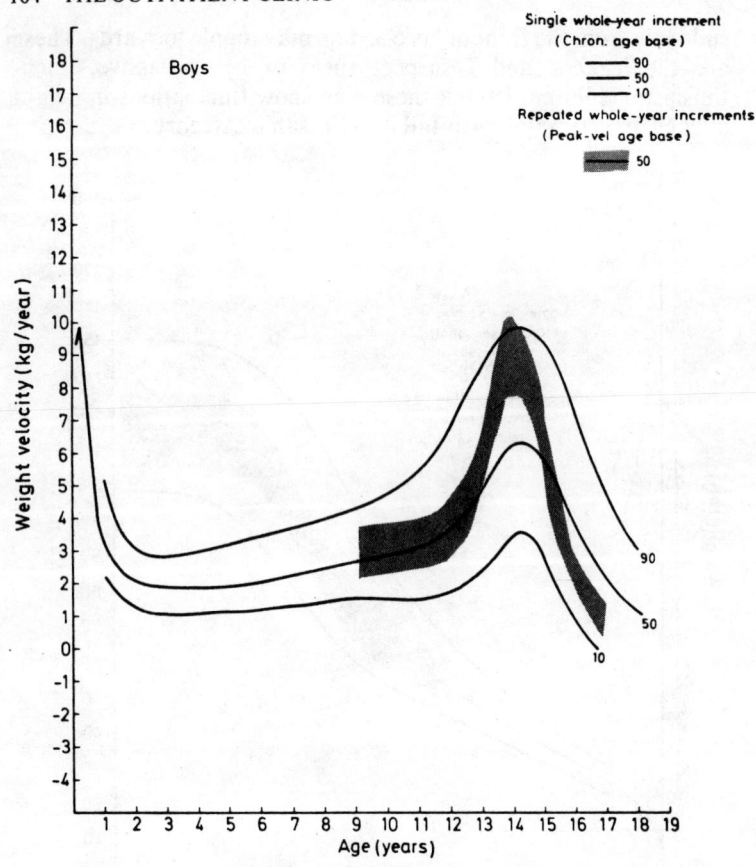

Figure 6.5. Velocity chart: Height of boys

periods. One might, for example, be anxious to see how the height was responding when a badly controlled diabetic had been admitted to a home, or one might want to see if the rate of drift of a drifter was accelerating or slowing down. For the velocity chart to be of value the basic data must be precisely accurate. Even the best apparatus for measuring height in hospitals soon develops 1 or 2 cm of wobble in the cross-bar, and the more efficient anthropometer is expensive.

Weight

There are much greater week-to-week fluctuations in weight than there are in height, and weight therefore becomes a more useful

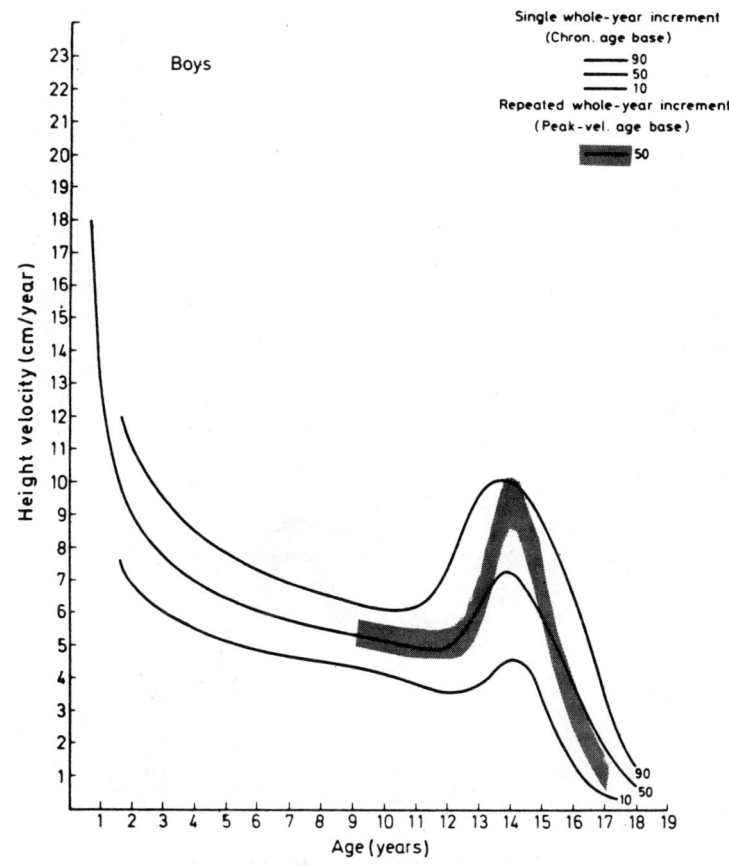

Figure 6.6. Velocity chart: Weight of boys

measure of diabetic control than height. One expects to see a gain of about 2.2 kg per annum. Certain variations fall within the normal range.

(1) There is a laying down of fat at puberty following the prepubertal spurt in height. The gain in weight does, however, begin in the prepubertal period.
(2) Height and weight do not proceed smoothly together. They advance by a series of asynchronous jerks in the same direction, the 'shooting up' and 'filling out' phases. These phases are prolonged and easily seen around puberty. In childhood they are shorter and difficult to detect without extremely accurate measurement.
(3) Some children show a seasonal variation, gaining in winter and

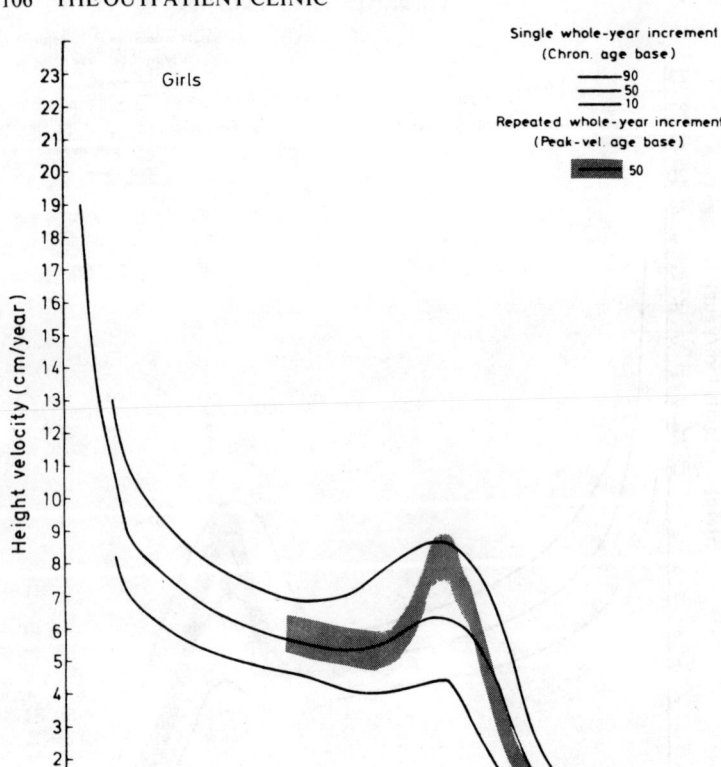

Figure 6.7. Velocity chart: Height of girls

remaining static in summer, possibly due to increased activity in the summer months.
(4) As with height, there may be familial variations in weight increase. All children in one family may put on weight at a certain age and lose it later, quite apart from puberty. The commonest pattern is for the normal peaks of fat deposition (i.e. at around one year, and again at puberty, possibly the only ages at which one can fairly talk of 'puppy fat') to be exaggerated.
(5) The weight lost in illness is rapidly restored by a weight gain on recovery.
(6) Although one regards weight gain as a favourable sign, the weight gain accompanying a change from poor to good control

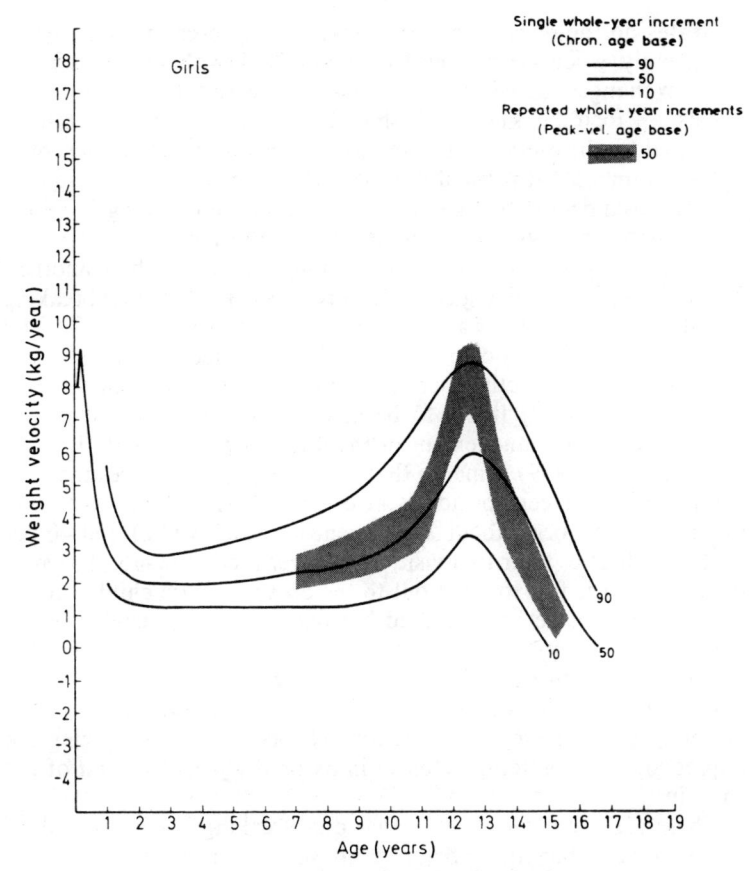

Figure 6.8. Velocity chart: Weight of girls

may in part be due to oedema. This situation is considered more fully in Chapter 12 (p. 253). It may also be due to overtreatment.

Even after taking these normal variations into account, there remain cases in which the gain or loss in weight appears excessive.

Excessive weight gain

Excessive weight gain may be due to gaining good control over a poorly-controlled diabetic (which will not be discussed further here), to over-eating and to overtreatment. The effects of overtreatment are discussed in a separate section on p. 117. The present section concentrates on the obesity of diet-breaking. Diet-breaking may occur unwittingly, when the mother is making mistakes about the carbohydrate exchanges, or wittingly when the child is deliberately taking sweets or food he knows he should not have. The first can be corrected by the dietitian, but in practice the mother often responds to the comment that her child's weight has been rising rather quickly with the comment 'I thought as much, she's been breaking her diet'. The diabetic child who becomes obese is usually a girl.

Recognizing the problem is one thing, dealing with it another. There is no point in giving the child a row. She may well be breaking her diet because she wants to be like her contemporaries and 'rejection' by her physician may only drive her deeper into the arms of her friends. Restrictive dieting, though possible, is not easy with a diabetic, and is not likely to be effective either. Stunkard, in a discussion on the management of the difficult patient with diabetes (Hinkle et al., 1959) remarks that everybody gets poor results with obesity. Five per cent of adults at certain obesity clinics lost 40 lb (18 kg) at their best, about 20 per cent lost 20 lb (9 kg) and 40 per cent default after their first visit. The longer the follow-up, the worse the results. It is fair to point out to the obese diabetic child that her transgressions have been spotted but one should not seek to blame her. She is unhappy enough as it is, if one accepts that some children over-eat as a substitute for love. A little gentle urging is probably best. If one can relax other restrictions slightly, for example the time of going to bed, so much the better; but one must avoid giving the impression of bargaining or one will assuredly get the worst of the bargain.

There are some who believe that diet-breaking is encouraged by giving extra carbohydrate before exercise, so that the child comes to believe that he has a licence to change his carbohydrate at will. Doctors with this belief will cut insulin before exercise instead of giving extra carbohydrate, but giving carbohydrate allows for greater elasticity of management and personally I do not regard it as an invitation to diet-breaking provided the child has been given an explanation, and his understanding of it and cooperation are checked from time to time.

Rarely, the onset of hypothyroidism may be the cause of excessive weight gain (p. 241). It is worth keeping this thought at the back of one's mind.

Excessive weight loss

Excessive weight loss indicates loss of diabetic control, *however good the urine charts may be.* This implies that some urine charts may be incorrectly filled in, a matter which will be discussed.

The urine chart

At the time the figures in this section were first drawn up we were using the five-drop urine test, which is why the top readings are 2 per cent, but the figures remain valid as examples so have not been changed.

The urine brought by the patient is tested at the clinic for sugar, ketones and albumin. This serves as some sort of check on the testing being done at home. The urine chart is the least reliable information given to the doctor at the clinic. One wonders if the chart *really* represents what has been happening at home. Some urine charts look particularly suspicious.

(1) There is the very neat chart, with all the markings so uniform that they have obviously been blocked in at a sitting. The patient should be asked if the results are first written down in a notebook or on the Clinitest chart. If the answer is 'No' the chart should be disbelieved unless it is enclosed in a home-made polythene case, which argues a passion for neatness and cleanliness.

	March								April	
Date	28		29		30		31		1	
	M	E	M	E	M	E	M	E	M	E
2%									X	
1%										
0.75%										
0.5%					X					
0.25%		X	X			X		X		
Nil	X			X			X			

Figure 6.9. *A urine chart; twice daily sugar testing. M = morning; E = evening*

(2) There is also the type shown in *Figure 6.9* which is presented

110 THE OUTPATIENT CLINIC

with the comment 'Isn't it odd how it's always up when he comes to the clinic? I think it's his nerves'. The trouble is that it *might* be his nerves, but it is more likely to indicate the presence of a smart operator (because the clinic always agrees with the home findings). The common fear of hypoglycaemia may result in the production of a falsely low chart so that the doctor will not raise the insulin, thus averting the risk of hypoglycaemia.

	March								April	
Date	28		29		30		31		1	
	M	E	M	E	M	E	M	E	M	E
2%										
1%				X		X	X		X	
0.75%		X	X							
0.5%	X				X			X		
0.25%										
Nil										

Figure 6.10. Another urine chart

(3) It is just not credible that a long succession of readings should all be between 0.5 and 1 per cent *(Figure 6.10)*. Readings of 0, 0.25 and 2 per cent are common, the middle ranges are not. When I say that such charts call for a vigorous revision course in urine testing and a random blood sugar, I cannot help thinking of Mrs Watson. What should I do about her?

Some years ago Mrs Watson, who lives in a tenement, had five children under the age of seven and a half years, three of these being diabetic. They all had *Figure 6.10* charts. There was no point in looking at the names on the tops of the charts as they were interchangeable. But at least they were filled in which showed that Mrs Watson was trying. When they were younger, the Watsons could be heared approaching the clinic at a range of 200 yards (184.6 metres), and they would burst into the consulting room shouting, pushing, but above all laughing, all with charts showing 0.5 per cent of sugar for the past month. Now that Jeannie the eldest is 11, they often arrive under her care ('James went all skelly eyed coming out the Underground, so I gave him a packet of crisps. Was that right Doctor?').

Mrs Watson is splendid and how she copes I do not know. Who am I to harry her? Would things be any better if I did? The children might stop laughing. There is a time for turning a blind eye.

	February								March	
Date	28		29		30		31		1	
	M	E	M	E	M	E	M	E	M	E
2%										
1%			X							
0.75%		X								
0.5%						X		X		
0.25%			X		X					
Nil	X						X		X	

Figure 6.11. *A very original urine chart*

(4) The chart shown in *Figure 6.11* was presented to me last year. The reader may care to exercise his wits upon it. The clue is in the dates. I was more embarrassed than the mother.
(5) Some charts can never be shown at all. These are:
 (a) 'Left it on the bus'.
 (b) 'Put it in the pillar-box by mistake'.
 (c) 'My house got burned down'.
 (d) 'It was above the stove and the chip pan went up'.

Perhaps it should be said at this point that nothing in this section has been invented for effect, and that every word quoted was really spoken. One develops a jaundiced outlook on urine charts. The only one which I now accept as authentic is tattered, dog-eared, blotched, and scribbled on; its changing symbols are rendered in multicoloured crayon, and most of the readings are 3 per cent or more.

Blood sugar

At some clinics the patient's blood is taken for sugar analysis at every visit. I do not follow this routine, partly because I doubt its value and partly because I do not want a child to feel that every visit to the clinic inevitably means a prick. A random sugar may be a help in disclosing a faker of urine charts or in confirming that management is erratic, for example when a child has a blood sugar of 2.7 mmol/l (50 mg per cent) at one visit and 27.7 mmol/l (500 mg per cent) at the next, under theoretically constant conditions. The reflectance meter is of value in giving quick results (p. 54).

A good chart and a falling weight

When faced with this state of affairs, one can carry out certain quick checks. One suspects that the urine specimen is basically water or that urine testing is not supervised and that the blood sugar is high. One starts by probing the history. It is always worth finding out whether the urine specimen is obtained and/or tested behind a locked bathroom door. One father assured me that there could be no possible error, particularly as the boy was so obviously pleased with a good result, and then went on to give the game away by saying 'You can hear it in the tone of his voice when he shouts down the stairs'. The situation in which a child tests his urine in the bathroom and then, like a leadsman in the bows shouting information to the captain on the bridge ('By the mark, a quarter per cent'), shouts the result to his mother in the kitchen is diagnostic of faking. One should also be very wary of the word 'embarrassed', as in 'He's too embarrassed to let me watch him test his urine'. He might possible be embarrassed about supervision in passing his urine, but when it comes to testing the urine, it is neither embarrassment nor pride that is drawing the veil, but anxiety. One should then investigate the testing materials and the urine itself.

(1) The storage and appearance of the Clinitest tablets should be reviewed but this is a very rare cause of false test results.
(2) 'Tap-water has a pH of 7' is a popular but inaccurate belief. The pH of Glasgow tap-water is 6, and in the south it may well be on the alkaline side. The pH may not help much, but it is worth doing as it gives an immediate answer.
(3) All urine contains urea and creatinine. A specimen with no urea is not urine.
(4) A random blood sugar can be done. The reflectance meter gives

an immediate answer, accurate enough for the present purpose. It is possible to have a sugar-free fasting urine followed by a blood glucose of 24.9 mmol/l (450 mg per cent) in mid-morning, but it is unlikely.

(5) If one is dealing with traces of a reducing sugar, sugar chromatography can supply helpful information indicating that the sugar is not glucose. When one suspects strongly that urine is being faked there must be a discussion, which is not always friendly. The physician should be braced to hit the mat as soon as he enters the ring, because the tests being done may indicate to the mother what is coming next. 'I was wondering ...' says the doctor. 'Let me tell you!' says the mother. 'I *know* my child, and she would *never* do what you're thinking.' It's a wise mother who knows her own child, and one must not give way completely on such a point. It is seldom that a definite explanation of the mechanism of the faking is found, but often charts become realistic once the matter has been given an airing. At such a time one can reassure the mother that it does not really matter if there is 2 per cent of sugar in the urine *at times* as long as one knows it is there. Faking is more likely to have been caused by over-anxiety than the primal evil of deceit (although the latter may sometimes occur) and a general chat aimed at releasing anxiety over the whole diabetic spectrum is to be preferred to the stormy approach. There is no need to have a row about it. Only once (and it was very recently) has a parent come into the consulting room and said 'I don't think these charts are right, Doctor. You see, he's passing a lot of water and I think he must be getting his tests wrong. I'll watch him closer from now on'. If such cooperation is not forthcoming and the problem persists at the next clinic visit (which should be an early one), the child should be readmitted for investigation.

One should not underestimate the intelligence of a determined 12-year-old faker. One of my patients was found to be adding diabetic orange squash to water to make her 'urine' the right colour. Dr J. W. Farquhar has told me of an even more cunning manoeuvre carried out by one of his patients. This enterprising lad got hold of a plastic squeeze bottle with a swan neck, filled it with water, held it inside his pants by a hand in his pocket, and ejected a stream of pure water through his fly-buttons, the other hand disguising the tiny plastic 'penis'.

A bad chart and a falling weight

Faking may be used to make a good chart into a perfect one or a bad chart into a good one, so anything said in the previous section could also apply here. The children discussed in this section may simply be one degree more forthright than the fakers, and no different in the control of their diabetes.

What should one do when faced with a chart which is frankly bad and a weight which is falling? One should ask questions, which are best supplied in the form of a check-list, the basis of many of the points having already been discussed in Chapter 3.

(1) *Insulin.* Is it the right type? Error has been known in writing the first prescription or issuing the first supply. Bring it to the clinic next time. Is it kept between 4 and 10 °C? It almost certainly is.
(2) *Injection sites.* Is he injecting into a fatty tumour? Is the injection too superficial? Angle of injection? Is the measuring accurate? One may ask for a demonstration. Any trouble with bubbles? Any leak back from injection site, or from needles? A point like this can be very important. One must remember that the error of a moment can result in a week's loss of control. If the insulin is improperly given or improperly absorbed (for example from a fatty tumour) the blood sugar will rise and Providence will not intervene to wipe the slate clean the next morning, which the patient will begin with a blood sugar higher than his usual. Compensatory adjustments of insulin may be needed.
(3) *Urine testing.* Are the tablets stored in a dry place, for example *not* above the bath or the kitchen sink, and are the caps screwed on the bottles? Is the testing technique correct? *Figure 6.10* is the type of poor chart which should lead to doctor, parent and child testing the urine together. If the chart is all 2 per cent there is no need to check the testing.
(4) *Diet.* Is it too high in sugar (for example milk, fruit, the sweeter biscuits, ice cream, etc.) at the expense of starch? It is banal to repeat that starch causes less fluctuation in the blood sugar than sugar itself, yet this is a point which may be overlooked in practice. Are reserve stores of energy (protein and fat) being taken adequately?
(5) *Exercise.* Has any change been forced on him, for example by the closing of a swimming bath? Or has he taken up a sedentary life at school after an active holiday? Some children seem much more sensitive to exercise, or the lack of it, than others. Indeed, one mother found this out for herself and made so much use of the fact that she virtually controlled the child's diabetes by exercise rather than insulin or diet. If she had a high urine sugar the child was sent to run three times round the block. Intrigued, I watched this system for a number of years. It seemed to work.

(6) *Nervous stress.* In its simplest form, this could be something like school examinations. Many children show a sharp rise in urine sugars at such times. A more serious psychological upset may appear in a diabetic as in any other child.

> Mrs McKay arrived one day with a six-inch cut down her face. 'Nothing really, doctor,' she said, 'It's not deep. It's the woman across the road, she's always at it. She's told Henry it's his turn next. Oh yes, she's been had up but she's out on bail, and I've pled with the house-factor for a move, but I can't get one.' Henry's diabetes was out of control, probably in part due to direct fear, and in part indirectly as his fear prevented him leaving the house so that he got no exercise.

The tendency for blood sugar to be high and for ketoacidosis to recur at times of nervous stress have been referred to in Chapter 4 and will be mentioned again in the section on recurrent ketoacidosis (p. 176). However, stress may not always raise the blood sugar. Chance (1969) mentions that *sudden* anger and fear may cause a fall in the blood sugar particularly if it is initially high.

(7) A simple *infection,* such as a febrile cold or a furuncle, is unlikely to be missed. One must also be prepared for subtle infections, such as pyelonephritis or tuberculosis. Tuberculosis has long been linked with diabetes, and in the past was a common cause of death in the diabetic. In Western countries it seldom shows itself by specific signs and is most often detected by the Mantoux test, activated by a high degree of suspicion. It may show itself by diabetic deterioration in a formerly well-controlled child, but equally it may appear insidiously in a child who was badly controlled in adverse social circumstances. In Britain at present, tuberculosis is most likely to be found in the immigrant population.

The Somogyi effect

Somogyi (1959) investigated patients with juvenile onset diabetes so severe it was virtually uncontrollable. Hyperglycaemia and ketosis alternated with hypoglycaemia. His findings were startling. Two of his main conclusions should be quoted:

(1) There was complete lack of parallelism between the amount of insulin injected and the amount of carbohydrate utilized. Even when insulin and carbohydrate intake were held constant under hospital conditions the sugar in blood and urine was found to vary over a very wide range.

(2) Barring other physiological and emotional stresses, *conspicuous fluctuations in glycosuria are unmistakable evidence of excess insulin action* (his italics).

A few children may often be clinically hypoglycaemic towards the end of the morning, yet if the urine is then tested it is found to contain much sugar and probably ketones. This phenomenon, the virtual coincidence of hypoglycaemic attacks with ketosis and hyperglycosuria, is a manifestation of the Somogyi effect. The body over-responds to the fall in blood sugar produced by the morning dose of insulin and produces hyperglycaemia with sugar spilling into the urine. Classically, the child appears to be hypoglycaemic but when the urine is tested almost immediately it is found to contain sugar and ketones. The physician, faced with undoubted glycosuria, and possibly rather doubting the mother's story of hypoglycaemia, unthinkingly raises the dose of insulin. The hypoglycaemia is accentuated and so is the subsequent hyperglycaemic reply. This initiates an escalation by which the urine continues to show much sugar despite increasing doses of insulin, and the child has frequent hypo attacks. Any insulin with a fast-acting component may produce the attacks. The children who are thus affected may have minor inborn metabolic irregularities by which they react more briskly than others to insulin, or show the effects of hypoglycaemia more readily, and respond too quickly with a hyperglycaemic response to a hypoglycaemic threat.

The Somogyi effect is not uncommon and physicians must be aware of it. The typical case may be easy to recognize, but there can be difficulties.

(1) The fluctuating sugar levels of a child under nervous stress. However, these children seldom show the hypoglycaemic phase as clearly.
(2) In some there may be chemical hypoglycaemia with little or nothing in the way of clinical signs, such children being clinically resistant to the physical signs of hypoglycaemia: but they too can become involved in the escalation of insulin.

The Somogyi effect may be stumbled over by mistake, as in a child seen recently.

A girl of eight years who had been moderately well controlled began to show 2 per cent of sugar in her morning urine. She was therefore asked to carry out double voiding, in the expectation that the first specimen would show 2 per cent sugar and the second might be clear. The reverse was the case. The girl got up in the morning and passed a clear urine specimen but 20 minutes later it showed 2 per cent sugar, without any food having been taken. This appears to have been a Somogyi effect, possibly in this case mediated by a brisk adrenalin flow on waking.

This girl also showed a rise in urine sugar and ketosis after exercise (another manifestation of the same phenomenon), and we have seen two boys doing the same thing. It is unwise to dismiss an unexpected finding as faulty observation.

Overtreatment with insulin

It has been assumed that the Somogyi effect is the result of an out-pouring of glucagon and adrenalin, and possibly glucocorticoids and growth hormone, in response to hypoglycaemia. The controversy over this classic view has been summarized by Campbell (1976), and most recently Gale and Tattersall (1979) have failed to find a rise in these hormones of a degree sufficient to cause the hyperglycaemia of the Somogyi phenomenon. Whatever the cause may be, there is no doubt that the Somogyi effect exists as a very important clinical entity.

I recently had the care of 18 diabetics aged 12 to 16 years at a diabetic camp where the emphasis was on the outdoor life—canoeing, sailing, camping and hill-walking. On arrival, the 18 were taking a total of 1090 units of insulin daily. On the first day at camp I cut all insulins by 10 per cent on the grounds that the children would be taking more exercise than usual. The matter did not stop there. On the 13th and last day of camp the total requirements were down to 650 units, a drop of 43.7 per cent from the original dosage. The type of insulin was not changed.

Some of the individual falls in insulin were striking. One boy dropped from 148 to 40 units, and had at least one hypo attack each day while doing so. He had a brisk nocturnal hypoglycaemic convulsion when passing 60 units on the way down. Another dropped without major upset from 60 to 8 units. Nine of the 18 children had their insulin reduced to half or less than half of their original dosage. It is true that they were living a different life, with plenty of exercise, carefully supervised injections, little opportunity for diet-breaking and freedom from the tensions of home, and it is true that the total numbers are small. Nevertheless, 50 per cent of these children were having at least twice as much insulin as they needed under optimal conditions. How many of our clinic patients are being grossly overtreated with insulin?

Rosenbloom and Giordano (1977) found that 90 per cent of children referred to them specifically for unstable diabetes were being overtreated with insulin, though the standard taken for overtreatment (10 per cent reduction in insulin) was perhaps rather low. The list of symptoms found in these children is worth giving in full.

In 40–50 per cent of the children they found frank hypoglycaemic episodes; polyuria, nocturia, enuresis; excessive appetite.

In 20–40 per cent, hepatomegaly, headaches, weight gain, exercise intolerance; marked variations in glycosuria; frequent ketosis, ketoacidosis; mood swings, irritability.

In 10–20 per cent, absence of rationale for dose increase; ketonuria without glycosuria; worsening of symptoms with dose increases.

In 4–10 per cent, decreasing school performance or attendance; dizziness, weak spells; growth failure, maturational delay; abdominal pain, constipation; improvement of symptoms with illness: nightmares, night terrors, night sweats; oedema of extremities; visual problems; weight loss.

Some of these symptoms may cause raised eyebrows. Polyuria, indeed! 'Everyone knows' that these are symptoms of too *little* insulin! And so they are, even during the relative insulinopenia of the hyperglycaemic phase of the Somogyi phenomenon. Excessive weight gain is due to overeating, 'everyone knows' that. But is it so in the case of the diabetic child, particularly when there has been no change in his diabetic habits over the years? He and his parents may be lying, I agree. But why not try reducing the insulin and see what happens?

Some signs of overtreatment have already been mentioned:

(1) The co-existence of hypo attacks and high urine sugars, and possibly ketosis.
(2) The unexpected appearance of heavy glycosuria just after rising in the morning, or after exercise.

Two other very important signs are:

(3) An unexplained gain in weight.
(4) An insulin dose of more than 1 unit/kg body weight/day.

Insulin resistance does exist but we have in the past too readily accepted it as the cause of all high insulin doses. The child having more than 1 unit/kg/day should always be regarded as a possible case of overtreatment. Having had one's suspicions aroused, what is one to do about it? The aim is to see if one can get down to 1 unit/kg/day in the course of two weeks. If one is dealing with intelligent stable parents with a telephone this may be done without admission to hospital. The primary concern at this stage is the general well-being of the child rather than the urine sugars, and one should remember that hypo attacks are not uncommon during the reducing phase. The urine sugars may not improve until a week or two after the reduction has been made. If one's relationship with the parents is tenuous, as it may be even after numerous clinic visits, it is best to admit the child for observation while cutting the insulin.

Attaining control of overtreatment in hospital is relatively easy. I usually begin by cutting down the short acting insulin which seems more likely to cause swings in blood sugar. Maintaining control when the patient has left hospital is more difficult, and I am not sure that I have the answer to this. At present I modify the existing 'rules' *(see next section)* for raising insulin by suggesting either that they wait for five successive high urine sugar readings or that they raise only when ketones of two or three pluses are present for two successive readings, but I think I only say this because the parents expect me to say *something*. I also say that the suggestions for lowering insulin should be unchanged—three successive blue readings or a hypo attack. It may be necessary to advise against any rise in insulin. The really important thing is to keep in close touch with the parents, even by daily telephone calls. Urine sugars are relatively unimportant at this stage. The key question is 'Is he any worse?' referring both to urine tests and his general state. If the child is active and well, reassure and press on!

Somogyi wrote, it will be remembered, that gross fluctuations in glycosuria were due to too much insulin 'barring other physiological and emotional stresses'. Emotional stress may have been the main factor in starting the child on his course of escalation, but on the other hand the major alterations in management proposed to combat overtreatment may themselves create stress in a family where stress did not exist before. This means that reducing the insulin may be ineffective unless one regards the child as a person who may have been or who may now be under stress. Practically, it means that one has to keep in very close touch with the child and his family, to give constant support.

The concept of overtreatment has been based on work with children. It is now being realized that the same thing can happen with adults (*Lancet*, 4.8.79).

This diatribe may be in part due to the guilty knowledge that I have in the past done my fair share in overtreating diabetics. I do not withdraw one word about the importance of overtreatment, but at the same time it must be admitted that a high insulin dosage may have several causes.

(1) The presence of insulin antibodies.
(2) The presence of antagonists, particularly at puberty.

(3) The injection of insulin into fatty lumps.
(4) Emotional stress, because it is easier to raise insulin than lower emotional tension.
(5) The Somogyi effect, which has just been discussed.

These causes seem definite. There are others which I only suspect. That adolescent boy who dropped from 148 to 40 units, what about him? Did he always take his insulin, or did he sometimes forget? At any rate, I am not saying that *all* children on a high dose of insulin are being overtreated. I *am* saying that if the dose is more than 1 unit/kg/day the possibility of overtreatment should be seriously considered. It is more common than we used to think, when urine sugar tests were taken as the sole basis of treatment.

Adjusting the insulin

The information that can be obtained at a clinic visit has been discussed. It is now desirable to consider how best to use this information. The majority of visits call for little action from the doctor. The insulin dosage seems satisfactory, there are no problems with diet and the child is thriving. This happy state of affairs is probably due largely to the mother adjusting the child's insulin when necessary, though ideas differ on what these adjustments should be.

(1) Some have joined my clinic, usually from an adult clinic, with instructions not to change the insulin unless the doctor at the clinic says so. This scares me. Children are prone to infections and I have visions of them lapsing into ketoacidosis if the insulin is not raised. This is not a system I would recommend for children.
(2) Our patients are usually instructed to raise the insulin by 10 per cent if there are three or four successive readings of 3 or 5 per cent, assuming that they are on a single daily injection, that they are testing only twice a day and that the sugar is still high in the morning when insulin is to be given. 'Three or four' is not a vague phrase, it depends on whether the first high reading appears in the evening or the morning. This applies to children who are still on one injection a day. If they are on two injections it would become three successive morning or evening readings.

If the child is on a single injection of mixed short- and long-acting insulins the principle is the same. On a Semilente–Lente mixture, three high evening readings would indicate an increase in the Semilente, three low mornings readings would indicate a decrease in the Lente. On the other hand, if the child is on a single dose of Leo Neutral and Retard it may be difficult to decide if blue readings in the late afternoon indicate rather prolonged action of Neutral or early action of Retard, and it would then be desirable to check a few midday urines to elucidate the point.

(3) If one looks at a large number of urine charts it will become apparent that many children will have spells of a week or so when the chart is low alternating with similar spells when it is high, there being no obvious reason for either of these phases. It may be for this reason that some prefer to wait for longer runs of blues or 2 per cent levels than suggested above and then to adjust the insulin by more than 10 per cent. It is for the individual physician to decide. My own view is that the low runs indicate his ideal diabetic state and that he *should* be able to run on that dose semipermanently. A cause for the high runs should be sought and even if no cause is found I tinker with the rules to prevent too marked an increase in insulin. However, the rule about raising insulin during infection remains inviolate.

A further rule which should be discussed with the parents before the child is first discharged is that an *unexplained* hypoglycaemic attack calls for a drop in insulin. Whichever set of rules is chosen from those give above, it can only be taken as a general guide. The physician has the opportunity at the outpatient clinic of modifying the rules to suit the individual child. Some common modifications are now discussed.

Some common modifications

(1) If it becomes apparent that a certain child invariably needs a rise in insulin of 20 or 30 per cent whenever he gets a fever, then that rise can be given as one increment at the onset of infection, perhaps after only one high reading if the signs of infection are obvious. As soon as fever subsides the insulin can be lowered sharply by the same amount.

(2) A persistently high urine sugar chart, interspersed with just enough readings of 0.5 per cent to preclude raising insulin by rule, is usually indicative of the parent's fear of hypoglycaemia. A rise in insulin is advised at the clinic, particularly if there is ketosis or the gains in height and weight are poor.

(3) A persistently high urine sugar chart in the absence of ketosis, or even with ketosis, should make one wonder if the child is showing the Somogyi effect. (The reader is warned against the current popular usage of the verb 'to Somogyi'. The present participle

causes laryngeal spasm.) The action to be taken is discussed above in the section on overtreatment.

Reasons for readmission

If one excludes obvious reasons such as severe ketoacidosis and intractable hypoglycaemia, the remaining indications for readmission may be summarized as follows.

(1) *The need for a change in type of insulin.* Classically, this would be represented by the pre-pubertal girl who can no longer be controlled on one injection a day; but there are also younger children who cannot be kept on one injection without showing undesirable hypo- or hyperglycaemic effects at some time of day. A somewhat recherché reason for converting to two injections a day is that it is proposed to take a child to America or Australia by air; the time changes involved are more easily managed if the child is on frequent doses of a short-acting insulin.

(2) *Chaos in the mind of the physician.* This is a regrettably common reason in my clinic. There are times when I do not know if a hyperglycaemic child is failing to get her reputed insulin, is developing insulin resistance, is showing the Somogyi effect, is becoming emotionally unstable or is approaching puberty. Or all at once. When a child is readmitted under such circumstances her reputed insulin dosage should be maintained for a day or two. If one made a change from beef to pork insulin on the first day and she immediately improved, one would not know if the improvement were due to the change in insulin, an improved measuring and injecting technique in hospital or separation from home worries. In practice it is not uncommon to find that a child readmitted because of high urine sugars goes home on the same type of insulin at a significantly lower dosage. This means that the instructions given have been satisfactory but either they are not being carried out or they are not applicable in the home situation (for example because of nervous stress in the child).

(3) *In adverse social circumstances.* If control is bad in a poor home it may be difficult to decide whether this is due to poor management or inherently unstable diabetes. If admission suggests that the cause of the trouble is poor management it may then appear that the parents have virtually opted out of their responsibility towards the child. With older children one should try to ensure that at least one member of the family takes responsibility,

the child himself. This may be easier said than done (*see* p. 85), but one should not give up.

I remember talking to a priest in Glasgow's East End about a diabetic boy, known to both of us, from a very poor, unstable home. I said there were times when I felt like packing it in. 'Don't, he said, 'You may be the only connection with what we call reality that that boy has. He may just be hanging on to the clinic by the crook of his little finger, but if you give way, he's gone.' 'But,' said I, 'There are a number of people, and you must have seen your share of them, who seem impervious to civilization. When do they get so fixed in their ways that you can do nothing about them?' 'Certainly not before the age of 17', he replied. 'You may see a sense of morality developing up till then.' The boy of 11 or 12 still has his imagination and can look forward to living his own life. It is a possibility that the moderately ordered life of a medical ward, with set times for doing things and a recognized code of behaviour, may have some appeal for him and encourage him eventually to break from his home surroundings and live a different kind of life of his own. The alcoholic may seem hopeless till he suddenly breaks the habit. One cannot convert the 'hopeless' diabetic child with a string of words; one can only show him without comment, that there is a better way of doing things and a spell in hospital may help him to realize this. As with the alcoholic, such realization must come from inside himself. One's attitude to the 'impossible' case should be to stick with it, even if it makes one feel useless for years on end. The words of Richard II at his deposition come to mind:

> 'Though some of you, with Pilate, wash your hands,
> Showing an outward pity; yet you Pilates
> Have here delivered me to my sour cross,
> And water cannot wash away your sin.'

This is good strong stuff well worth a 'Blam!' or 'Zowie!' scribbled in the margin of anybody's Shakespeare. The lines are easy to remember and paediatricians should not forget them.

The 'impossible' child with a personality defect and inadequate backing at home is the biggest problem in the clinic. It may be worth giving him a rest, by which I mean that he tests his urine on only two days a week and is allowed considerable latitude in his diet. After all, stricter measures of control have been tried already and have failed. I do not put this forward as a sovereign remedy, simply as something worth trying. If one can gain his confidence one can tighten his control again later.

(4) *The need for a psychiatric opinion.* There are some who main-

tain that the parents of every new diabetic should have a consultation with a psychiatrist. This may be possible in a children's hospital but it is doubtful if it is even desirable. Perhaps one should not speak until one has tried the routine for oneself, but so far I have shied away from it. The competent mother faced by a psychiatrist may wonder just who is getting scared.

There are certainly cases where psychiatric care is needed from the start, for example with a genuinely needle-shy mother, but the generally accepted approach is to ask for psychiatric help only when it is definitely indicated. When is it indicated? There is no straight answer to this as it is largely a matter of the doctor's own personality, but if he feels he is making no headway with a behavioural problem he should seek psychiatric advice. I think a child should be admitted to hospital when such advice is wanted. A referral as an outpatient to a psychiatric department may fill a patient with foreboding and, still worse, hostility. Admission has several advantages: the psychiatric approach is seen in perspective as one of many investigations, the parents can be gradually eased into the situation and the psychiatrist, by dropping in for a couple of minutes at lunch time or the end of the day, can see more of the child than he would at outpatient visits.

The major psychiatric problems which accompany recurrent ketoacidosis and attempted suicide are dealt with elsewhere, but one cannot leave the subject without mentioning what seems to me another major psychological problem, the case of the doubting and questioning parents (Coppolillo, 1965). These parents are good parents in that they try to have everything just right, but bad in that 'just right' is a measure of perfection unattainable in diabetic control. Probably due to their own upbringing they can only live life according to strict rules. Their thirst for knowledge about diabetes in unquenchable. A hypoglycaemic attack is illegal, immoral and to be regarded with indignation. It must not be allowed to happen, and this leads to odd new rules appearing, for example one complaint of headache = 2 Mars bars. Nuance means nothing to them. Things cannot be played off the cuff or as they come, they must be foreseen, and the rules settled beforehand. They can never shrug their shoulders.

Conversations like this imaginary one quickly get out of hand:

Mother: You said he was to have a quarter of a Mars bar before he went swimming.
Doctor: I said he could have, or something like it.
Mother: He swims for half an hour. What do we do if it's threequarters?

Doctor: Give him three-eighths of a Mars bar.
Mother: That would be very difficult to measure.
Doctor: Not if you mark off a half, then a quarter, and cut between the two.
Mother: He's a very good swimmer, what if he wanted to swim across the Firth of Clyde on a sponsored swim, for example?
Doctor: Is he going to?
Mother: No, but supposing he did.
Doctor: He would need a lot of Mars bars.
Mother: But you said he wasn't to have a lot of Mars bars, they put his blood sugar up too quick. Should he have bread instead?
Doctor: I don't think that would be a good thing.
Mother: Why not?
Doctor: Well, you can't very well swim across the Firth of Clyde chewing bread.
Mother: If you put it in a homogenizer with some milk you could suck it through a tube when you felt like it.
Doctor: So you could.
Mother: What speed should I set the homogenizer at?

The example is a shade facetious but it does give an impression of the tone of such conversations. From the start one knows one is heading for an imbroglio of unreality where one is expected to play the twin roles of judge and prisoner in the dock. Talking to a doubting parent is like flamenco dancing in a bath of mud.

If one accepts Coppolillo's suggestions, which I do, these parents see themselves as in a state of defeat, for which they feel guilt and shame*. They are looking for justification. They need support and the admission that their problem is difficult. It may give the physician better insight if he asks the mother what *she* thinks about a problem and sees how far off the mark she is. It may also help if one stops telling these patients what to do. Instead, one suggests that they might try something and let the doctor have their opinion on the outcome: or keep a certain point under observation and tell the doctor what their conclusions are. This gives them the feeling that they are running things. They like that! These brittle parents do not worry about everything, and are probably mustard when it comes to

---

* They may take this out on the doctor, and have an active dislike for him. Perhaps they regard him as a heterodox usurper of an authority he is unfit to wield. This dislike may escape notice, as sometimes the way of life of the doubting parent includes being polite to doctors.

putting in Income Tax Returns, but they are at something of a loss with the non-conforming diabetic child. One should keep calm, forget about one's own lunch and do one's best to be considerate and patient. They will still be at it two years later.

HYPOGLYCAEMIA

It is probably true that the diabetic is not as well controlled as he might be unless he is having occasional hypoglycaemic attacks. Hypo attacks are manifested by pallor, sweating, confusion, irritability or drowsiness, headache, hunger, abdominal pain, weakness, ataxia, visual disturbances and bizarre behaviour. Tingling of the lips, commonly quoted as a symptom in adults, is uncommon in childhood but may occur, as may other odd sensory phenomena. Pallor and sweating, which are caused by the increase in adrenalin production induced by the hypoglycaemia, are the classic signs, but in young children irritability may be the predominating early feature, and in nearly all children confusion is prominent so that few of them remember to abort an attack by taking sugar even although they are word perfect on the necessary action before the attack begins. If the attack is prolonged, as is most likely to be the case if it occurs overnight, it may proceed to coma and vomiting or convulsions. The longer an attack has lasted the more difficult it is to stop. The shorter acting the insulin, the shorter will be the attack.

The pattern of the attack may vary from child to child, but is usually constant for each child. Some children become hypoglycaemic more readily than others, presumably because they do so at a higher level of blood sugar, while some have more severe attacks than others, presumably because they are more sensitive to a given low level of blood sugar. The attacks may be alarmingly sudden, and alarmingly difficult to treat.

> One child would get up in the morning apparently well and within minutes collapse on the bathroom floor. She clenched her teeth against sugar, responded poorly to Glucagon when she got it (her mother would drop the ampoule in her excitement) and usually vomited. After a while she made bizarre demands for food (ryebread, in fact) and recovered in hours rather than minutes. A considerable rise in her evening carbohydrate was ineffective, and the attacks were so severe that she was changed from Rapitard to Semilente to allow a degree of hyperglycaemia in the mornings, as it was feared that two injections of soluble might produce the same early morning or overnight effect as the Rapitard. We eventually obtained good control with Leo Neutral and Retard.

Usually, however, an attack can be averted by giving 20 g of glucose or sugar in a very little water. Glucose tablets weigh 3.3 g, large lumps of sugar 5 g, the common small lumps 2 g and a rounded teaspoon of cane sugar 5 g. If there is no obvious improvement after 5 minutes, the dose of sugar is repeated. This sugar is, of course, given in addition to the daily carbohydrate intake and is not subtracted from the next meal. If a child has frequent hypo attacks, or if the attacks are infrequent but severe, a supply of Glucagon should be given.

The attacks can be expected at certain times of day, particularly before a meal, depending on the insulin being used. With soluble insulin the attacks occur before lunch, with Semilente before tea and with Lente before breakfast. However, if large doses of insulin are being used, implying a degree of insulin resistance, the hypo attacks may come later, e.g. in the afternoon after a morning dose of soluble.

Gale and Tattersall (1979) found nocturnal hypoglycaemia (blood glucose < 2 mmol/l) in 22 of 39 badly-controlled insulin-dependent diabetics. Even mild symptoms (night sweats, morning headaches) were important clues to diagnosis. Many patients seemed to have become adapted to nocturnal hypoglycaemia with the passage of time, so that the nocturnal hypoglycaemia went unnoticed and the insulin dose escalated because of the high day-time sugars. This is another example of overtreatment. The writers found these cases very difficult to treat. Moore, Smith and Asplin (1979) found that estimating the cortisol/creatinine ratio in a morning urine was a help in diagnosing overnight hypoglycaemia, in the same way that insulin-induced hypoglycaemia is used to test the pituitary–adrenal axis.

Differential diagnosis

The diagnosis of hypoglycaemia may sometimes be difficult. Some common instances are appended.

(1) 'Nightmare'. A half-waking, confusional state in the middle of the night may represent a hypo attack, or may represent a half-waking, confusional state. It seems to me that half-waking and indeed sleep-walking occur in tense, conscientious, slightly obsessional children, rather than in frankly neurotic children who are more prone to nightmares. Even by trial and error a diagnosis may not be evident, as the non-diabetic child in a half-waking state may come round convincingly if given some sugar. Certainly it is always safer to give sugar, in keeping with the general rule that *if there is doubt about whether a child is having a hypo or not, sugar should always be given*. Nevertheless, it is desirable to

try to determine the cause of the nightmares. An appraisal of the child's temperament may give a hint, but a change in insulin may give a diagnosis.

(2) A child may pretend to have a hypoglycaemic attack in order to be given sugar or to manipulate his environment in some other way. At times the diagnosis may be obvious, as quoted elsewhere in this book about a mother who cured hypo attacks by walking her daughter up and down until they wore off. Those were not hypo attacks. However, the diagnosis may be difficult particularly when, as is usually the case, the performance is staged for non-medical persons such as school teachers. An attack occurring before lunch is more likely to be a hypo than one after lunch. Occasionally, the offender may be a bit too explicit about his symptoms ('Can't see the blackboard, Miss. Now my head's going queer') but often the physician is left in some doubt because of the lack of a clear history. It may help if the physician expresses his doubt by saying 'I wonder if that really was a hypo attack'. 'You're kidding us on, my lad' is not really necessary.

(3) The casualty officer may be confused by a child brought in reputedly in a hypo attack but with a blood glucose of 6.7 mmol/l (120 mg per cent). Such a finding is quite consistent with a hypo attack, particularly if the child has been in coma. The blood sugar can rise spontaneously without the administration of glucose or Glucagon. Recovery from coma may be delayed after the blood sugar has been raised to normal by the combined action of the body defences, the waning of the effect of insulin and the re-assertion of the diabetic state. Any child with a hypoglycaemic attack which has not responded quickly to oral sugar or to glucagon should be referred to hospital.

(4) Acute anxiety attacks, which seem to be becoming more common in children over the age of ten, may perfectly simulate hypoglycaemic attacks. I was sure that a boy at a recent diabetic camp was having a hypoglycaemic attack, so I talked to him kindly and stuffed him with sugar and he quickly recovered. He did it three times more but within range of Dextrostix and the blood glucose was never less than 7.2 mmol/l (130 mg per cent). He was a highly-strung boy, and the final diagnosis was acute anxiety attacks in a diabetic. One should be aware of the possibility, particularly if hypo attacks occur at unexpected times, and arrange for the blood glucose to be tested by the parents in the home when indicated.

The danger from repeated severe hypo attacks is cerebral impairment, commonly appearing as mental retardation, epilepsy or behaviour disorder of the cerebral dysfunction type. The children most at risk are the very young, and the younger they are, the worse the outlook. Infant diabetics, in whom frequent hypo attacks may be missed during their long hours of sleep, are most at risk of permanent cerebral damage. The parents of diabetics who get hypo attacks when they are of school age can, however, be assured that hypo attacks will cause no lasting harm.

It has been argued that a child who convulses during a hypo attack has an epileptic tendency independent of his diabetes. It is difficult to be dogmatic about this without a follow-up for decades, but certainly many children who have convulsed in a hypo attack show no other sign of epilepsy during the childhood years. Eeg-Olofsson (1977) discusses EEG findings in relation to hypoglycaemic convulsions in the diabetic.

When dealing with hypo attacks in the outpatient clinic, one should first enquire about late or missed meals or undue exercise, excitement or late nights. It is surprising how often such questioning reveals the answer. One would expect that a mother briefed in the causation of hypoglycaemic attacks would volunteer the relevant information but, in fact, she seldom does. Questions are necessary. However, there will always remain a hard core of unexplained hypo attacks, probably best dealt with by an increase in carbohydrate. Another phenomenon for which one should be prepared is the previously well-controlled child who suddenly produces a run of several hypo attacks in the course of a week or two, with little or no alteration in the urine sugar charts. Usually the attacks stop as mysteriously as they began, leaving the physician to wonder what it was all about, but in one of our patients it indicated the onset of auto-immune thyroiditis (p. 241).

SOME TALKING POINTS IN THE CLINIC

There are certain other matters which are raised by parents at the outpatient clinic, and these are discussed below.

Holidays

Holidays in Britain present little problem. Advice on fitting a hotel menu to a diabetic is given in Chapter 13. What most concerns the parent is the action to be taken when an early start is planned. For example, they plan to start at 6 am, and it will not be convenient for the child to have his usual insulin and breakfast at 8 am. If he is on a single daily injection, he can have his insulin and breakfast at 6 am, his mid-day meal one hour earlier than usual and his later meals at the usual time. This assumes that he will reach his destination the same day and that he will be able to revert to his usual routine the following morning. Fears of hypoglycaemia induced by the longer gap between main meals could be stilled by giving an extra 10 g of carbohydrate at mid-morning and mid-afternoon, but it seems preferable to stand by to treat hypoglycaemia in the hour before meals. Hypoglycaemia is not very likely to occur as sitting in a car all day is a hyperglycaemic situation, which could be potentiated by giving extra carbohydrate. If the child is on two injections a day the risk of hypoglycaemia caused by delayed meals is greater, but on balance it is still probably better to abort hypoglycaemia when it arises. If the child is known to be difficult to treat in a hypo attack, giving extra carbohydrate at the snacks would be safer.

Touring holidays are to be discouraged for all children and particularly diabetics. It is one thing for adults to spend most of their waking hours in a car, but it is not good for children. Taking a day or two to get to the destination and the same time to come back is acceptable, provided the child has a good active holiday in between.

Holidays abroad, for example a package deal to Majorca, present snags which are easily overcome. Enough measured carbohydrate in snack form should be carried to cover unforeseen delays on the journey. The insulin should be carried in the hand luggage in case it is frozen in the unheated luggage compartment. Virtually all the holiday hotels have a windowless shower room or bathroom attached to the bedroom, and the stone floor of the bathroom will keep insulin at a satisfactory temperature. Unexpected vegetables such as chickpeas, which can be scored as ordinary peas, may turn up, but if they are too baffling they can be left aside. Crisps, ice cream and hot dogs are freely available for the snacks. One father said 'He was running about so much I just let him take as much Coke as he wanted, because I thought that would take care of his fluids and his energy', and this seems a very sensible holiday outlook. Insulin needs may be less in hot climates and the parents should be forewarned of this but often there is no obvious change.

Holiday health insurance for diabetic children is unlikely to be given under the routine travel agency arrangements (diabetes being a pre-existing disease) but can be obtained by consulting Messrs. Stewart Wrightson (Southern) Ltd., 20 Station Road, South Norwood, London, SE25 5AJ. At present there are three scales, the allowance for medical expenses ranging from £1500 to £5000, the premiums for a two-week holiday ranging accordingly from £6 to £16.50. The one policy includes the usual benefits for personal accident, loss of luggage, etc. *Balance,* the newspaper of the BDA, will keep parents up to date in these matters.

Dependence and independence

The dangers of undue dependence of the diabetic child on his parents on the one hand and of undue independence on the other, are discussed on p. 81. They are mentioned here to remind the reader that the management of diabetes is not simply the adjusting of insulin and diet. Throughout all his conversations with the mother and child at the outpatient clinic the physician must have one ear cocked for the psychological overtones, because it is in these overtones that the solution to many problems will be found. It is not true of all children but it is true as a generalization that the main psychological problem facing the physician is to ensure that the child develops gradually a mature independence and self respect. This will happen only when the family have a realistic approach to diabetes and are ready to accept the limitations it imposes. Some children are by nature passive and wait for everything to be done for them, often by elderly doting parents. Others have passivity thrust upon them by parents so anxious they are afraid to let the child do anything for himself. Some children are by nature self-assertive and rebel against their diabetes by assuming complete independence of all attempts at diabetic control.

When the physician is faced with a poor urine chart he should ask himself not only if the insulin dosage is correct but also if the psychological balance between dependence and independence is satisfactory. Either extreme is almost invariably associated with unsatisfactory control. The over-protecting parent need not be scolded, for emphasis can be laid on what the boy should do rather than what the parent should not do. The passive child should be encouraged into hobbies, perhaps at first sedentary but later more active, because a hobby can enhance a personality. The child who is too independent may be reacting against his diabetes through fear of the future and the physician can indulge in a little pre-emptive phrase-dropping like 'When you leave school you will do so-and-so' or 'When you have children of your own, you will do the other' rather than a head-on attack of the 'Test your urine when I say so' type. There is admittedly a place for being a bit sharp at times, particularly if there is disagreement between parent and child, but sharpness should not become a routine response to any problem of behaviour.

With the very rebellious older child there may be a case for temporary relaxation of the management regime. One must not be short-sighted in management. It is of great importance to maintain good support for the young diabetic. They have enough trouble later as it is, which is brought out clearly in the valuable paper by McGregor (1977).

The eyes

The one thing that almost all parents know about diabetes is that blindness may supervene, and they, therefore, tend to worry about the child's eyes. The child may realize this and play up a little, so it is necessary for the diabetic clinic to have a good liaison with an ophthalmologist. All our patients are referred to a consultant ophthalmologist and are reviewed yearly. This system is of great help to the diabetic clinic and physicians may well consider making use of similar facilities in their own neighbourhood. Diseases of the eye are discussed in the chapter on complications.

Smoking

It is easier never to start smoking than to give it up and young diabetics should be so advised. In addition to the probable increased risk of cardiovascular disease it may have a bearing on diabetic retinopathy (Paetkau, 1978) and possibly on other complications of diabetes.

The teeth

Glasgow is rightly proud of its water supply which may be bottled and sent to America as 'Loch Katrine Water' (which indeed it is). It mixes well with whisky, but due to its softness, slight acidity and rather low fluorine content it does not mix so well with the teeth of diabetics. Glaswegians have bad teeth and extractions of the primary dentition are common.

All but well-controlled diabetics are at a disadvantage in maintaining good oral hygiene. It is true that they should not be taking sucrose by mouth, and it is true that glucose is less harmful than sucrose, but the constant secretion of glucose in the saliva puts at risk the teeth of the moderately or poorly controlled diabetic. Sterky *et al.* (1971) found that the teeth of diabetics passing less than 30 g of glucose in the urine daily were as good as the teeth of non-diabetics, but most adolescent diabetics lose more glucose than 30 g.

Glucose is converted by the bacteria present in dental plaque to acids, which demineralize the teeth. One thing the diabetic can do is to ensure, by meticulous cleaning of the teeth, that plaque does not form and that bacterial action is thus minimized. A pamphlet produced under the auspices of the Health Education Council (1979) gives excellent practical advice. The following points are important:

(1) The teeth should be brushed thoroughly at least once a day, preferably in the evening when there is less hurry. If it can be done twice a day, so much the better, but one good brushing is better than two perfunctory sluicings.
(2) The best method of brushing is the old-fashioned rotary scrubbing action. The vaunted up-and-down ('roll') brushing has not worked out well in practice, probably because it is very difficult to do.
(3) Despite their reputation, crunchy foods like apples and carrots do nothing to prevent plaque formation.
(4) Tablets are available which disclose the presence of plaque and can be brought across the counter. In Britain, Colgate's tablets 'For Better Brushing' are good. Similar tablets are produced in the USA by the Pacemaker Corporation, PO Box 16163, Portland, Oregon, 97216. A tablet is chewed and the mouth rinsed out. Plaque which has been there for 24 hours is stained blue, or pink if it has been there for 12 hours. Plaque is most likely to be found at the gum margins, and the molar and lingual surfaces of the lower teeth are likely to to be extensively involved. The dye brushes off easily so the child can quickly work out an efficient brushing technique.

Sometimes a parent announces out of the blue that a child has just had three teeth out. There has been no special preparation related to the diabetes and no harm has ensued, but dental extraction should be taken seriously. There is no reason why a dentist should not remove the teeth of a stable diabetic in his own surgery, but some dentists do not like to do this and certainly all unstable diabetics should have their extractions done in hospital. The dentist working in his own surgery should have the services of a trained anaesthetist and it is desirable that there should be consultation between dentist and doctor, directly or through the mother.

Ideally, the operation should be done about 9 to 9.30 am. If this can be arranged, both insulin and breakfast can be withheld till after the operation. If the child is on a depot insulin, for example Lente, there may be a fear that its continuing action will lead to hypoglycaemia in the absence of carbohydrate, and indeed if he has constantly negative urines in the morning this may be a risk which would indicate admission to hospital, but on the whole the risk is exaggerated. It was pointed out in Chapter 1 that there is a tendency for blood sugars to be higher after operation than before it, and there does seem to be a built-in defensive mechanism in the body (probably mediated through Glucagon, p. 149) which covers short operations. On the other hand, there is no tendency to an excessive rise in blood sugar after a short operation. If the operation is to be done at mid-morning, the child can be given his usual insulin covered with breakfast carbohydrate as sugar, washed down with one or two mouthfuls of water. This can be spread over an hour, as long as two hours are left before operation. The rule is often quoted that nothing should be taken by mouth for four hours before operation, but sugar with a little water does not seem to overload the stomach. *The one thing to be avoided is giving insulin without carbohydrate cover.* As soon as he is round from his anaesthetic the mid-morning snack can be given as sugar. If the operation is to be done in the afternoon the child starts his day normally but takes his lunch as sugar. If it is done in the early afternoon, say 2 pm, lunch can be brought forward to 12 noon, and if he is on Semilente insulin, of which the maximal action is in the afternoon, an extra 10 g of carbohydrate can be given. If the anaesthetist has been warned he can have a supply of intravenous glucose at hand in the unlikely event of it being needed.

It has already been mentioned that it is better for unstable diabetics to have extractions done in hospital. If they have a tendency to produce ketosis, ketosis may well be precipitated by withholding insulin and carbohydrate in the morning. In hospital they can be given about two-thirds of their carbohydrate requirements intravenously about half to one hour before operation, assuming it is done in the morning. If it has to be done later in the day, it may be advisable to convert to soluble insulin beforehand. However, in hospital it should be easy to monitor blood and urine sugar (Dextrostix is useful in such a situation) and to adjust the balance by giving soluble insulin or intravenous glucose as the circumstances warrant.

Surgical operations

The regime given for dental extraction can be applied to any short operation, and, although it is not strictly a matter for the outpatient clinic, a further word on surgery in the diabetic is not out of place here. In long operations the blood sugar should be monitored frequently. Such a patient is probably already on an intravenous drip, so intravenous glucose or subcutaneous insulin can readily be given. Even in emergency operations, for example for a road traffic accident, the diabetic should be at no greatly increased risk and the immediate need for operation over-rides consideration of his diabetic state. On the other hand, a lesion like a ruptured appendix may have produced severe ketoacidosis with dehydration, in which case hydration should be corrected before operation is attempted.

The use of a mini pump to infuse insulin throughout an operation is described by Barnett *et al.* (1980).

Careers

To be frank, the physician in a children's hospital is seldom consulted about careers for diabetics, although he may be asked for his advice if he follows his patients into adolescence. The child's future occupation will depend largely on his own intelligence. He is best suited to a profession, the business world, a trade, clerical work or working in a shop. He should choose a job which calls for the same output of physical effort every day, not one in which he is in an office one day and scrambling up and down hills the next, although the average diabetic could adjust his diet to cover such variations in activity. If he is going into banking or clerical work he should make sure that the company's pension scheme includes diabetics. If he is not gifted academically he may become a labourer, but he should not work at heights for fear of hypoglycaemia. Strolling across a plank a hundred feet above ground with a hod full of bricks is not for the diabetic.

Girls who have diabetes are fit for almost all the jobs usually filled by women, whether on the factory floor, or in shops, offices or the professions. Shift work can be a problem, as with the men, but the problem can usually be solved by soluble insulin.

A list of *occupations not suited to diabetics*, and from many of which diabetics are barred, is as follows.

(1) The services—the armed forces, police, merchant navy and fire brigade.
(2) Driving public service vehicles, buses, trains, heavy lorries.
(3) The control of potentially dangerous machinery, e.g. cranes.
(4) Flying duties (other than steward).

These are the obvious ones. There are doubtless more. The most depressing feature for the diabetic, however, is that if two men are equally qualified the non-diabetic is likely to get preference over the diabetic—and for the wrong reason. The word 'diabetes' is taken as a synomyn for 'absenteeism' by some employers, whereas the work record of the diabetic, who may take better care of himself than does the average man, is good. It is relatively easy for the man who develops diabetes while in a job to convince his employer that diabetes has not impaired his efficiency. It is much more difficult for the young diabetic to get a start, so much so that many diabetologists believe that the new worker should at first conceal his diabetes. I cannot accept this view whole-heartedly, but advance it as an opinion strongly held by others.

Car driving

A last word on *car driving*. Diabetics may hold driving licences, but a doctor is required to give a certificate of their fitness to drive. In the well-controlled diabetic of relatively late onset there is little problem—the average man is probably as likely to have a coronary at the wheel as the experienced diabetic is to have a sudden severe hypo attack—but the unstable, unreliable diabetic is a different matter, and the doctor may advise against the granting of a licence. A car is, after all, potentially dangerous machinery. The diabetic must declare his diabetes or his insurance will be invalid.

ENVOI

Despite the great mass of literature on diabetes very little has been written about the outpatient clinic. Now I know why. An exception was Chance (1969), and even he found that his account of outpatient care had to be 'somewhat idealized'. It is virtually impossible to describe the chiaroscuro of circumstances that envelops each diabetic. Who am I, still puzzled by many of my patients, to give advice to others?

> The Watson family come back to mind. Despite their interchangeable charts, they have seldom required re-admission except for Elsie, the middle one. She had a bad spell in 1972–73, being re-admitted five times in six months with ketoacidosis. She has now had diabetes for over five years, and has been re-admitted at no other time. Jeannie has had to be re-admitted once in eight years, James not at all in five years. What went wrong with Elsie that did not affect the others? And why is it that Elsie is growing very well, but the other two are not?

It is questions like these which give such an interest to the diabetic clinic. If we knew all the answers, how dull life would be!

REFERENCES

Barnett, A. H., Robinson, M. H., Harrison, J. H. and Watkins, P. J. (1980). Minipump: method of diabetic control during minor surgery under general anaesthesia. *Br.med.J.,* **1,** 78

Born to Fail? (1973) by Peter Wedge and Hilary Prosser. Arrow Books, London

Campbell, I. W. (1976). The Somogyi Phenomenon: a short review. *Acta diabet.lat.* **13,** 68

Chance, G. W. (1969). Outpatient management of diabetic children. *Br.med.J.,* **II,** 493

Coppolillo, H. P. (1965). The questioning and doubting parent. *J.Pediat.,* **67,** 371

Eeg-Olofsson, O. (1977). Hypoglycaemia and neurological disturbances in children with diabetes mellitus. *Acta paediat.scand.,* Suppl. 270, 91–95

Gale, E. A. M. and Tattersall, R. B. (1979). Unrecognised nocturnal hypoglycaemia in insulin-treated diabetics. *Lancet,* **I,** 1049.

Gale, E. A. M. and Tattersall, R. B. (1979). Brittle diabetes.*Br.J.hosp.Med.,* **22,** 589

Health Education Council (1979). *The scientific basis of dental health education.* Ed. Holloway, P. London

Hinkle, L. E., Fischer, A., Knowles, H. C. and Stunkard, A. J. (1959). The role of environment and personality in the management of the difficult patient with diabetes mellitus. *Diabetes,* **8,** 371

MacGregor, M. (1977). Juvenile diabetics growing up. *Lancet,* **I,** 944

Moore, R. A., Smith, R. R. and Asplin, C. M. (1979). Simple test for nocturnal hypoglycaemia in diabetic patients. *Lancet,* **I,** 409

Paetkau, M. E. (1978). Diabetic retinopathy and smoking. *Lancet,* **II,** 1098 (also *Lancet* editorial (1978), **I,** 841)

Rosenbloom, A. L. and Giordano, B. P. (1977). Chronic overtreatment with insulin in children and adolescents. *Am. J. Dis. Child.* **131,** 881

Schwandt, R., Richter, W. and Wilkening, J. (1979). Chronic insulin overtreatment. *Lancet,* **II,** 261

Somogyi, M. (1959). Exacerbation of diabetes by excess insulin action. *Am. J. Med.,* **26,** 169

Sterky, G., Kjellman, O., Högberg, O. and Löfroth, A–L. (1971). Dietary composition and dental disease in adolescent diabetics. *Acta paediat. Scand.* **60,** 461

CHAPTER 7

Insulin and Metabolism

'God bless my soul, sir!' exclaimed the Reverend Doctor Folliott, bursting, one fine May morning, into the breakfast room at Crotchet Castle, 'I am out of all patience with this march of mind. Here has my house been nearly burned down, by my cook taking it into her head to study hydrostatics, in a sixpenny tract, published by the Steam Intellect Society, and written by a learned friend. ...

My cook must read his rubbish in bed; and, as might naturally be expected, she dropped suddenly fast asleep, overturned the candle, and set the curtains in a blaze. Luckily, the footman went into the room at the moment ... she is a greasy subject, and would have burned like a short mould.'

T. L. Peacock, *Crotchet Castle.*

Growth hormone, it has been said, is a self-contained glucoregulatory system, involving ACG, an acceleratory polypeptide which promotes glucose uptake, and ING, an inhibitory polypeptide which discourages it. So much for that. I shall not refer to it again.

Rows of filing cabinets could be filled with the papers written on the metabolism of insulin and its related hormones and on the several factors controlling the action of every enzyme. This chapter could be infinite in length. In the simplified account which follows much has been left out, but it is hoped that what remains will help the clinician to understand his patients, particularly if they do not behave according to the approved rules of thumb.

CARBOHYDRATE METABOLISM

An understanding of carbohydrate metabolism in an uncomplicated form is a good basis from which to start. It may be helpful to consider

CARBOHYDRATE METABOLISM

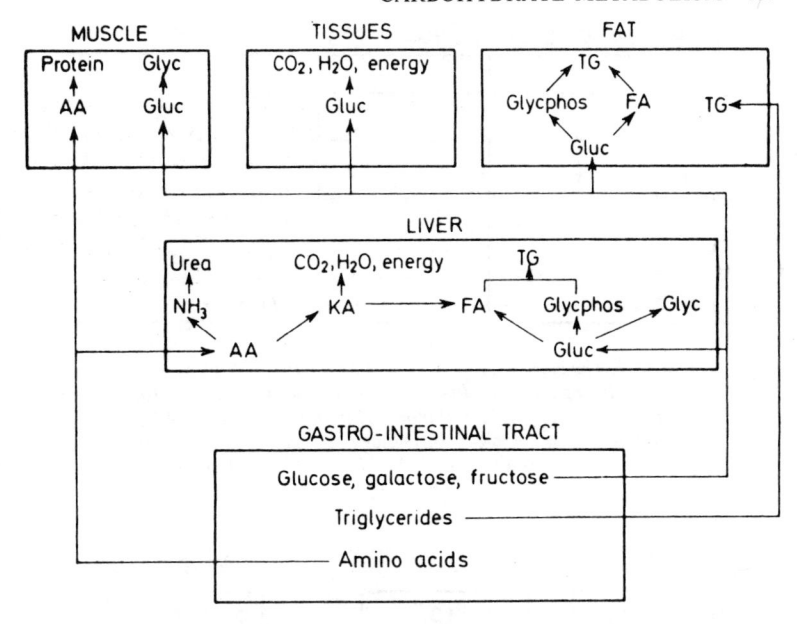

Figure 7.1. Pathways of the absorptive phase of carbohydrate metabolism (from Human Physiology *by* Vander, Sherman and Luciano, 1975, McGraw-Hill: New York)

AA = amino acids
FA = fatty acids
Gluc = glucose
Glyc = glycogen
Glycphos = glycerophosphate
KA = ketoacids
TG = triglycerides

carbohydrate metabolism as being composed of an absorptive and fasting phase, the latter resembling in many ways the diabetic state.

The absorptive phase is outlined in *Figure 7.1*. Glucose enters the blood from the intestinal tract. In the liver it is stored as glycogen but it is also used in the production of triglycerides which are conveyed to adipose tissue and there stored as fat. Adipose tissue is not inert, and makes its own fat from glucose by a similar process, on site. In muscle also, glucose is stored as glycogen, but in other tissues it is used as an immediate source of energy.

The connection between protein and fat metabolism on the one hand and carbohydrate metabolism on the other is rather tenuous in the absorptive phase, but they become closely linked in the fasting phase. In the absorptive phase, amino acids taken up from the gut are carried to the muscles, where protein may be formed, and to the liver, where they produce ketoacids, from which in turn are derived fatty acids and energy. Urea is produced as a by-product in the alanine

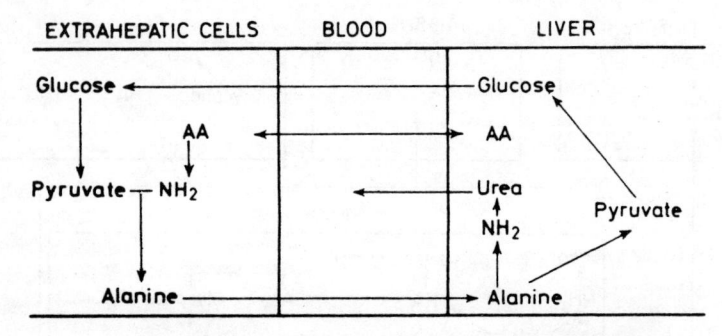

Figure 7.2. The alanine cycle. This avoids the toxic action of ammonia produced during the breakdown of protein to amino acids by attaching NH_2 to pyruvate to produce alanine. Glutamine has the same function as alanine (from Medical Physiology *by H. M. Goodman (Ed. Mountcastle) 1974, C. V. Mosby Co.: St. Louis)*

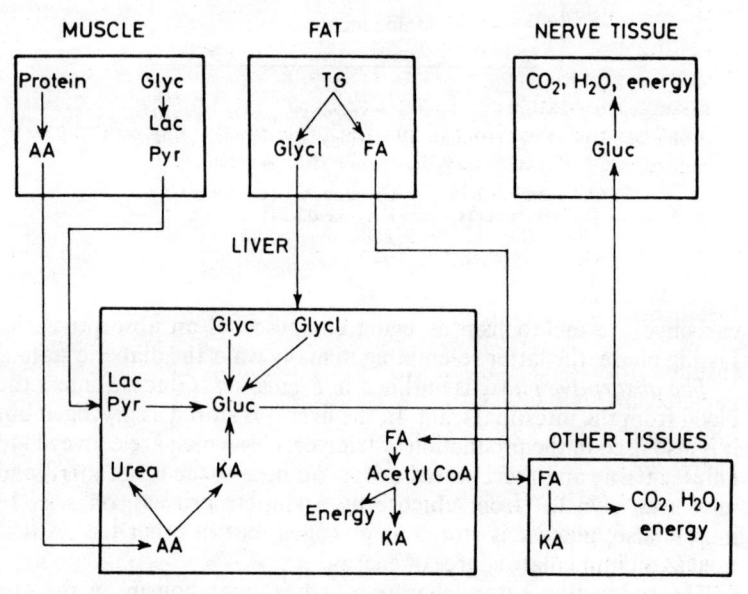

Figure 7.3. The fasting phase of carbohydrate metabolism (from Human Physiology *by Vander, Sherman and Luciano, 1975, McGraw-Hill: New York)*

AA = amino acids
FA = fatty acids
Gluc = glucose
Glyc = glycogen
Glycphos = glycerophosphate

Glycl = glycerol
KA = ketoacids
Lac = lactate
Pyr = pyruvate
TG = triglycerides

cycle *(Figure 7.2)*. Triglycerides are transported directly to the adipose tissue.

The fasting phase (Figure 7.3) is essentially a reversal of the absorptive phase, but certain divergencies exist. A few notes may elucidate the diagram.

(1) Muscle cannot convert glycogen to glucose, but produces lactate and pyruvate instead.
(2) In the liver there is virtually no conversion of fatty acids to glucose and certainly no net synthesis of glucose from fatty acids, but glycerol is converted to glucose and in the moderate fasting state produces all the glucose needed by the body. After several days of fasting glucose is produced by the kidney. The liver itself uses fatty acids for energy during fasting, instead of amino acids.
(3) However, the major source of blood glucose during fasting is indirectly the muscles, which supply amino acids to the liver for gluconeogenesis (the production of sugar from amino acids).
(4) In the early stages of a fast, the nervous system can obtain energy only from glucose. Other tissues do not use glucose during fasting but derive their energy from fatty acids instead, thus sparing glucose for the brain. However, after four or five days of fasting, the brain begins to use ketones. This unexpected development has the side effect of sparing protein catabolism, and can be regarded as a last desperate attempt at survival.

INSULIN

Insulin action

Insulin, or the lack of it, plays a large part in the metabolic activity depicted in *Figures 7.1* to *7.3*. Its actions may be summarized as follows:

(1) It facilitates the diffusion of glucose into cells, particularly those of muscle and adipose tissue. It does not, however, control glucose uptake by the brain, nor does it affect the transport of glucose across the renal tubule or the intestinal epithelium.
(2) It stimulates glycogen synthesis
   (a) by increasing the glucose in the cells, and
   (b) by increasing the activity of cyclic nucleotide phosphodiesterase, which degrades cyclic AMP, an inhibitor of glycogen formation. Insulin may also stimulate glucokinase, which is involved in phosphorylation and is much reduced in starvation and untreated diabetes.

(3) It stimulates triglyceride formation by a similar double effect, increasing the glucose substrate and inhibiting the enzymic breakdown of triglycerides. It also inhibits the release of glycerol from adipose tissue.
(4) Almost all the enzymes involved in the utilization of insulin in the liver are potentiated by insulin, and the synthesis of glucose is inhibited, the mechanism involved not being fully understood.
(5) Insulin facilitates the transport of amino acids, particularly into muscle, and is involved in protein synthesis. It inhibits the release of amino acids from muscle, thus depriving the liver of the substrate needed for gluconeogenesis. Further, the enzymes involved in gluconeogenesis fall when insulin is in good supply.

It will be seen that if insulin is absent or reduced, as in diabetes, the result will be very similar to the fasting phase, the high blood sugar being a notable exception which gives rise to the description of diabetes as 'starvation in the midst of plenty'. A more detailed account of the effects of insulin lack is given in the section on ketoacidosis (Chapter 8).

Insulin synthesis and secretion

In a typical secretory cell is a reticulum of canals on the walls of which are small patches of ribonucleic acid, known as ribosomes. Such areas can be separated off by differential centrifugation, the ribosome and its immediately surrounding tissue being known as the microsome. The microsome is particularly concerned with the synthesis of protein which, in the beta-cell of the pancreas, is insulin.

Insulin is synthesized through its precursor, pro-insulin, which can be represented as a long curved single chain, the ends linked by disulphide bonds. The loss of a connecting peptide (C-peptide) produces insulin with its A (glycyl) and B (phenylalanyl) chains *(Figure 7.4)*.

C-peptide is produced in a 1:1 ratio with insulin and passes through the liver unchanged. This fact can be used clinically in detecting deliberately induced hypoglycaemia in non-diabetics (insulin high, C-peptide low) and most insulinomas (high C-peptide, low blood sugar). It may also be useful in assessing the results of pancreatectomy for carcinoma, when the bulk of insulin produced may be taken up by the liver (Horwitz, Rubinstein and Steiner, 1978). In addition, C-peptide gives a measure of remission in the early stages of diabetes (Ludvigsson and Heding, 1977).

Insulin is stored in combination with zinc in the beta-granules, each of which is contained by a membrane. Secretion of insulin is brought about by the granule migrating to the cell surface, where the membranes of granule and cell fuse, insulin then being spewed forth by a process known to the genteel as emiocytosis. It has been estimated that the time from synthesis to secretion of insulin is three hours. The 'quick release' of insulin comes from the stores in the granules. The mechanism of slow release is uncertain but presumably involves further synthesis.

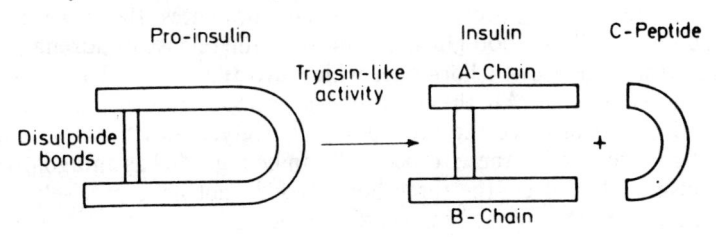

Figure 7.4. The genesis of insulin

The main stimulus to insulin secretion in man is glucose, particularly when its concentration in the blood rises above 5 mmol/l (90 mg per cent). The higher the sugar level, the quicker is insulin synthesized. Experimentally, mannose can be shown to have a similar but lesser effect, but galactose and fructose are inactive. Glucose presumably assists in conveying the insulin to the cell surface, but its specificity among sugars in so doing raises the question of how it does so. It might have a specific ability to cross the cell membrane in entering the cell, but it is more likely that it has its effect by phosphorylation through the pentose pathway. D-Mannoheptulose, a sugar which occurs naturally in the avocado, is known to inhibit phosphorylation, and it inhibits the stimulus of glucose to insulin secretion.

As has been noted above, amino acids appear to cause the rise in plasma insulin after a protein meal. The ability of arginine to raise the circulating insulin level is used in research techniques. Lysine, phenylalanine and, as paediatricians will remember, leucine have a similar effect. Undue sensitivity to leucine can produce post-prandial hypoglycaemia and convulsions in the child. The amino acid stimulus to insulin secretion is in fact the dominant stimulus in fish, but how it brings about its effect within the cell is unknown.

Insulin is secreted into the portal system and anatomically compelled to pass through the liver, where 40 per cent of the insulin may be taken up before the remainder passes into the systemic system and on to the periphery. The route taken by insulin may have importance in causing non-ketotic hyperosmolar coma (p. 181). The uptake of insulin by the liver is high in the fasting state, lower after a meal. This means that more insulin reaches the periphery after a meal, allowing for glycogen and triglyceride synthesis.

INSULIN ANTAGONISTS: SOME GENERAL CONSIDERATIONS

A rise in blood glucose concentration stimulates the release of insulin. A fall in blood glucose stimulates the release of adrenaline, glucagon and growth hormone, which are therefore all increased during starvation. All these hormones promote gluconeogenesis in the liver, all produce the breakdown of triglycerides to fatty acids and glycerol, and in these respects all can be regarded as antagonistic to insulin. However, the three hormones do not have precisely the same effects throughout carbohydrate metabolism. Adrenaline and glucagon antagonize insulin by their involvement in the breakdown of glycogen to glucose, but growth hormone does not exhibit this effect. On the other hand, growth hormone does exhibit primary antagonism to insulin by decreasing glucose uptake by muscle, which the other two hormones do not.

It has been said that adrenaline, glucagon and growth hormone show the same response to blood glucose levels, a response which is opposed to the action of insulin. The same cannot be said of the response to high plasma amino acid levels, glucagon and growth hormone rising in the same way as insulin. A carbohydrate meal leads to a rise in insulin alone, a protein meal to a rise in insulin, glucagon and growth hormone. The rise in glucagon and growth hormone allow gluconeogenesis and the production of glucose from glycogen after a meal high in protein and low in carbohydrate, whereas if insulin were left on its own the amino acids would be stored in muscle, the conversion of glycogen to glucose would be reversed and the blood sugar would be lowered, possibly to hypoglycaemic levels. Briefly, if insulin were the only hormone, a high protein meal would cause hypoglycaemia.

During starvation circulating insulin is low and insulin is not available for protein synthesis, but at such times growth hormone acts as a brake on protein catabolism.

The response of the diabetic to *exercise* leads to a reconsideration of the action of insulin. It has been shown that if insulin is present in small amounts it will inhibit both glucose production by the liver and free fatty acid (FFA) production at the periphery before it has any direct effect on peripheral glucose uptake. FFA inhibits peripheral insulin usage, so a small amount of insulin will therefore affect muscle uptake of glucose more by reducing FFA (which it does in the presence of the greatly increased blood flow supplying extra glucose to exercising muscle) than by any *direct* effect on peripheral uptake. This sheds new light on the old saying that 'the exercising muscle uses glucose without the benefit of insulin'. It should also be remembered that exercise may speed absorption of insulin from its depot site. A review covering this and related subjects has been written by Sönksen and West (1978).

Other hormones are involved in carbohydrate metabolism. It is well known that the prolonged administration of steroids may be diabetogenic in man, through the action of the *glucocorticoids*, cortisol and corticosterone, the former being the more important. Excess of cortisol produces hyperglycaemia, insulin resistance (which in the normal person can be compensated for by an increase in insulin secretion) and an increase in liver glycogen. Cortisol promotes gluconeogenesis in the liver and inhibits peripheral glucose uptake, which leads to increased blood pyruvate from which glucose is resynthesised in the liver, these two actions of cortisol thus combining to increase the liver glycogen. The glucocorticoids have another action which may be of clinical value. If the recovery from severe hypoglycaemia has been delayed despite the blood sugar having been returned to normal (by the injection of glucose or glucagon) glucocorticoids may prove effective in restoring consciousness, presumably by helping the neurones to utilize glucose. *Thyroxin* may cause diabetes in animals in whom the pancreas has been damaged, and may increase gluconeogenesis as well as affecting the pancreatic cells themselves. An analogous situation may occur in man, as it has been suggested that the insulin needs of a diabetic are increased by the onset of thyrotoxicosis. However, though glucocorticoids and thyroxin play a part in carbohydrate metabolism, they are not directly affected by blood glucose levels in the way that adrenaline, glucagon and growth hormone are affected.

INSULIN ANTAGONISTS CONSIDERED SEPARATELY

Although one talks of insulin antagonists, it will have been realized that insulin and its so-called antagonists work harmoniously together in the healthy subject. It is only when insulin production fails that the moderating effect of other hormones appears as antagonism. Factors antagonistic to insulin will now be discussed in greater detail.

Insulinase

The half-life of insulin injected into the human has been calculated as 40 minutes. Insulin is inactivated and degraded by 'insulinase', an unfortunate term in that at least two enzyme systems are involved. One is an insulin-specific protease which appears to break insulin into amino acids and small peptides, although the mechanism is not clearly understood; the other is glutathione–insulin transferase, which reduces the disulphide bonds between the A and B chains, thus separating the chains. The higher the concentration of the transferase in a tissue the lower is its sensitivity to insulin, so the enzyme may in part dictate the extent to which cells of different types utilize insulin. However, the situation is more complicated than has just been implied, as in certain circumstances the transhydrogenase appears to be capable of joining up the A and B chains once more. It is also possible that the catabolic action of the transferase paves the way for another enzyme to split the chains into their constituent amino acids, but the transferase would remain as the important rate-controlling enzyme.

It has been claimed that insulin breakdown is increased in diabetics when the plasma insulin level is high, reduced when it is low (Frost *et al.*, 1973). The main site of insulin degradation seems to be the liver. In fasting and diabetic animals there is a fall in the amount of insulin inactivated by liver cells, so presumably there is a fall in 'insulinase'. There certainly seems to be a fall in the transhydrogenase (Thomas, 1973). The level of circulating insulin may control the level of liver transhydrogenase, implying that insulin signs its own death warrant. The kidney, however, plays an important part in degradation and its action is independent of the level of circulating insulin.

It will have been noted that, in theory, diabetes could be caused by the over-action of 'insulinase', but such a situation has not been demonstrated in the human. Indeed, a lack of one of many enzymes or the excess of another, the lack of one hormone or the excess of another, could all theoretically cause diabetes. In practice, however, the cause of juvenile diabetes is a failure in insulin production.

Growth hormone

The idea that growth hormone and insulin are opposed to each other stemmed originally from clinical observations on abnormal subjects. Acromegalics are prone to develop diabetes. Diabetic retinopathy may improve if hypopituitarism supervenes. Animals may be rendered diabetic if given anterior pituitary extract for long periods. Growth hormone raises the blood sugar in hypophysectomized diabetics. All these statements are true, but mask certain physiological characteristics of the two hormones.

The primary action of growth hormone seems to be by increasing lipolysis, breaking down stored fats and releasing free fatty acids. It also encourages nitrogen retention and promotes protein synthesis, in which actions it mimics insulin and may indeed act through insulin. In this respect the two hormones are acting towards the same end, the retention of nitrogen.

The links between the metabolism of carbohydrate and fat stands out clearly when one looks at the effect of growth hormone on carbohydrate metabolism. It has already been said that the uptake of glucose by muscle is inhibited by growth hormone; but it may take hours before this effect is seen. The rise in blood sugar after a large injection of growth hormone is considerably delayed. This delay suggests not so much direct neutralization of insulin action or suppression of insulin production as a cause of the hyperglycaemia as some more subtle interference with the ability of insulin to promote the utilization of sugar. This mechanism appears to lie in the peripheral lipolytic action of growth hormone. The ketone bodies and non-esterified fatty acids produced by lipolysis have both been shown experimentally to diminish the uptake of glucose by muscle. The reactions involved are shown in *Figure 7.5*.

The key substance in *Figure 7.5* is acetyl coenzyme-A, which holds an important position in the metabolism of both fat and carbohydrate. It is produced by the beta-oxidation of fatty acids. It also comes indirectly from glucose by oxidative decarboxylation of pyruvate. The increased catabolism of fat produced by growth hormone results in a rise of acetyl CoA, and such a rise inhibits the oxidation of pyruvate. The rise in acetyl CoA is also important directly and in the production of citrate in inhibiting phosphofructokinase, and indirectly hexokinase. This leads to a damming back in the glycolytic pathway, phosphorylation and utilization of glucose by the cells are inhibited, and glucose rises in the blood.

A concept helpful to the reader may be *'the glucoregulatory state'* in which three main hormones are involved, insulin being concerned with the storage of glucose when it is in good supply, glucagon and growth hormone being the hormones of glucose lack, mobilizing glucose from other sources (protein and fat) while at the same time inhibiting the action of insulin at the periphery, thus permitting available supplies of glucose to reach the brain where it can be used without insulin (Unger and Eisentraut, 1964).

In the normal individual with small amounts of circulating growth

148 INSULIN AND METABOLISM

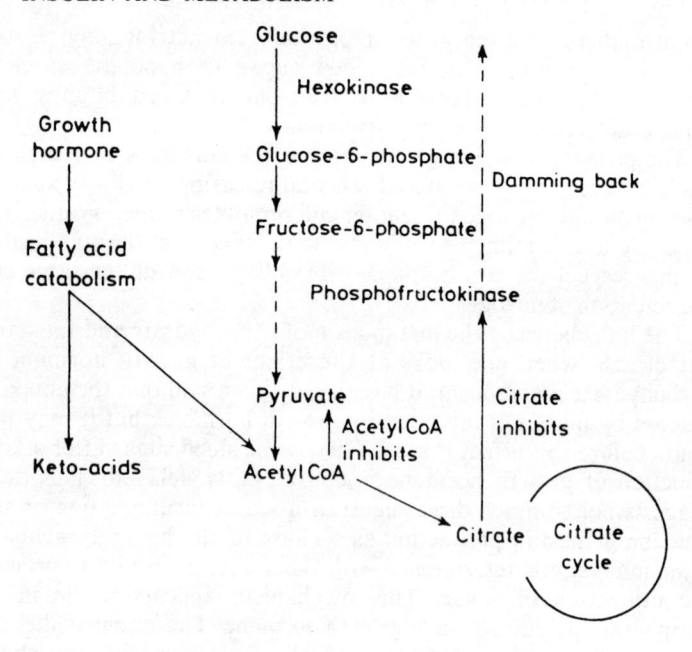

Figure 7.5. The role of growth hormone in fat and carbohydrate metabolism

hormone the system depicted in *Figure 7.5* remains in balance, but an increase in growth hormone can unbalance it and cause hyperglycaemia with ketosis. It must be stressed that the action of growth hormone in doing so takes some hours, and it is only a sustained rise in growth hormone, as may be found in the presence of an abnormality such as acromegaly, that will produce the diabetic state. It is an observed fact that children appear to have had a slight growth spurt before the onset of clinical diabetes (p. 196). Could this spurt and the onset of diabetes be produced by a common factor, excess of growth hormone? The point is interesting, and has been discussed by Chiumelli *et al.* (1971) and Baird, Hunter and Smith (1973). There is a clash of opinion on whether newly diagnosed untreated diabetic children do or do not show rises in growth hormone after glucose loading, and a similar clash on whether growth hormone is or is not raised in potential diabetics who have had a glucose load. In a number of cases of pancreatic insufficiency studied by Baird, Hunter and Smith one is of particular interest in the present context. When first studied after a glucose load he had a normal growth hormone response, peaking at three hours, and normal non-esterified fatty acids, but he showed very low insulin responses throughout. Six months later he developed insulin-dependent diabetes, by which time the level of growth hormone was high throughout, as it is known to be in poorly controlled diabetes. In this diabetic insulin deficiency preceded the rise in growth hormone, and the rise in growth hormone appeared to be secondary to insulin lack and not vice versa. This is only one case, but it is suggestive, and there is no evidence pointing firmly in the opposite direction.

Catecholamines (p. 153) appear to be involved in growth hormone control. Blackard (1973) has investigated the possibility that nearly all the stimuli for a growth hormone response (physical and emotional stress, hypoglycaemia, vasopressin) could be mediated through the catecholamines. His conclusions indicate that alpha-catecholamines stimulate and beta-catecholamines depress growth hormone secretion. This is the opposite of the mechanism of insulin secretion in response to catecholamines. The control may be exerted solely at hypothalamic level (where catecholamines are more concentrated than anywhere else in the CNS) or may come directly from the adrenals themselves.

Islet cells

Our knowledge of islet cells is increasing and it is now known that insulin and glucagon are not the only products of the islets. The islets are composed of roughly 50 per cent beta-cells (insulin), 25 per cent alpha-cells (glucagon), 10 per cent each of D-cells (somatostatin) and F-cells (pancreatic polypeptide), with the remaining 5 per cent divided between D_1-cells (vasoactive intestinal polypeptide) and EC-cells (serotonin). There has been considerable recent interest in the presence of somatostatin in the pancreas and the major hormones will now be discussed.

Glucagon

Glucagon is a polypeptide produced in the alpha-cells of the pancreas. Its role in raising blood sugar is well known, and it is widely used in the treatment of hypoglycaemic coma. It produces sugar from glycogen in the liver. It also activates lipases in the liver and in adipose tissue, all three actions being mediated through cyclic AMP. This results in glucagon producing hyperglycaemia and ketosis, in both of which activities it is more powerful than insulin lack, so when there is no insulin glucagon will 'run wild' (Raskin and Unger,

1978). It does not appear to be active on muscle glycogen but does activate hepatic gluconeogenesis.

Until recent years, glucagon and insulin have been supposed to have diametrically opposed actions in their response to blood sugar. If blood sugar were to fall, glucagon would be released by the alpha-cells to raise the glucose level. Conversely, if blood sugar were to rise plasma insulin would rise, while glucagon would lie dormant. It is now accepted that the interplay of insulin and glucagon is more complicated than was first believed. Samols, Marri and Marks (1965) observed that glucagon stimulated insulin secretion, and it has since been shown that glucagon receptor sites exist in beta-cells. Thus, when glucagon raises blood sugar a built-in governor system between alpha- and beta-cells is brought into play, whereby insulin is liberated in pursuit of the rising blood sugar.

Buchanan (1973) has described work in Belfast on glucagon and insulin responses in normal and diabetic subjects. In normal controls, plasma insulin rises and glucagon falls after oral glucose is given, implying that glucagon is not a factor in insulin secretion within the normal hormonal balance of healthy persons. On the other hand, if oral glucose is given to untreated diabetics the opposite happens, and there is a relatively poor rise in insulin but a marked rise in glucagon even in the presence of hyperglycaemia (and the poorer the insulin response the greater the rise in glucagon) as if the glucagon were trying to raise the insulin to deal with the hyperglycaemia; which it cannot do, as there is not enough insulin available in the diabetic. In short, the hyperglycaemia of severe insulin deficiency may in fact promote glucagon activity. On the other hand, Alberti *et al.* (1975) showed that stopping insulin in juvenile onset diabetes led to hyperglycaemia and ketosis but not hyperglucagonaemia; but Raskin and Unger suggest that such a sudden fall in insulin allows the unchanged level of glucagon to exert a maximal effect. One must consider the possibility that an upset in the insulin–glucagon balance could be a factor in the aetiology of diabetes, but primary insulin deficiency seems more likely to be the cause of any upset in glucagon as the same glucagon response can be seen in 'true' diabetes, experimental insulin deficiency and some cases of chronic pancreatitis, in all of which the common factor is insulin deficiency.

There is obviously a potential role for glucagon in conditions of stress, defined by Bloom (1973) as a state of potential energy requirement. Although resting levels of glucagon do not seem to be under sympathetic nervous control, abnormal states can be created in which nervous control of glucagon seems definite. For example, splanchnic nerve stimulation in adrenalectomized calves can raise the plasma glucagon 20-fold in some 12 minutes, the speed of reaction suggesting direct nervous control. Further, artificially induced pain in monkeys has given a five-fold rise within two minutes. Psychological factors have also been considered and sudden noise has given a similar four-fold rise in monkeys. In humans, major surgery is not associated with a noticeable glucagon rise, but postoperative fever is. Infants who have suffered fetal distress have higher glucagon levels than the normal.

Although much of this work has been done on animals it is very suggestive of glucagon release being increased under stress. This mechanism may well play a part in the instability of the diabetic under nervous tension, though probably not the major part as rises in cortisol, catecholamines and growth hormone have been demonstrated in acute states of diabetic ketoacidosis. The role of the catecholamines in stress will shortly be discussed. At present it can be said that the importance of stress as a cause of loss of diabetic control has a firm physiological foundation.

The part played by glucagon in the production of hyperosmolar nonketotic coma is discussed on p. 181.

Somatostatin

Somatostatin (Rizza and Gerich, 1978) was first found in the hypothalamus and called 'growth hormone release inhibiting hormone' (GHRIH) or 'somatotropin RIH' (SRIH) because this was its first recognized form of activity, but since then it has been found to have an inhibitory effect on the release of many hormones so that 'somatostatin' seems a better name. Somatostatin has been found at other sites, for example in the pancreas and gastro-intestinal tract. It has a short half-life (about one minute) which makes it reasonable to assume that it is active at the sites where it is found. The same short half-life has so far prevented its therapeutic use.

Most substances which release insulin release somatostatin and insulin inhibitors inhibit somatostatin. On the other hand, somatostatin appears to inhibit both alpha- and beta-cells in the pancreas, slightly favouring beta-cells on balance, so that somatostatin given intravenously to a normal person produces mild hypoglycaemia. In the diabetic it is probable that somatostatin has a modifying effect (but not a dominating one) on falls in insulin and rises in glucagon. The D-cells (containing somatostatin) are increased in the diabetic islet not just as a percentage but absolutely, so the hormone may be more important than we realize at present. We still do not understand why it appears to lower the blood sugar in juvenile onset diabetes whereas it raises it in maturity onset diabetes, and we do not know to what extent, if any, its action may be through growth hormone inhibition, but the very presence of this short-lived hormone in the islets suggests that its role in diabetes is of considerable significance.

Gastro-intestinal hormones and the entero-insular axis

It has been shown that when glucose is given by mouth there is a rise in serum glucagon, but there is no such rise if it is given intravenously. This suggests that there is a hormonal link between the stomach and intestine on the one hand and the pancreatic islets on the other ('the entero-insular axis'). The part played by the gut in carbohydrate metabolism is less passive than once thought. Several hormones appear to be involved—gastro-intestinal polypeptide (GIP), vasoactive intestinal polypeptide (VIP), pancreozymin, secretin and probably others. At the same gastro-intestinal sites may be found somatostatin, glucagon and a substance with glucagon-like immunoreactivity (GLI) which is composed of molecules larger then glucagon and which may be a precursor of smaller polypeptides.

Pancreatic polypeptide (PP), coming from the F-cells of the islets, appears to have a further effect on digestion, possibly acting through the gall bladder. At present one has the impression that there are almost too many enzymes involved in the entero-insular axis and it is not surprising that their individual actions remain to be clarified. What is certain is that the entero-insular axis cannot be ignored in anything related to carbohydrate metabolism.

Insulin receptors

For insulin to be utilized by cells there must be appropriate receptors on the cell surface. The receptor is situated on the cell membrane and is specific for one hormone, in this case, insulin. Once formed, the receptor-hormone complex is 'internalized' into the cell, so the receptor may have further metabolic action. In theory, the receptor system may be upset outside, at or within the cell membrane. Insulin antibodies may create an insulin complex which is not taken up by the receptor. The receptor itself may be affected in three ways.

(1) Receptors may be defective in number, probably as a response to preceding hyperinsulinism as in obese maturity-onset diabetics. When over-eating stops hyperinsulinism disappears and the number of receptors returns to normal.

(2) The receptor may be 'deformed' as in excess glucocorticoid action. Resistance to steroid action in leukaemia is caused by normal cells being killed and replaced by a new group of lymphocytes with mutant receptors which do not accept steroid.
(3) Antibodies to receptors may appear. The most striking example is myasthenia gravis, where the great majority of patients have antibodies to acetylcholine receptors.

It will be seen that so far it has not been demonstrated that defective receptor activity plays a major role in childhood diabetes (though it may do so in some rare conditions, for example acanthosis nigricans). However, one cannot forecast what may be found in the future. The reader who wishes to go further into this complicated subject is referred to the papers of Flier, Kahn and Roth (1979) and Baxter and Funder (1979).

Catecholamines

The catecholamines are also regarded as insulin antagonists. The two main catecholamines, adrenaline and noradrenaline, come from the adrenal medulla. There is a marked species-variation in the ratio between the two. Humans produce 20 per cent noradrenaline, in which respect they fall between rabbits (4.5 per cent) and hens (80 per cent)*. The human fetus produces only noradrenaline. Catecholamines are quickly inactivated in the body into metanephrine and normetanephrine and are excreted in the urine as 3-methoxy-4-hydroxymandelic acid (VMA). The action of adrenaline in producing the 'fight or flight' reaction is now so well known that it has entered lay speech.

Adrenaline increases the blood sugar primarily by its effect in producing glycogenolysis in the liver and muscles, though it has indirect effects through growth hormone (see p. 146). Adrenaline also tends to produce lactate, a by-product of rapid glycogenolysis, and free fatty acids from fatty tissue. Noradrenaline is similar in action to adrenaline, but is more effective in raising the blood pressure and less effective in relaxing smooth muscle, so it is the hormone which produces the physical signs of anxiety.

There is a theoretical possibility that increased adrenaline, due to chronic anxiety, recurrent bouts of acute anxiety or a severely traumatic psychological experience could cause diabetes in a predisposed subject, and several clinical papers suggest that this has

* This fact is totally irrelevant to the present discussion, but a humbling thought is timely, particularly when it can lend sparkle to the dullest conversation.

happened at times. Of greater clinical importance are the observations of Baker *et al.* (1969) on the measurable production of catecholamines in diabetic patients subjected to nervous stress, which show that the catecholamines, though not necessarily involved in the onset of a given case of diabetes, can cause havoc in its clinical development. I do not think it possible to deal adequately with child diabetics without having this concept always in mind. The matter is considered in greater detail in the section on recurrent ketoacidosis (p. 176).

THE PRODUCTION OF KETOACIDOSIS IN DIABETES

It was said at the beginning of this chapter that the diabetic state and the fasting phase of carbohydrate metabolism had much in common, though it was added later that diabetes represents an unusual form of fasting, 'starvation in the midst of plenty'. With some knowledge of carbohydrate metabolism and the actions of insulin we can now consider the appearance of ketoacidosis in uncontrolled diabetes.

When insulin is deficient in quantity, or is being countered by antagonists or antibodies, the cells of the body are unable to take up and utilize glucose. The body responds to this by raising the blood glucose, as if trying to force glucose into the cell. The production of large quantities of glucose is made possible by an increase in the activity of certain quiescent mechanisms which also produce ketoacidosis more or less as a side effect.

Fat

Glycerol can be used by the liver as a substrate in producing gluconeogenesis. It is produced in adipose tissue along with free fatty acids (FFA) by the breakdown of tryglyceride under the influence of a lipase. The lipase is activated by catecholamines, glucagon and cortisol acting through cyclic adenosine monophosphate (cAMP) and is inhibited by insulin. Catecholamines, glucagon and cortisol are demonstrably high in ketoacidosis and insulin is lacking, so glycerol and FFA are produced *(Figure 7.3)*. Under normal conditions these substances would be re-esterified within the cell, but with the insulin lack re-esterification is inadequate. The net result is an increase in lipolysis and a resulting increase in glycerol and FFA.

Glycerol is conveyed to the liver and by conversion through phosphoglyceraldehyde to fructose-1,6-diphosphate enters the carbohydrate pathway as a source of gluconeogenesis. FFA are initially oxidized in the liver to produce acetyl coenzyme-A (AcCoA). This may be converted to acetoacetate in two ways;

(1) by condensation of two molecules of AcCoA, or
(2) through the 3-hydroxy-3-methyl glutaryl CoA pathway. This is probably the more important.

Acetoacetate in turn is reversibly convertible to beta-hydroxybutyric acid, the ratio between the two being determined by the ratio between NAD and NADH (nicotinamide-adenine dinucleotide and its reduced form). These ketone bodies enter the blood stream in excess. Ketones can be used as fuels but production exceeds utilization. Unfortunately ketone utilization depends on a high ketone level in the blood, so ketones are perhaps best regarded as undesirable by-products in the manufacture of glucose from fat.

In addition to entering the carbohydrate pathway glycerol may be carried to the liver and converted back to triglyceride particularly when the diabetic state improves. It has been suggested that this has produced the fatty liver found in some diabetics who, although not necessarily needing admission to hospital, have frequently developed a moderate degree of ketosis.

Protein

It is an important concept that body proteins are in a constant state of change. If a single amino acid with labelled nitrogen is fed to an animal several different amino acids containing the labelled nitrogen may soon after be recovered from the animal. There is thus a constant interchange of nitrogen atoms between amino acids, and the concept of 'dynamic equilibrium' in protein easily follows.

Insulin depresses gluconeogenesis (the formation of sugar from proteins) so where there is insulin lack gluconeogenesis is increased. In addition, cortisol, which is increased in severe diabetes, activates the relevant liver enzymes thereby increasing gluconeogenesis.

The basis of gluconeogenesis is that amino acids shed their NH_2 ions, leaving behind a carbon structure which can be converted to glucose. This process is complicated. The amino acids lose their NH_2 groups by deamination or transamination. The nitrogen-free moieties are then easily converted to substances involved in the tricarboxylic acid cycle, entering it at different points *(Figure 7.6)*.

The cycle is unidirectional and the products of amino acid breakdown pass round the cycle till they reach oxaloacetate, where they leave the cycle as phosphoenol pyruvate which is on the carbohydrate pathway. It will be noted that three of the amino acids

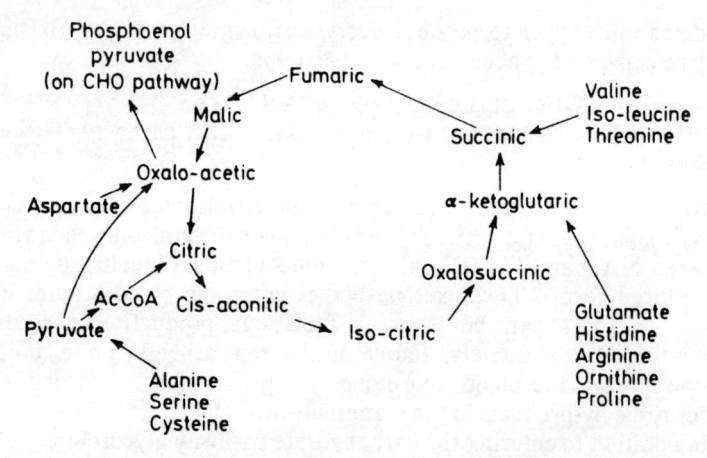

Figure 7.6. Amino acids and the tricarboxylic acid cycle, also known as the citrate cycle and the Krebs cycle

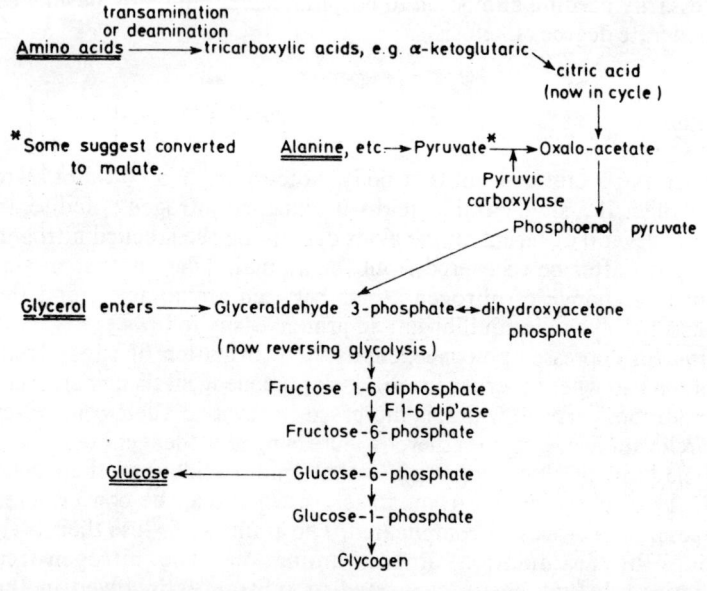

Figure 7.7. Gluconeogenesis and the utilization of glycerol

Enzymes controlling gluconeogenesis are:
(1) Fructose diphosphatase inhibited by fructose diphosphate and high intracellular AMP
(2) Pyruvate carboxylase stimulated by acetyl coenzyme-A. Thus ketosis can stimulate gluconeogenesis
(3) Activity of enzymes involved in converting small molecules to glucose

(alanine, serine, cysteine) are converted to pyruvate which is also on the carbohydrate pathway *(Figure 7.7)*. The reaction phosphoenol pyruvate to pyruvate is not easily reversible, and is reversed indirectly through oxalo-acetate with the assistance of adenosine triphosphate. The pathway to glucose is now clear. Most of the NH_2 ions are converted to urea in the liver, which raises the blood urea, but some are salvaged to take part in the making of new amino acids by means of the alanine cycle *(Figure 7.2)*.

Causes and effects of ketoacidosis

With these biochemical considerations in mind it is now possible to link the causes and clinical manifestations of ketoacidosis together in a simplified form as a diagram *(Figure 7.8)*.

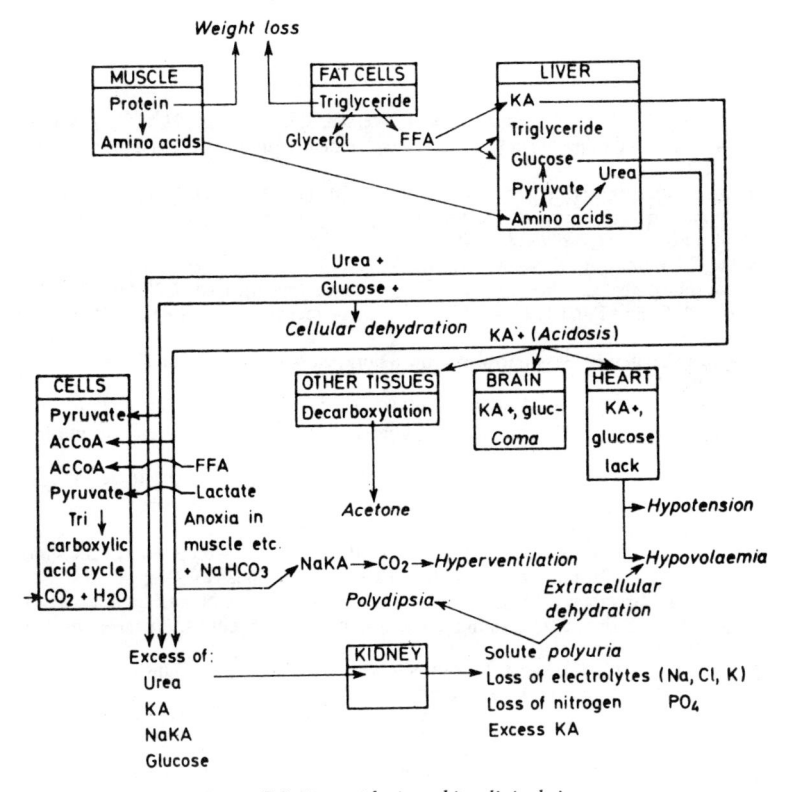

Figure 7.8. Ketoacidosis and its clinical signs

Notes on Figure 7.8

(1) Gluconeogenesis also takes place in the kidney. This has not been shown, in the interests of simplicity.
(2) Acetone is formed from acetoacetate only. Beta-hydroxybutyric acid is not strictly speaking a ketone, though usually referred to as such.
(3) Urea is formed solely in the liver.
(4) The three ketogenic amino acids (leucine, phenylalanine and tyrosine) are omitted. They increase the KA load.

In the next chapter, ketoacidosis will be considered as a clinical entity.

REFERENCES

Alberti, K. G. M. M., Christensen, N. J., Iversen, J. and Orskov, H. (1975). Role of glucagon and other hormones in the development of diabetic ketoacidosis. *Lancet*, **I,** 1307

Baird, Joyce, Hunter, W. M. and Smith, W. M. (1973). The relationship between human growth hormone and the development of diabetes mellitus and its complications. *Postgrad. med. J.*, **48,** 132

Baker, L., Barcai, A., Kaye, R. and Haque, N. (1969). Beta-adrenergic blockade and juvenile diabetes: acute studies and long-term therapeutic trial. *J. Pediat.*, **75,** 19

Baxter, J. D. and Funder, J. W. (1979). Hormone receptors. *New Engl. J. Med.*, **301,** 1149

Blackard, W. G. (1973). Control of growth hormone secretion in man. *Postgrad. med. J.*, **48,** 122

Bloom, S. R. (1973). Glucagon, a stress hormone, *Postgrad. med. J.*, **49,** 607

Buchanan, K. D. (1973). Pancreatic glucagon in diabetes mellitus and chronic pancreatitis. *Postgrad. med. J.*, **49,** 604

Chiumelli, G., Del Guercio, M. J., Carnelutti, M., Devetta, M., Rossi, L. and Caccamo, A. (1971). The role of growth hormone in the pathogenesis of diabetes mellitus in childhood. *J. Pediat.*, **79,** 768

Flier, J. S., Kahn, C. R. and Roth, J. (1979). Receptors, anti-receptor antibodies and mechanisms of insulin resistance. *New Engl. J. Med.*, **300,** 413

Frost, D. P., Srivastava, M. C., Jones, R. H., Nabarro, J. D. N. and Sonksen, P. H. (1973). The kinetics of insulin metabolism in diabetes mellitus. *Postgrad. med. J.* **49,** 949

Horwitz, D. L., Rubinstein, A. H. and Steiner, D. F. (1978). Proinsulin and C-peptide in diabetes. *Med. Clin. N. Am.*, **62,** 723

Ludvigsson, J. and Heding, L. G. (1977). C-peptide in juvenile diabetes. *Acta paediat. Scand.*, Suppl. 270, 53

Raskin, P. and Unger, R. H. (1978). Glucagon and diabetes. *Med. Clin. N. Am.*, **62,** 713

Rizza, R. A. and Gerich, J. E. (1978). Somatostatin and diabetes. *Med. Clin. N. Am.*, **62,** 735

Samols, E., Marri, G. and Marks, V. (1965). Promotion of insulin secretion by glucagon. *Lancet,* **II,** 415

Sönksen, P. H. and West, T. E. T. (1978). Carbohydrate metabolism and diabetes. In *Recent Advances in Endocrinology and Metabolism.* Ed. J. L. H. O'Riordan. Edinburgh; Churchill-Livingstone.

Thomas, J. H. (1973). The role of 'insulinase' in the degradation of insulin. *Postgrad. med. J.*, **49,** 940

Unger, R. H. and Eisentraut, A. (1964). Studies of the physiologic role of glucagon. *Diabetes*, **13,** 563

CHAPTER 8

Ketoacidosis, Pre-Coma and Coma

Ketoacidotic coma is difficult to define accurately, particularly if one tries to link it with the clinical state. Hockaday and Alberti (1972) found that the main indications of a poor prognosis in adults were low blood pressure, the age of the patient and the depth of the coma. The degree of coma was not related directly to the biochemistry. However, in describing various types of coma it is helpful to include certain objective biochemical standards, and Hockaday and Alberti suggested two: a serum bicarbonate of less than 9 mmol/l (60 mg per cent) or ketone bodies (acetoacetate and 3-hydroxybutyrate) of over 3 mmol/l (54 mg per cent) as standards of severity.

The various chemical states, excluding hypoglycaemia, which may lead on to diabetic coma can be classified as follows:

(1) *Ketoacidotic coma* with hyperglycaemia, ketone bodies over 3 mmol/l (54 mg per cent) and a reduced pH is the common form. Perhaps best classed as a variant of this is: *Euglycaemic diabetic ketoacidosis* (Munro et al., 1973) in which the blood sugar may be normal or more commonly slightly raised; less than 16.7 mmol/l (300 mg per cent).

(2) *Non-ketotic diabetic coma*
  (a) *Hyperosmolar and hyperglycaemic* with ketone bodies less than 3 mmol/l (54 mg per cent) and osmolality over 300 mmol/l. 'Non-ketotic' is perhaps a misnomer in that a slight excess of ketones may be present. The level of ketones is the main distinction between this form and ketoacidotic coma, although the blood sugar is usually higher than in ketoacidotic coma.
  (b) *Hyperglycaemic, non-ketotic, non-hyperosmolar coma* is

rare. There is little increase in osmolality as sodium is low and uraemia mild.
(3) *Diabetic lactic acidosis*. The criterion of diagnosis is a blood lactate of 7 mmol/l (126 mg per cent) or more. If ketoacidosis is also present it is classified as ketoacidotic coma. If ketoacidosis is slight but associated with a low pH, lactic acidosis should be suspected.
(4) In *diabetic uraemic coma* there is acidosis and a blood urea of over 33 mmol/l (200 mg per cent). Hyperglycaemia, if present, is moderate, and so is ketoacidosis. There is no lactic acidosis or hyperosmolality.

CLINICAL KETOACIDOSIS

The biochemistry of ketoacidosis was discussed in the previous chapter, but the clinical aspects are discussed here.

Diagnosis

Diabetic ketoacidosis should be regarded as a medical emergency. If a diagnosis of diabetes has not been made previously and the child is left untreated, he will die. The most important signs are: dehydration, with loss of skin turgor and sunken eyes; hyperventilation, with acetone on the breath; peripheral vasodilation and flushing; drowsiness, pre-coma or coma; and subsidiary signs are abdominal pain and possibly distension; muscular weakness; a feeling of coldness; and possibly hypothermia or hyperthermia.

Non-diabetic ketoacidosis (for example, aspirin poisoning) has been discussed in the first chapter, where the importance of taking a history of urinary function as a guide to diagnosis was stressed. All diabetics have had polyuria. Certain snags in diagnosing ketoacidosis remain.

A *weak positive reaction* to Ketostix does not exclude ketoacidosis. Ketostix reacts with acetone and acetoacetate but not with 3-hydroxybutyrate. The ratio between acetoacetate and 3-hydroxybutyrate is normally 1:2, but in ketoacidosis it becomes 1:4 and sometimes higher. This high 3-hydroxybutyrate is not detected by Ketostix, and acetone itself, which is picked up by Ketostix, does not produce ketoacidosis; so Ketostix is not a completely reliable guide and marked ketoacidosis may show only a weak reaction to Ketostix. If the pH of the blood confirms the response to Ketostix no further action need be taken, but if the drop in pH is marked and the

Ketostix result is weak or moderate it is advisable to have the lactic acid and 3-hydroxybutyrate levels measured in the laboratory. It is also possible to have ketoacidosis present with a negative urinary response to Ketostix, presumably due to defective kidney function.

Piqûre diabetes was originally named because it was first demonstrated by experimental puncturing, but it can be produced by various lesions irritating the hindbrain, for example head injury or subarachnoid haemorrhage. It is characterized by varying muscle tone, irregular respiration and possibly rapid alterations in pupil size, and non-ketotic hyperosmolar diabetes may imitate it to a certain extent, as may ketoacidosis at times while under treatment. If a known diabetic suffered a severe head injury, confusion could lead to ignoring the head injury. The findings are essentially those of head injury+hyperglycaemia, and the history should give the initial clue. There is nothing to be lost in examining the skull in 'diabetic coma'.

Hypoglycaemia may be mistaken for ketoacidosis in a known diabetic, possibly with disastrous results if larger doses of insulin are given, but it takes a great effort of the imagination to diagnose ketoacidosis as hypoglycaemia, which shows characteristic pallor and sweating.

Suicide attempts are not unknown among teenage diabetics and, although I have never seen it happen, a suicide attempt with aspirin could obviously set a diagnostic poser. The initial treatment with intravenous fluid and possibly bicarbonate would be similar for both conditions, and there might be a suggestive, though not diagnostic, history of sudden onset after aspirin ingestion.

The causes of ketoacidosis

The ways in which ketoacidosis may arise during the treatment of a known diabetic are many.

(1) *Diet-breaking* is frequently regarded as a cause of diabetic ketoacidosis but, if one takes 'diet-breaking' in the popular sense of occasionally eating illicit sweets, I doubt if it is an important one. It is true that sweets are high in carbohydrate, higher than many perhaps imagine. The typical bar of chocolate or similar confectionery may contain 40–50 g of carbohydrate, enough for a major meal. It would certainly cause hyperglycaemia, but the average diet-breaker breaks his diet in minor well-spaced episodes and a rise in insulin can well forestall ketoacidosis. If, however, 'diet-breaking' is taken to mean a complete failure to adhere to a diet, that is a different matter altogether; but when that happens it

is usually accompanied by inaccurate urine testing and the abuse of insulin, and I would regard it as 'collapse of management' rather than simple diet-breaking.

(2) *Failure in insulin administration* seems more important. The child who consistently injects into a fatty tumour, the child who has falsified urine results and so is taking too little insulin, the parent too irresponsible to check that insulin is given correctly, they all may cause ketoacidosis. These faults may be very difficult to track down. A child may be admitted to hospital out of control and in ketoacidosis on a theoretical 40 units of insulin a day, and may be discharged a week later balanced on 20 units a day. That he was admitted in relative insulin lack there is no doubt, but the lack was not in the prescribed dose. When he goes home, his insulin dosage and ketosis may drift up again. It is disturbing to me how many parents seem to regard this situation with equanimity and never feel inclined to investigate it on their own. Perhaps they are unwilling to face what they think they may find. There is a longer description of lines of investigation in Chapter 6.

(3) *Infection* is certainly a common cause of diabetic ketoacidosis, but it may not be present quite as often as it is diagnosed. 'It was probably just some upper respiratory viral thing' may be said when there are no respiratory symptoms and the ESR, temperature and blood picture are normal. If the physician's conscience lets him take this way out, so much the easier for him. He will be saved weary searching for some social or psychological factor as a cause. However, infection frequently does lead to loss of diabetic control, and children frequently get infections. A febrile enteric infection such as dysentery where there is rapid fluid loss from the body may be particularly difficult to manage, and the difficulty may be compounded by the well- meaning nurse or practitioner who advises withholding insulin as the patient is not eating. The rule for such cases is 'follow the urine sugar', a rule which must be clearly impressed on the parents. I write it down, I underline it, I jab my ball point through the page and sometimes I rap hard objects on the desk, but still insulin is withheld in the presence of febrile infection. This is most likely to happen if there is a long interval between leaving hospital and the first infection which gives the parents time to forget. It is true that most infections, which are minor febrile respiratory infections, can be dealt with at home. On the other hand, a child with diarrhoea and fever should be admitted to hospital as he can deteriorate very rapidly.

(4) *Prolonged vomiting*, with or without obvious infection is a reason for readmission.

(5) *Nervous stress* may precipitate ketoacidosis. Nervous stress is difficult to eradicate, so one can go further and say that nervous stress may cause *recurrent* attacks of ketoacidosis. This is almost a clinical entity on its own, and is given a separate section later in this chapter.

THE TREATMENT OF KETOACIDOSIS

'The treatment of diabetic coma is based on the triad of intravenous fluid, insulin and gastric lavage.' So I was taught as a medical student and the advice is good, for it reminds one of the importance of gastric lavage, of which more later.

FLUIDS

The type of fluid to be given

One need not stress the importance of intravenous fluids. When blood volume has been restored one can be sure that insulin will be absorbed, that the kidneys can work normally and that metabolic improvement will be transmitted to the tissues throughout the body.

In diabetic ketoacidosis the brain cells have a high content of sugars. Their osmolality is further increased when insulin is given, as Na^+ and K^+ enter the cells. It is therefore argued that isotonic solutions should be given intravenously, not hypotonic solutions which could cause cerebral oedema. It has been noted clinically that cerebral oedema does not occur above a blood glucose level of 13.9 mmol/l (250 mg per cent). Cerebral oedema is thus a complication of the correction of ketoacidosis.

Cerebral oedema causes death and treatment is ineffective. It usually occurs about four or five hours after beginning intravenous therapy but it has been observed as late as 16 hours. All seems to be going well and consciousness is improving when the child suddenly lapses back into coma and dies within minutes rather than hours. In treating diabetic ketoacidosis in children one thought should be paramount in the physician's mind—avoid cerebral oedema.

It is quite likely that all cases of diabetic ketoacidosis on intravenous therapy suffer a degree of cerebral oedema; one investigation showed a steady increase in CSF pressure in the first hours of treatment in *all* patients, despite outwardly satisfactory clinical progress. The degree to which a disturbance of the polyol pathway is involved, producing a rise of sorbitol in the brain, is not certain but it may not be as important as once thought.

In deciding the type of infusion fluid to be used two factors have to be balanced. Normal saline may contribute to hypernatraemia and hypotonic saline is more likely to cause cerebral oedema. Some, as the result of intricate metabolic calculations, have recommended giving half-normal saline as a routine (though this was to be accompanied by a relatively high intake of sodium bicarbonate) and stray remarks scattered through the literature indicate that half-normal saline is the routine in some clinics. Again, paediatricians may be afraid of hypernatraemia which they tend to equate with hypernatraemic dehydration of infants and its serious complications. My own opinions have tended to vacillate through the years as various cases have seemed to suggest now one thing, now the other (*see* p. 184), but I have finally settled for normal saline. I do not now believe that hypernatraemia is the bogey it is made out to be; and I would add that, as even low-dose insulin therapy can lead to a very rapid fall in osmolality in the first two hours of therapy, maintaining the sodium level is a buffer against cerebral oedema, probably even in the treatment of hyperosmolar coma.

When the blood glucose has fallen below 14 mmol/l (250 mg per cent) glucose should be added to the intravenous fluid and I favour half-strength saline with 5 per cent glucose. This solution is slightly hypertonic at the moment it enters the body but this does not seem important as the glucose is soon utilized, losing its osmolar effect. The figure '14 mmol/l' should be used only as a guide, for example if a report is received that half an hour earlier the blood sugar was at 15 or 16 mmol/l and was falling, and further insulin had already been given, then sugar should be introduced into the intravenous fluid at that point. The blood sugar should be monitored and bolus injections of glucose can be given to prevent too rapid a fall in blood sugar, although that expedient is very seldom necessary.

Quantity of fluid

Complicated methods of calculating fluid requirements from theoretical electrolyte loss do exist, but simpler methods are just as effective. One method has been concisely tabulated by Farquhar (1973) as shown in *Table 8.1*.

A child in prolonged severe ketoacidosis may lose up to 10 per cent of his body fluid, the maximum loss consistent with maintaining life. Any greater loss in weight is due to wasting of solid tissues. In practice, as part of the fail-safe regime, I now suggest allowing for a

TABLE 8.1
Quantities of intravenous fluid to be given at various ages

Age (years)	Weight (kg)	10 per cent dehydration	Fluid/kg maintenance	Total maintenance	Total volume	First hour	Hourly thereafter
1	10	1000	120	1200	2200	200	85
5	18	1800	100	1800	3600	360	140
10	30	3000	75	2250	5250	600	200
15	50	5000	50	2500	7500	1000	280

Fluid allowances in ml

(From Farquhar, 1973, by permission of the publisher)

(1) Do not use this table without reference to the text.
(2) The table implies that the same amount of fluid is given in each hour after the first. I do not use precisely this regime *(see text)*.

5 per cent loss of fluid at the most. I have seen two cases of cerebral oedema in which the instruction 'up to 10 per cent' was taken to mean '10 per cent for all' which can produce drastic results in a child who is only moderately dehydrated, particularly if hypotonic fluid is used. It is also advisable to stress that the paediatrician who sets up drips more often on babies than on bigger children must remember that the infant figure of 120–150 ml/kg/day for maintenance does not hold throughout childhood.

The oft-quoted instruction 'Do not give more than 20 ml/kg in the first hour' is certainly true, indeed possibly over-generous. If 20 ml/kg *has* been given in the first hour the rate of flow should be decreased very markedly in the second. I suggest two other rules.

(1) Having estimated the 24-hour requirement, cut it by at least 25 per cent to protect against cerebral oedema. Furthermore, any 'squaring off' of figures should be downwards rather than upwards in the first few hours. I am a cautious therapist, preferring to nudge the patient towards recovery rather than seeking to cure him out of hand, because heroics may go too far and leave the patient worse off than before. If you kill your patient at the start your chances of a subsequent cure are nil.

(2) Having decided on the total amount of fluid to give, I then give one-third equally spread through the first four hours, one-third in the second eight hours and one-third in the last 12 hours. Should 'extra' fluids be given (for example intravenous plasma or oral fluids) they are subtracted from the total.

An example follows:

The case of a boy aged ten years, weight 30 kg approximately.

Maintenance: 30 kg×75 ml/kg/day   = 2250 ml
Replacement: 5 per cent of 30 kg=1.5 kg   = 1500 ml
                                  Total   = 3750 ml

To avoid cerebral oedema use 75 per cent of total=2813 ml, call it 2800 ml.

Fluid spread during day as follows:
 One-third in first four hours   = 900 ml or 225 ml/hour
 One-third in next eight hours   = 110 ml/hour
 One-third in next 12 hours   = 75 ml/hour

Note that assuming 10 per cent weight loss rather than 5 per cent would have raised the first total by 1500 ml.

Other writers suggest an initial flow rate rather faster than that suggested in *Table 8.1*, for example 500 ml in the first hour for children aged 2–5 years (Moseley, 1975). I think it prudent to use the slower rate. There is a therapeutic dilemma here. The child to whom one would like to give a rapid infusion because of hypovolaemia and hypotension is also the child whose heart is most likely to succumb to overloading. In such a situation, mercifully rare, where the systolic blood pressure might be down to 60 mmHg, the extremities cold and oliguria present, one could consider giving dextrans of relatively low molecular weight (for example Dextraven 110 in saline, possibly diluted to reduce the salt content though this, indeed, I have never used). Whole blood or plasma could be used instead. If hypotension is marked one should also consider the possibility of a serious undiagnosed infection, such as septicaemia. One should also be careful about giving potassium supplements in the presence of hypotension, because if hypotension is not responding to intravenous therapy the cells may continue to lose potassium to the blood, even after insulin is given, and adding potassium to an already high serum potassium could be lethal. Admittedly, in this situation the prognosis is poor at the best of times.

Oral fluids

Oral fluids may be given as soon as the child shows an inclination to take them. They may be offered without being pressed from about four hours after the setting-up of the drip, depending on the level of consciousness. They should be given in 10 ml quantities at first. It may well be more than 12 hours before the child is ready to drink but he is usually drinking within 24 hours, and it is therefore seldom that the first day's fluid requirements will all be given intravenously. The amount taken by mouth is deducted from the calculated requirements and the drip-rate slowed accordingly. Even when the total requirements are being taken by mouth, it is advisable to leave the drip in the vein running just quickly enough to keep it open until one is satisfied that the child is retaining his oral fluid. Vomiting occasionally recurs if the stomach has not been washed out, and this may radically upset one's calculations.

The giving of oral fluids is likely to be followed within a few hours by a change to the subcutaneous route for insulin, and certainly within the first 24 hours one would hope to be giving the child's carbohydrate requirements (*see* p. 39) by mouth. This will involve converting from water to milk and sugar. Two hundred ml of milk contain 10 g of lactose, to which can be addded 10–20 g of glucose, depending on the age of the child. If this is given four-hourly, a range of 120–180 g of carbohydrate per 24 hours is available and could be begun as smaller quantities given more often. Children seem to find this acceptable. An alert child who is unwilling to drink may have been slightly overhydrated intravenously, and may drink if the drip rate is reduced. The giving of oral fluids is a virtual guarantee against overloading the circulation. During the second day it should be possible to introduce more solid starchy food.

INSULIN

Until very recent years it was accepted that a child in diabetic pre-coma should be given, as an initial dose, 2 units of soluble insulin per kg of body weight, half being given intravenously and half intramuscularly. For a ten-year-old weighing 30 kg the dose would then be 30 units intramuscularly and 30 units intravenously, and if a student did not say something close to this in an examination he was in danger of being failed. Now one might be in danger of being failed if one said anything remotely like it. The reader may here impose on himself a two-minute silence to ponder on the mutability of medical laws.

A change in ideas about insulin dosage has come from the recognition of certain facts:

(1) Insulin exerts its optimal effect at a blood level of 20–200 μunits/ml (Sönksen *et al.*, 1972). When all insulin receptors are saturated extra insulin is no help.
(2) The half-life of insulin given intravenously is four to five minutes, of intramuscular insulin about two hours.
(3) A large intravenous dose of insulin will give a rapid fall in blood sugar, possibly to hypoglycaemic levels, or to moderate levels sufficient to produce symptoms of hypoglycaemia if the fall in blood sugar is very fast, but this effect wears off very soon. Even if large doses of intravenous insulin are given hourly, there will be periods during each hour when the insulin activity is both too great and too little, because of the very short half-life of insulin.

It is of considerable interest that in 1932 Priscilla White advocated treating diabetic coma with small doses of insulin given *half-hourly*. More recently Sönksen again advocated the treatment of pre-coma with repeated small doses of insulin; Alberti, Hockaday and Turner (1973) elaborated the intramuscular treatment; and Moseley (1975) described the application of the method to children. The rationale of the method is that small hourly doses of insulin given intramuscularly will, after about two hours, keep the blood insulin within the range of maximal therapeutic effect without sudden fluctuations, and thus lead to a steady fall in blood glucose. In practice, this worked out so well that the blood glucose level could be forecast some four hours ahead with a good degree of accuracy.

The rate of fall after the first two hours was about 90 mg (5 mmol) per hour, infection being the only factor to interfere with this to any great extent. In particular, previous treatment with insulin had no adverse effect, as it might have been expected to do by having produced insulin antibodies. Another remarkable feature is that small doses of insulin appear to be active during ketosis, apparently belying the belief that ketosis is a cause of insulin resistance. Growth hormone rises less than with conventional therapy and lactate falls from the start of treatment, instead of showing an initial rise. The initial dose of soluble insulin is 0.25 units/kg body weight intramuscularly, then 0.1 units/kg hourly. Five to ten doses usually bring the blood sugar below 16.6 mmol/l (300 mg per cent).

The method seemed simple and effective, and fitted in with a clinical impression that high doses of insulin were not particularly beneficial in childhood.

> Our first fumbling approach to the new method was with a girl of ten years, a new patient. She had a three-week history of thirst, polyuria and nocturia, proceeding to lethargy, headache, coldness and shivering. Aspirin was given on her practitioner's advice. When seen by him two days later she was severely dehydrated. Diabetes was then suspected but could not be confirmed in her home as she was anuric. On admission she was severely dehydrated and a chest x-ray showed microcardia. The blood pressure was 90/60 and the heart rate was 150 per minute. Overbreathing was marked. There was tenderness in the right hypochondrium. Further investigations and treatment are shown in *Table 8.2*.

This table calls for a number of comments.

(1) We were still wary of omitting intravenous insulin. The timing of intramuscular insulin was irregular, as a busy receiving day was interfering with a precise timetable. It has since been realized that it is perfectly safe to write up the first four doses at the outset, so that the sister or nurse can give the insulin if the doctor is delayed. Even so, the irregular timing, which resulted in intramuscular insulin being given about every one and a half hours, did not seem to interfere with the child's progress.
(2) The fluid given was half-strength saline and no sodium bicarbonate was added (*see below*). Even so, there was a slight rise in serum sodium. The rise in pH without bicarbonate should be noted.
(3) The quantity of fluid given in four hours was not great. Nevertheless the child passed urine one and a half hours after the drip was begun.
(4) Considering the child's state on admission it was surprising to

find her asking for, and retaining, oral fluids three-and-a-half hours after treatment began.
(5) Potassium (*see below*) was at first withheld because of anuria, a normal T-wave on the ECG and (as was known soon after) a slightly high potassium in the blood. A small amount (0.5 g potassium chloride) was given when the child had passed urine and the serum potassium had fallen slightly. As far as it went, this course of affairs supported the claim that the new method tended to normalize potassium rather than drive it down, although Alberti *et al.* had given potassium supplements.

TABLE 8.2

Progress of a case of ketoacidosis

Time (hours)	Insulin (units)	Blood glucose	Biochemistry (mmol/l)	Remarks
0	10 i.v.	920 mg (51 mmol)	Na 141, K 5.2, urea 14, bicarb. 8.5, pH 7.12, base deficit 21 Calculated osmolality 358	Very ill
¾	6 i.m.			
1¾	4 i.m.			Passed urine, 150 ml
2		660	Na 145, K 4.4, urea 15, bicarb. 9.5, pH 7.27, base deficit 19, Calculated osmolality 341	Hyperpnoea less
3¼	4 i.m.			
4				Total i.v. 975, 150 ml orally, asked for
4½	6 i.m.			
6¼	6 i.m.			
7½	6 i.m.			Oral fluids continued. Hyperpnoea gone
9	6 i.m.			
12	20 s.c.	290		Total i.v. 1580 ml, oral 1100 ml

(6) Biochemistry was not repeated after the second specimen as the child was obviously improving and it was by then out of normal laboratory working hours.

(7) A summary of present practice (Moseley) will be given shortly.

Initial qualms about giving repeated injections to a child quickly died away. The precomatose child does not seem to remember this as a traumatic period.

Intravenous insulin

The use of a steady infusion of intravenous insulin has more recently been advocated, and certainly appears effective. There were early reservations about such therapy as insulin tended to be absorbed on the walls of the apparatus unless combined with human albumin, a costly and complicated business. Page *et al.* (1974) made up 24 units of soluble insulin to 20 ml in a plastic syringe which was fitted to a mechanical pump for slow infusion. This relatively strong solution loses little by absorption, and is renewed every four hours, the rate being 6 units per hour for adults. This has the advantages of keeping the insulin concentration in the blood even more constant than that obtained by hourly intramuscular injections and of allowing the insulin supply to be stopped instantly, but has the disadvantage of employing extra expensive equipment. The more complicated the apparatus used, the greater is the chance of something going wrong. Present experience suggests that both hourly intramuscular injection and continuous intravenous infusion of insulin are effective.

ELECTROLYTE THERAPY

Sodium bicarbonate

The use of intravenous sodium bicarbonate to correct acidosis has been a matter of debate, with opinion now swinging to the view that too much bicarbonate has been given in the past. When dehydration has been corrected and insulin therapy begun the kidneys are able to help in correcting the acidosis.

The debate on bicarbonate has been well summarized by Kaye (1975). The arguments against giving bicarbonate are:

(1) There will be impairment of oxygen supply to the tissues as the dissociation of oxygen from haemoglobin decreases as pH rises. This would be particularly important in hypovolaemia.

(2) A self-regulating mechanism comes into action as soon as insulin is given. Glucose is utilized, and the ketoacids are now oxidized in the citric acid cycle to produce carbon dioxide, with an increase in endogenous bicarbonate.
(3) A relative acidosis remains in the brain cells as the blood pH rises, creating a pH gradient. This mechanism merits further comment. Cessation of hyperventilation leads to retention of carbon dioxide, which easily crosses the blood–brain barrier, thus tending to increase acidosis in the CSF, which mirrors the pH in the brain cells. Consciousness is more closely related to the pH of the CSF than the pH of the blood. Bicarbonate does not cross the blood–brain barrier as readily as carbon dioxide, and so tends to alkalinize the blood. Stopping hyperventilation quickly could thus cause a harmful pH gradient between blood and CSF.

The arguments in favour of giving bicarbonate are:

(1) The respiratory centre is not mechanically perfect. Hyperventilation is most effective between pH 7.1 and 7.2. Below pH 7.1 the minute volume of air to the lungs decreases. Correction up to pH 7.2 therefore hardly affects (3) above.
(2) A low pH adversely affects
　(a) the respiratory centre
　(b) myocardial contractility
　(c) cardiac rhythm (producing arrhythmias).

The balance of evidence therefore suggests that bicarbonate should be given below a pH of 7.1, but carefully, in small quantities.

A formula, potentially lethal, which may lurk in the heads of paediatricians is that the number of mEq of sodium bicarbonate to be given is the base deficit × weight in kg × 0.3 which is now accepted as giving an answer about 100 per cent too high. As the base deficit in severe ketoacidosis is commonly 22 or greater, i.e. off the Astrup scale, the dose often works out as 7 mEq/kg (1 mEq is contained in 1 ml of 8.4 per cent sodium bicarbonate). It was the custom to give half to three-quarters of the calculated dose in the first three to six hours of treatment. Even so, an initial dose of 3.5mEq/kg would now be considered high. Alberti *et al.* now use the pH as an indicator of the need for alkaline therapy. If the pH is less than 7.1 they give 50 mmol (50 mEq) to an adult, repeating 30 minutes later, a total of approximately 1.5 mmol/kg. Any further therapy depends on monitoring. If the pH was below 7.0 the initial dose was 125 mmol, repeated as above, and giving a total of about 3.5 mmol/kg. My practice in children is to give less, e.g. 0.5 mmol/kg repeated in an hour if pH is under 7.1, 0.75 mmol/kg for those with a pH of less than 7.0. Further doses may be given after monitoring, but are seldom necesssary.

Potassium

An easily remembered blanket rule for giving potassium is to add 1 g of potassium chloride to the first bottle of intravenous fluid. This automatically means that the smaller the child the more slowly he gets his potassium. Until recently potassium was given unless:

(1) there was anuria, or
(2) ECG monitoring suggested the existing potassium level was very high, or
(3) hypotension was failing to respond to treatment, in which case serum potassium may continue to rise spontaneously from further diffusion from the cells.

There was a tendency for potassium to fall dramatically with treatment (i.e. with correction of acidosis), particularly if sodium bicarbonate was given, and adding potassium to the infusion fluid was designed to prevent this. The rule was that it was obligatory to supply potassium if sodium bicarbonate was given.

The hourly intramuscular insulin method has cast some doubt on the absolute value of some of these rules. Alberti *et al.* comment that the regime tends to edge the potassium towards normal, high levels falling and low levels rising, but not with the speed seen when using the older insulin schedule. From our experience this seems to be true and we would now only give potassium at the outset if we knew the level to be so low as to put the heart at risk; and children stand low levels of potassium well. Thereafter, potassium would be given if the serum potassium fell below 3 mEq/l.

GASTRIC LAVAGE

This should be carried out early in treatment, as soon as the drip is running and insulin has been given. A stomach tube is not necessary: a nasogastric tube of the largest convenient bore is satisfactory. Lavage is carried out with warm tap water.

Lavage is of particular value if the child has been vomiting, because otherwise he may vomit again when oral fluids are introduced. Ketoacidosis may cause dilatation of the stomach and sometimes bleeding from a hyperaemic mucosa. All that need be

SOME OTHER CONSIDERATIONS

written about gastric lavage can be written in a small space, but that is no reason for underrating its importance.

SOME OTHER CONSIDERATIONS

Fructose and phosphate

If fructose is given to ketoacidotic patients the ketones fall and the glucose rises. Clinically, however, there seems to be no benefit and there is potential for harm. Pyruvate, lactate and uric acid rise and acidosis is increased. Phosphate and ATP are lowered. Fructose has fallen out of fashion, the real answer to the problem being the adequate administration of insulin. The giving of phosphate is also out of fashion, though there is a loss of inorganic phosphate in ketoacidosis.

Treatment on a shoestring

The above summary of the treatment of ketoacidosis should not deter those called upon to treat ketoacidosis at the back of beyond with minimal equipment. The essentials are physiological saline, a drip set and a supply of soluble insulin, and a few Dextrostix would be a help.

Few children will become hypernatraemic if normal saline is used in the amounts previously suggested. Most will get on perfectly well without sodium bicarbonate or potassium supplements. The hourly intramuscular use of small doses of insulin makes one much less dependent on laboratory help than did the previous large-dose intravenous and intramuscular regime, the fall in blood sugar being steady. Hypoglycaemia can be detected by Dextrostix or clinical observation, or prevented by switching to subcutaneous insulin as soon as the child is moderately alert. If transfer to hospital is going to take four or five hours, it would be well worth the delay of initiating this simple regime before starting the child on his journey. It is true that some patients would die, but some patients die in hospital also.

Monitoring

Reference has been made to the 'monitoring' of progress. This is done biochemically and clinically. The frequency of monitoring the biochemistry will depend on the severity of the case, but might be done hourly at first in those who are severely ill. It is desirable to know the blood sugar, sodium, potassium, urea and standard bicarbonate and, from the Astrup apparatus, the pH and base deficit. It is useful in the very serious cases to know the arterial pO_2. If this is less than 80 mmHg, oxygen should be given, but if it cannot be estimated in a child it is worth giving oxygen in the presence of severe acidosis and hypotension, where tissue anoxia and increasing lactic acidosis are potential risks.

Whereas clinical and biochemical monitoring will usually go hand in hand there are times when they diverge. If a child's state of consciousness is improving he is getting better, even though the biochemistry shows little change. Where there is clinical improvement there should be no heroic change in treatment. On the other hand, if a child remains unconscious after a few hours of treatment one should suspect that a full diagnosis has not been reached, even though the biochemistry shows some improvement. Has he, for example, a severe infection such as septicaemia, or even meningitis?

Acetone in the urine is not a reliable guide to ketoacidosis. It is fat soluble, and its excretion may continue from transient depots in body fat after true ketoacidosis has been corrected.

RECURRENT KETOACIDOSIS

This state is sufficiently common to be regarded as a clinical entity. A child may be admitted to hospital every month for six months, each time in ketoacidosis. He, or more probably she, may have kept clear of hospitals for years before then, and may do so for years thereafter. The state is seen most often in pre-pubertal girls but may occur in either sex at any age. The problem is best illustrated by a case history.

A girl of 11 years and two months was first admitted in March, 1973 with a typical history of polyuria and polydipsia for three weeks, leading on to lethargy and abdominal pain. At her first admission she seemed reasonably controlled on one injection of Lente insulin, and when she was discharged it was hoped that she might enter a short remission period before needing the twice daily injections which her age suggested. Her diabetic control was poor from the beginning, although it could have been called a remission by her own standards in that she stayed out of hospital for ten weeks, which was to prove a record for the next six months. Her admissions and changes of insulin, are shown in *Figure 8.1*. She might have been admitted more often, but strenuous efforts were made to keep her at home by frequent use of the telephone and by giving extra glucose and extra insulin injections which were often moderately successful in

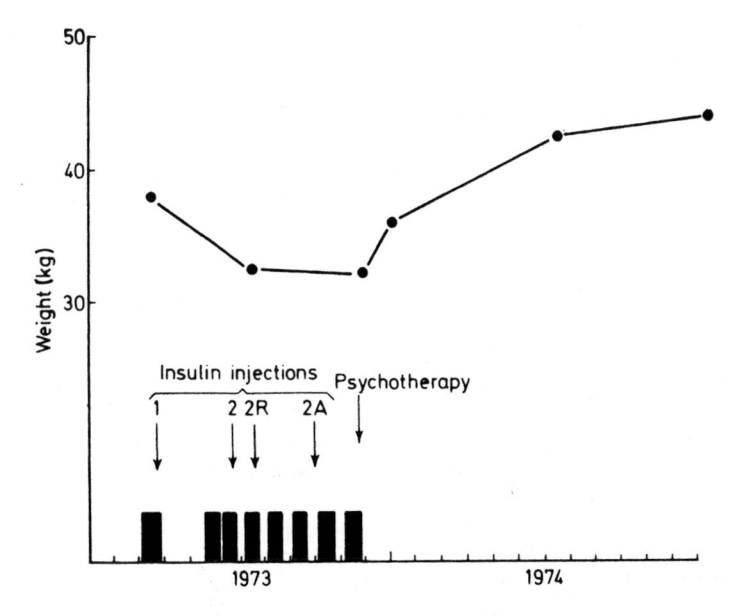

Figure 8.1 Progress of a girl with recurrent ketoacidosis. Hospital admissions shown as black rectangles. Note gross changes in weight. Insulins given, in order, were; a Semilente-Lente mixture, two injections of soluble, two of Rapitard and two of Actrapid. (We do not use these insulins now)

combating ketoacidosis. Changes of insulin are shown in the diagram at each readmission. A summary of the biochemical findings is given in Table 8.3.

Only on 7th July and possibly 2nd August, was the biochemistry really seriously disturbed, yet on all occasions she was ketotic and dehydrated, looked very ill and needed intravenous fluid.

The monthly pattern will be noted. One admission has been omitted (21.9.73) as it was planned in order to change from Rapitard to Actrapid. It is of interest that in October, while in the ward, she suddenly went into severe ketoacidosis (glucose 30.4 (548), Na 134, bicarbonate 9.5, urea 10.3 (62), pH 7.19, base deficit 18.5) and needed a drip. This is the only time I have seen a diabetic child deteriorate so sharply as to need a drip while under ward conditions. Was the trouble being caused by suppressed menstrual periods? It is well known that insulin requirements may rise before menstruation. However, this girl had not menstruated by the end of 1974, and during that year she did not require readmission.

Hormonal causes were considered. Her father was on drug therapy for thyrotoxicosis. He gave a positive antibody test for thyroid microsomes, but his thyroglobulin tanned red cell titre was negative. The mother was negative to both tests. The patient was also negative to both, and to the

TABLE 8.3

Date	True glucose (mmol/l) (mg%)	Sodium (mmol/l)	Bicarb.	Urea (mmol/l) (mg%)	pH	Base deficit
29.5.73	18.1 (326)	132	10	6.7 (40)	—	—
7.6.73	33.7 (606)	132	22	7.7 (46)	7.29	12.5
7.7.73	40.0 (720)	142	9	10 (60)	7.14	22
2.8.73	22.4 (404)	137	10.5	10 (60)	7.23	17.5
4.9.73	31.7 (570)	138	13	5 (30)	7.30	16
6.11.73	23.6 (424)					

precipitin test. Other tests (Dr W. Hamilton) showed that adrenal androgens increased with stimulation, but there was an inadequate glucocorticoid response which was difficult to fit into the clinical picture. Growth hormone varied between 1.8 and 18.0 (four estimations) but the variations again did not seem related to the clinical picture.

Attention then settled on possible psychological factors. Her parents seemed sensible and stable, remarkably so considering their violent introduction to the problems of childhood diabetes, and the girl appeared to be a pleasant and honest child. However I found, with a sense of shame, that the notes made at her first admission contained a pertinent observation by the house officer, 'Likes to sit on her mother's knee throughout the interview' (she was 11 years old). I myself had written the next morning 'Early breast development, dignified by a brassiere'. There was a suggestion in these two contrasting comments that the conflicting pulls towards childhood and adult life were felt more keenly by her than by the average prepubertal child.

Further information quickly emerged, revealing a regrettable breakdown in communication in the past. The nursing staff observed that she would sit for an hour with the needle for her injection indenting her skin, yet she would allow nobody to give the injection for her. (As mentioned elsewhere, when she was given a 'gun' she sat for an hour with her finger on the trigger.) A psychiatric opinion was sought. She was found to be a very conscientious child who virtually lived with her diabetic management all day long, but who had great difficulty bringing her worries to the surface. It took some time before she contributed more than 'yes' or 'no' to an interview. After several interviews at a relatively superficial level she was discharged and has not needed readmission since. She had only four further psychiatric chats at monthly intervals. She still tends to become ketotic easily and worries at a new school seem to upset her balance at times, but it has been possible to maintain her as an outpatient. The weight chart in *Figure 8.1* gives a good indication of her overall progress. She has just begun to attend an adult hospital under Dr J. T. Ireland, who reports that her control is improving steadily and that she seems to be maturing psychologically.

The reader may feel that psychiatry, seated on the Throne of Coincidence, has received undue credit. Before reaching such a conclusion he should consider the work of Baker *et al.* (1969). They investigated two girls with histories very similar to that of the patient described above. They were each given three psychiatric interviews;

(1) a pleasant interview,
(2) a stressful interview,
(3) a stressful interview while on a β-adrenergic blocker (MJ 1999, Solatol: propranolol does not appear to be suitable).

It was found that after the pleasant interview the blood sugar had risen by 1.4 mmol/l (25 mg per cent), after the stressful interview by 10 mmol/l (180 mg per cent), and after the stressful interview under β-adrenergic blockade by only 0.5 mmol/l (10 mg per cent). Free fatty acids were similarly affected. Urinary adrenaline rose but quickly returned to normal during blockage, the other catecholamines being unaffected. The pathway is seen as emotional arousal → autonomic nervous system activation → excessive and prolonged lipolysis → increased free fatty acid concentration → excessive production of ketone bodies by the liver → diabetic ketoacidosis. The situation is rather more complicated than described and the reader is referred to the original paper, but it does appear that nervous stress may imbalance diabetes through catecholamine metabolism. Baker *et al.* point out that emotional arousal at home would not be terminated abruptly by the ending of an interview. It appears that a major factor in the family is inability of the members to communicate easily with one another. I think the patient may also be unduly inhibited in talking to her physician and will talk more freely to a psychiatrist who is not directly involved in the details of diabetic control.

One feature of recurrent ketoacidosis which must be stressed is the speed with which it can occur. The student is taught that ketoacidosis appears slowly, hypoglycaemia suddenly, and this is usually true; but recurrent ketoacidosis provides exceptions. One boy (in his earlier days the roller-skater referred to in Chapter 4), showed this feature very clearly. He had three sudden attacks, two just before he left us at the age of 13, one just after he left us. They were all the same. His diabetes appeared well controlled and on the morning of the attack he would seem well. At mid-day he did not feel like having his lunch, but his urine was free from ketones. By 4 pm he was vomiting and his urine was loaded with ketones, and by 6 pm he was in hospital on intravenous fluids.

This does not complete a survey of recurrent ketoacidosis. Although it is most often seen in pubertal girls it also occurs in the 'quiet' years of middle childhood. It is my experience that such cases occur more in good homes than bad, but this does not explain the fact, which would probably be attested by anyone with experience of childhood diabetes, that the attacks usually end as mysteriously as they began (as in the case of Elsie, p. 136). There is no reason why a transient emotional upset should not appear in a home where the diabetic management is poor. The very fact that recurrent ketoacidosis tends to be self-limiting suggests an emotional or hormonal cause, and its occurrence in eight-year-olds suggests that sexual maturation is not the only cause.

Rosenbloom and Giordano (1977) emphasize that over-treatment is a major cause of recurrent ketoacidosis. This does not invalidate the suggestion that the most important factor is psychological, because it may well be nervous stress that initiates the instability which leads to over-treatment.

Differential diagnosis

The differential diagnosis must be considered. First, recurrent acidosis may be produced by bad home conditions, the child's poor state being accepted by the parents without undue concern. Here one will have the general impression of a slipshod home, whereas with psychosomatic recurrent ketoacidosis the impression is often one of overanxious obsessionalism. In addition to that, it is surprising how seldom the badly managed child *has* to be admitted to hospital. I see them at the clinic and I say to myself 'I shall really have to admit him at his next visit if he is no better' and I go on saying this for months. They seem to become almost habituated to a state of ketoacidosis. The psychosomatic patients are entirely different. They plunge into ketoacidosis and have to be readmitted at once.

Secondly, one has to consider the possibility that recurrent ketoacidosis is being deliberately induced. This does not apply to children but does apply to teenagers, where it is a form of self destructive behaviour resulting from 'denial' of diabetes. They may omit insulin and thus suffer recurrent ketoacidosis. The behaviour may in some cases be no more than attention seeking, but in others it is an expression of hopelessness. There may be suicidal intent, but more often the attitude is 'I wouldn't care *what* happened' (Stearns, 1959).

Treatment

Baker, Minuchin and Rossman (1974) have carried their studies further. It could be that stress 'turned on' ketoacidosis too quickly, or 'turned off' too slowly, and in fact both mechanisms seem to apply. The child may be used in a family conflict in a way that precludes 'turn-off'. Beta-adrenergic blockade is more likely to prevent 'turn-on' then 'turn-off'. Isoproterenol has seemed effective with the relatively mild cases in a preliminary study, but the conclusion to be drawn is that β-adrenergic blockade should be regarded as an adjunct to psychotherapy, and not vice versa, as one is dealing with a family situation. My opinion at present is that the use of β-adrenergic blockade should be left to those who have experience with those drugs. Nevertheless, Baker and his group have done great service by drawing attention to these patients and by outlining the physiological and psychological mechanisms involved. As soon as we recognize this psychosomatic syndrome we should seek the help of a psychiatrist. One cannot take refuge in the thought that the attacks will stop some day. If a child were caught in a sudden, serious attack far from medical help, he might die.

NON-KETOTIC HYPEROSMOLAR DIABETIC COMA

The hyperglycaemia and ketosis of diabetic coma are not always closely related. The existence of two contrasting extreme clinical forms, non-ketotic hyperosmolar coma in which the blood sugar is high, and euglycaemic ketotic coma in which it is near to normal, make this clear.

Osmolality

The osmolality of the blood can be regarded as a function of sugar, sodium, potassium and urea. It can be measured directly, by the osmometer, or it may be calculated from the formula

$$2(\text{sodium} + \text{potassium}) + \text{sugar} + \text{urea}$$
(all figures in mmol/l)

Where sugar and urea are quoted as mg per cent, the figures should be divided by 18 and six respectively. The answers obtained by calculation are about 20 mmol lower than those given by the osmometer in the higher ranges, and rather higher in the lower ranges (Jackson and Forman, 1966; Collins and Harris, 1971). Although I realize that osmolality is linked to the blood sugar level, it seemed of interest to compare osmolality with acidosis, for which pH was used as an index. The results from 68 cases are set out in *Figure 8.2*. The osmolalities were calculated, not measured. The diagram is slanted towards the more severe cases, because in some of the milder cases the full biochemical tests were not done.

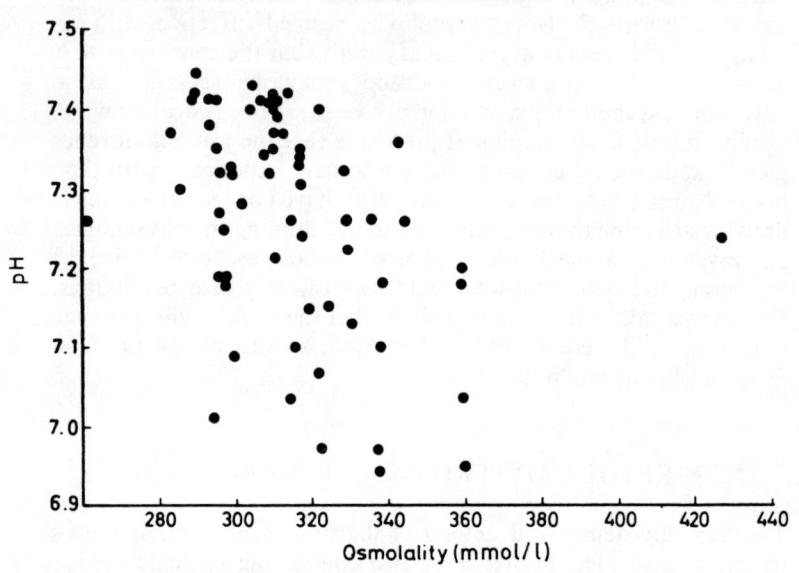

Figure 8.2. The relationship between plasma osmolality and pH

No attempt has been made to fit a line to the scattergram, as it is obvious that many cases would deviate far from the line which would therefore be of no clinical value. Few conclusions can be drawn. It can be said that absence of acidosis (i.e. a pH of 7.3 or above) and a relatively low osmolality (320 mmol or less) go together. It can also be pointed out that a very high osmolality need not be associated with severe acidosis (the isolated high osmolality of 427 is associated with a moderate acidosis of pH 7.24). A low pH may be associated with a high osmolality (pH 6.96 with osmolality 360) or with an almost normal one (pH 7.01 with osmolality 294). The dissociation between pH and osmolality helps to illustrate the different syndromes encountered, but does not explain the puzzles of diabetes. It would be much easier if acidosis and blood sugar were to walk decorously hand in hand.

Although it is the sugar which makes the major contribution to hyperosmolality, the role of sodium may at times be very important, as will be seen from *Table 8.4*.

TABLE 8.4

Variations in factors regulating osmolality

	Glucose (mmol/l) (mg%)	Sodium	Potassium	Urea (mmol/l) (mg%)	Osmolality
Normal	5 (90)	133	4.5	3.3 (20)	283
Case 1	78 (1400)	164	3.1	15 (89)	427
Extra mmol*	73	62	−3	12	144
Case 2	21 (380)	148	3.2	21 (126)	344
Extra mmol	16	30	−3	18	61

* The figures for sodium can be taken as an example of the calculation. In case 1, 164 is 31 mmol above the normal (133); but the formula given above requires that sodium be multiplied by 2, giving an excess of 62 mmol.

High though the sugar is in Case 1, the contribution from the sodium to hyperosmolality is almost as great. In Case 2, where the sugar is not very high, both the sodium and urea are more important than the sugar.

Treatment of hyperosmolality

I have said before that my opinions about the type of fluid to be used have vacillated and four short summaries are appended to show how doubts may arise.

(1) A boy of three and three-quarter years was admitted in 1966 with a four-day history of diabetes. He was severely dehydrated, glucose 77.7 mmol/l (1400 mg per cent), sodium 164, urea 15 mmol/l (89 mg per cent), pH 7.24, base deficit 11.5, osmolality 427 mmol. Before the biochemistry was known treatment was begun with normal saline and 40 mEq of sodium bicarbonate, in accordance with the practice of the time. When the sodium level was known he was changed to quarter-strength saline but he died two and a half hours after admission.

(2) (Treated at Stirling Royal Infirmary by Dr A. L. Speirs, several years ago). A girl of 13 months who was admitted with a three-day history of irritability had routine biochemical tests done on admission. This showed a blood glucose of 116 mmol/l (2080 mg per cent), urea 40 mmol/l (238 mg per cent), osmolality 470 and pH 7.04, but her urine was free from ketones four hours after admission. Quarter-strength saline was given (at that time we were even more uncertain about the treatment of hyperosmolar coma than we are now) and after four hours the sodium level (not done on admission) was 158 mmol/l. Twenty-five hours (very late) after admission she had some twitching of the limbs attributed to cerebral oedema, but she recovered to become a 'normal' diabetic.

(3) A girl of 12 years was admitted in deep coma with a one-week history of diabetes. Her blood glucose was unique in my experience, 180 mmol/l (3240 mg per cent), urea 40 mmol/l (238 mg per cent), sodium 134, pH 7.02. The case is described in Chapter 12 and the neurological state in particular by Stephenson and Byrne (1978). Normal saline was given, with low-dose intramuscular insulin. The blood glucose fell to 70.4 mmol/l in two and a half hours, falling more gradually thereafter.

(4) A boy of 11 years was admitted with a two-month history of diabetes. Blood glucose was 106 mmol/l (1908 mg per cent), sodium 154, urea 25 mmol/l, pH 7.18, osmolality (measured) 476. Treatment was begun with normal saline, changed to half-strength after two hours when the figure for sodium was known. Despite this the sodium ranged between 170 and 176 for six readings between the sixth and 23rd hours of treatment. Although he had no frank signs of cerebral oedema he was very obstreperous and foul-mouthed for three days after clinical recovery; this was attributed to a hypothalamic upset, but was transient.

All these cases were hyperosmolar, with relatively little acidosis—

a pH of 7.02 being chickenfeed compared with a blood glucose of 180 mmol/l (3240 mg per cent). The first case turned us against the use of normal saline as the initial fluid, but the third case came to no harm from a similar regime and may indeed have been protected by normal saline against cerebral oedema which could have resulted from a precipitate fall in blood sugar. (It should be noted here that the low-dose intramuscular insulin regime does produce a steady fall in blood sugar of about 5 mmol/l (90 mg per cent/hour), but *not* in the first hour or two.) The second case showed cerebral oedema on a weak saline solution. When the fourth case came along we decided to use half- rather than quarter-strength saline to offset any sharp fall in blood glucose. In the end, the boy seems to have been none the worse with a very high sodium level for the best part of a day. Was the outcome the result of good luck or good judgement?

One can suspect hyperosmolality on first seeing a diabetic patient if there is a very short history of diabetes and little over-breathing in the presence of dehydration and diminished consciousness. While awaiting the intial results it is safe to begin with normal saline but sodium bicarbonate should not be added. If there is hypernatraemia a change to half-strength saline can be made. There appears to be no great advantage and even some potential danger in using quarter-strength saline, even in the presence of gross hypernatraemia. Hypotonic solutions should not be used *in the stage of rapid rehydration*, and when they *are* used the infusion rate should be dropped by a further 25 per cent below that used in typical diabetic ketoacidosis. Experience has taught that these suggestions cannot be put forward as absolute rules but only as current opinions. The possibility of personal variation means that every patient must be assessed as an individual.

The prognosis for hyperosmolar non-ketotic coma is relatively poor, and the cause of the syndrome is not yet known for certain. Theories abound concerning hyperosmolality and the absence of ketosis. Hyperosmolality can be the result of dehydration, excessive sugar intake (for example Lucozade), impaired renal function leading to fluid loss but retention of sugar, and excess production of human growth hormone, thyroid, steroids or adrenaline. Lack of ketogenesis might be caused by the following.

(1) Failure to increase lipolysis in adipose tissue, which might be due to low cortisol or human growth hormone, or there might be enough insulin to block lipolysis but too little to cope with hyperglycaemia.

(2) Acetyl CoA formation may be poor, or it might in some way be diverted to form cholesterol rather than ketone bodies.
(3) Uptake of FFA by the liver from the blood might be poor.

These are all unsubstantiated theories, or guesses. The observations of Joffe et al. (1975) are very interesting. They postulate that in non-ketotic hyperosmolar coma a certain amount of insulin is circulating, enough to activate the liver but not the periphery, and there is experimental evidence that this is so; in non-ketotic coma the portal vein concentration of insulin was 33 µunits/ml when the peripheral vein concentration was 18 µunits/ml whereas in ketotic acidosis both were 13 µunits/ml. The insulin in the liver may be enough to suppress the intrahepatic oxidation of FFA, and thus to suppress ketosis, which contrasts with the older theories that ketosis might be suppressed by the suppression of peripheral lipolysis.

The increase in gluconeogenesis could be due to glucagon (Parrilla, Goodman and Toews, 1974), which is high in both peripheral and portal blood in non-ketotic hyperosmolar coma. The insulin in the liver may not be enough to counteract the stimulus given by the glucagon to hepatic gluconeogenesis. These newer theories could explain how non-ketotic hyperosmolar coma occurs, but not why it occurs in some patients and not in others.

EUGLYCAEMIC DIABETIC KETOACIDOSIS

This type of metabolic imbalance was described by Munro et al. (1973), and should be included here as the patients ranged from ten to 28 years of age. The criteria for diagnosis was a blood sugar of less than 17 mmol/l (300 mg per cent) and a plasma bicarbonate of less than 10 mEq/1. Young children may get a starvation ketosis overnight with acetone but no sugar in the morning urine, but that is a less severe upset, though there may be an aetiological link.

Of 211 episodes of diabetic decompensation, 37 fulfilled the criteria quoted above. These 37 episodes involved 17 patients, psychological stress being suspected in one who had 15 episodes. The average blood sugar was 11.4 mmol/l (205 mg per cent) (though it was below 5.5 mmol/l (100 mg per cent) in seven episodes) with an average for urea of 6.5 mmol/l (39 mg per cent), sodium 137, potassium 4.6 and a bicarbonate of 7.3. The blood chemistry was corrected in 24 hours by means of large doses of insulin and a dextrose drip. Monitoring was based on the bicarbonate level. Bicarbonate was not given for fear of producing disequilibrium between intracellular and extracellular pH.

Certain clinical features stand out:

(1) The patients are young.
(2) All except one had cut down their carbohydrate intake because of nausea and vomiting, which was the cause, aggravating factor and result of ketoacidosis.
(3) Most patients walked into hospital, suggesting that clouding of consciousness is due to hyperglycaemia and hyperosmolality rather than ketoacidosis.

Ireland and Thomson (1973) suggest that a low renal threshold may be involved in the syndrome, with massive loss of sugar in the urine. They point out that there is an ability to outgrow the tendency.

LACTIC ACIDOSIS

When sustained hard exercise is taken by a normal person there comes a time when hyperventilation and a vigorously pumping heart can no longer supply the body with enough oxygen for energy production. From that point much energy is obtained by the production of lactate in peripheral tissues, chiefly muscle, under anaerobic conditions. The normal blood lactate level of 1–2 mmol/l may be increased ten-fold during exercise. When exercise stops and positive oxygen balance has been re-established, the lactate is oxidized back to pyruvate, which finally produces water, carbon dioxide and glycogen. This reaction takes place in many tissues, but not in the blood. Much of the carbon dioxide is retained in restoring the blood bicarbonate level instead of being lost in hyperventilation. The production of glycogen takes place in the liver.

The mechanism of lactic acid production in diabetes is not fully understood. It is presumably due to tissue anoxia, and may be potentiated by temporary malfunction in the liver which is normally very able to deal with the products of lactate metabolism. Hypovolaemia and hypotension are likely causes of tissue anoxia in severe diabetes. Peripheral vasodilatation may make the situation worse, and is in part caused by lactic acidosis, so that a vicious circle may be set up. Acidosis and hypokalaemia also contribute to peripheral vasodilatation.

The arterial oxygen tension may fall in some patients in coma, and this can contribute to lactic acidosis. The enzyme 2,3-diphosphoglyceric acid (2,3-DPG) is involved in oxygen release to the tissues and is low in states of acidosis. However, acidosis itself increases oxygen release, and the fall in 2,3-DPG could be regarded as a secondary balancing factor in the presence of acidosis rather than a primary protection against anoxia. The matter is still open.

Severe lactic acidosis is uncommon in diabetes. Farquhar (1973) comments that he had for years used Ringer lactate in children as the basic rehydrating fluid without seeing adverse effects. It is a biochemical rather than a clinical diagnosis, which can be suspected if the blood pH seems lower than the degree of ketosis would warrant. A level of more than 7 mmol/l establishes a diagnosis of lactic acidosis, but the rare combination of lactic acidosis and severe ketoacidosis is best classified as ketoacidosis. In lactic acidosis the diabetes is treated in the usual way, but particular attention is paid to the blood pressure. Isoproterenol is to be preferred to the catecholamines in treatment.

The oral antidiabetic agent phenformin has been incriminated as a cause of lactic acidosis. This is unlikely to be a factor in childhood, when phenformin is hardly ever used.

OTHER MANIFESTATIONS OF KETOACIDOSIS

While this chapter was being written there appeared a patient who caused considerable head-scratching. Her history is appended as it served to bring home some problems of management in which the rules given above may be broken. If the patient breaks the rules there is no point in the physician being gentlemanly about it: he should break the rules too.

A girl aged 12½ years was a patient at another hospital who were unable to admit her on this occasion because of pressure on beds. She had been diabetic for three years during which time she had been readmitted six times in ketoacidosis or hypoglycaemia. Four of these readmissions had occurred close together early on. There was then a gap of a year to October 1974, when she first menstruated and had to be readmitted. She was again readmitted that December in euglycaemic ketoacidosis with a blood sugar of 16 mmol/l (285 mg per cent) and her seventh readmission was in March 1975 to the Royal Hospital for Sick Children.

On this occasion there was a two-day history of vomiting and abdominal pain. On the day before admission, though listlessly ambulant, she had eaten nothing and had drunk only one glass of milk. She was very drowsy on the morning of admission and was given no insulin as the mother was very busy trying to find a doctor.

On admission she was unconscious. She responded faintly to deep abdominal pressure but not to injections. Her pupils were unequal and did not contract to light. Her blood pressure was unrecordable. She was hyperventilating and her breath smelled of acetone. Her pulse rate was 50 per minute. ECG monitoring showed a rather high T-wave. Her progress is given on a time-scale, to which notes have been appended so as not to break the narrative.

Zero hour   Core temperature 31.2°C (86°F), skin temperature 25°C (75°F) (1). Begun on drip of half-strength physiological saline, 240 ml/hour, 20 mmol sodium bicarbonate added to first bottle. Blood pressure 90/50 after half an hour (2). Insulin 10 units intramuscularly, then 4 units hourly.

One hour   Biochemistry reported (all readings in mmol), sodium 123, potassium 5.7, bicarbonate 4.5, urea 15.5 (93 mg per cent), true glucose 33 (576 mg per cent), pH 6.83, base deficit >22 (3).

Three hours   pH still 6.83 and base deficit >22, but faint blinking of eyes (4).

Seven hours   Improved. Calls faintly for nurse, passed urine when held propped, urine loaded with ketones. Pupils equal and reacting. Core temperature 34.5°C. Has had 2 litres of fluid, containing 80 mmol of sodium bicarbonate.

Biochemistry subsequently reported as Na 135, K 4.6, bicarbonate 4, urea 16.5, true glucose 18 (324 mg per cent), pH 7.07, base deficit >22 (5).

Nine hours   Sodium 139, potassium 4.2, bicarbonate 6.5, urea 17, true glucose 11.1 (200 mg per cent) (6). Insulin 20 units subcutaneously, fluids tried by mouth, poorly taken and vomited.

21 hours   Sodium 140, potassium 3.4, bicarbonate 8.5, urea 10.5, pH 7.13, base deficit 19.5. Still overbreathing. Abdominal pain, vomited (7). Returned to hourly intramuscular insulin 4 units, six doses given. Hb 13 g per cent, WBCs 19 599, platelets 70 000 (8). Serum lactate subsequently reported as 0.8 mmol/l (low normal).

28 hours   Sodium 142, potassium 2.7, bicarbonate 14, urea 6.5, true glucose 14.6 (163 mg per cent), pH 7.33, base deficit 12 (9). Oral fluids tried again. Return to s.c. insulin, potassium chloride 2g/bottle.

36 hours   Sodium 144, potassium 2.8, bicarbonate 18, urea 7.0, true glucose 6.2 (112 mg per cent), pH 7.41, base deficit 6, platelets 57 000. Fragmented cells on film (9). Moving normally in bed, still drowsy. All urines still show acetone +++ (10). Her subsequent recovery was uneventful, and she was ambulant and alert after three days.

Notes

(1) A feeling of coldness may be a complaint in ketoacidosis and objective coldness of the extremities is quite a common finding. Here, however, there is severe hypothermia. She was nursed in a room at 28°C, and her trunk and limbs were wrapped in foil.

(2) A very slow start. (We would now begin with normal saline.) Drip rate was slow, but how a hypothermic child would respond was uncertain. There was a fear of pulmonary oedema or heart failure if a more rapid rate were used. Blood pressure fortunately rose very early which

seems more likely to have been due to slight warming and bed rest after admission than to the small volume of intravenous fluid given by then. Good nursing care may have saved her at this point.

(3) The sodium was low, so a change was made to physiological saline. The pH is very low, but the urge to give heroic doses of bicarbonate was resisted. One could say that the lower the pH the greater the risk of producing considerable pH imbalance between fluid and cells if doses of bicarbonate aimed at completely correcting the acidity are given. Potassium was high, so no potassium given.

(4) The pH is unchanged, an unwelcome surprise, but the child is still hypothermic so correcting mechanisms are possibly suboptimal and slow eye blinking and small head movements are not much, but they are a sign of clinical improvement, and it is probably wisest to accept this as the main criterion and leave treatment unchanged. One may not know exactly what one is doing, but getting excited is not going to help.

(5) Therapeutic inertia seems justified. Definite clinical improvement, and some biochemical improvement, though bicarbonate still very low and base deficit severe.

(6) Further improvement. Base deficit now registering and pH within a range where one would not normally give bicarbonate. To be tried with subcutaneous insulin, and small sips of fluid.

(7) Probably a misjudgement in changing too soon to subcutaneous insulin, also a failure of communication in not giving a second dose of subcutaneous insulin overnight. The net result is a slight deterioration. A return was made to the original hourly intramuscular regime.

(8) Diffuse intravascular coagulation (DIC) is suggested by the low platelet count. This complication is known to occur in septicaemia (particularly meningococcal, associated with adrenal failure), haemolytic uraemia and similar states. It appears to be due to sluggish blood flow through the small vessels, and an added defect in the vascular walls has been postulated. Possibly excess thromboplastin formation, which could occur in any tissue subjected to anoxia, plays a part. Timperley, Preston and Ward (1974) describe six deaths due to DIC in diabetic ketoacidosis, three of the cases being confined to the brain only, the other three being truly diffuse. Platelets, which form the basis of the clots, were low and other factors involved in clotting (fibrinogen, factor VIII and fibrin degeneration products (FDP)) were raised. There may be the associated phenomenon of intravascular haemolysis producing fragmented burr cells which, as well as the low platelet count, can be recognized on the blood film. DIC is thought to be particularly common in hyperosmolar non-ketotic coma. It is of interest that even when not in ketoacidosis diabetics may show raised levels of fibrinogen, factor VIII and FDPs, so the blood film by itself is useful in diagnosis. The problem in the present case was whether to give heparin or not. There was no evidence of kidney damage, the cerebral function was improving, the hypothermia might possibly have damaged small pulmonary vessels and heparin does not affect the vessels anywhere, so it was not given. It would,

however, be advisable to obtain the result of a blood-film as soon as possible, which was not done here.

(9) With acidosis almost corrected, the potassium begins to approach danger levels, so potassium chloride is given.

(10) The potassium level is held. There is still gross acetonuria, but acetone, being fat soluble, is still excreted after acidosis is corrected.

It has been suggested that frequent small doses of intramuscular insulin are insufficient to deal with the coma of ketoacidosis, but the prognosis in the present case, who had severe hypothermia and a pH of 6.83, was not very good and the child survived on a conservative regime.

REFERENCES

Alberti, K. G. M. M., Hockaday, T. D. R. and Turner, R. C. (1973). Small doses of intramuscular insulin in the treatment of diabetic 'coma'. *Lancet*, **11**, 515

Baker, L., Barcai, A., Kaye, R. and Hauque, N. (1969). Beta-adrenergic blockade and juvenile diabetes. *J. Pediat.*, **75**, 19

Baker, L., Minuchin, S. and Rosman, B. (1974). The use of beta-adrenergic blockade in the treatment of psychosomatic aspects of juvenile diabetes mellitus, *Excerpta medica*, **V**, 67

Collins, J. V. and Harris, P. W. R. (1971). Non-keto-acidotic diabetic coma. *Postgrad. med. J.*, **47**, 388

Farquhar, J. W. (1973). Diabetes mellitus. In *Text-book of Paediatrics*, p. 1136, Ed. J. O. Forfar and G. C. Arneil. Edinburgh and London; Churchill-Livingstone

Hockaday, T. D. R. and Alberti, K. G. M. M. (1972). Diabetic coma. *Clin. endocrin. Metab.*, **I**, 751

Ireland, J. T. and Thomson, W. S. T. (1973). Euglycaemic diabetic ketoacidosis. *Br. med. J.*, **II**, 107

Jackson, W. P. U. and Forman, R. (1966). Hyperosmolar non-ketotic diabetic coma. *Diabetes*, **15**, 714

Joffe, B. I., Goldberg, R. B., Krut, L. H. and Seftel, H. C. (1975). Pathogenesis of non-ketotic hyperosmolar diabetic coma. *Lancet*, **I**, 1069

Kaye, R. (1975). Diabetic ketoacidosis—the bicarbonate controversy. *J. Pediat.*, **87**, 156

Moseley, J. (1975). Diabetic crises in children treated with small doses of intramuscular insulin. *Br. med. J.*, **I**, 59

Munro, J. F., Campbell, I. W., McCuish, A. C. and Duncan, L. J. P. (1973). Euglycaemic diabetic ketoacidosis. *Br. med. J.*, **I**, 578

Page, M. McB., Alberti, K. G. M. M., Greenwood, R., Gumaa, K. A., Hockaday, T. D. R., Lowy, C., Nabarro, J. D. N., Pyke, D. A., Sönksen, P. H., Watkins, P. J. and West, T. T. (1974). Treatment of diabetic coma with continuous low-dose infusion of insulin. *Br. med. J.*, **II**, 687

Parilla, R., Goodman, M. N. and Toews, C. J. (1974). Effects of glucagon: insulin ratios on hepatic metabolism. *Diabetes*, **23**, 725

Rosenbloom, A. L. and Giordano, B. (1977). Chronic overtreatment with insulin in children and adolescents. *Am. J. Dis. Child.*, **131**, 881

Sönksen, P. H., Srivastava, M. C., Tompkins, Christine V. and Nabarro, J. D. N. (1972). Growth hormone and cortisol responses to insulin infusion in patients with diabetes mellitus. *Lancet*, **II**, 155

Stearns, S. (1959). Self-destructive behaviour in young patients with diabetes mellitus. *Diabetes*, **8,** 379

Stephenson, J. E. P. and Byrne, E. (1978). Prognostic value of oculo-vestibular reflex. *Br. med. J.,* **1,** 1346

Timperley, W. R., Preston, F. E. and Ward, J. D. (1974). Cerebral intra-vascular coagulation in diabetic ketoacidosis. *Lancet*, **I,** 952

CHAPTER 9

The Course of Childhood Diabetes

In discussing the course of diabetes during childhood it seems appropriate to begin with the first weeks or months of life. Of the two forms to be considered the first is neonatal diabetes, which has features peculiarly its own. The second is diabetes in the first year of life, a true diabetes mellitus which carries special dangers and needs special management.

NEONATAL DIABETES

Neonatal diabetes is transient, but is distinct from the transient diabetic states described on p. 15 in that it begins in the first week or two of life and lasts for weeks or months. A striking feature is that the affected babies are not ketotic. The clinical picture was described by Hutchison, Keay and Kerr (1962). The child has a waxy pallor and, despite increasing severe weight loss, remains active and alert. This syndrome is sufficiently definite and sufficiently different from that seen in other wasting diseases (for example gastroenteritis) to enable one to make an intelligent guess at the true diagnosis before testing the urine. The disease is rare, and the urine disappears in the nappy so that even with an experienced nursing staff the weight loss is likely to attract attention before the polyuria is noted. It is a true diabetes, but if one finds non-ketotic diabetes in the first week or two of life it is likely to be transient.

MacDonald (1974) found 41 cases in the literature, 30 of them being small-for-dates babies with poor placentas, and observed differences between the small babies and the large babies. In the small babies a family history of *neonatal* diabetes is common, in the larger babies it is not. In the large babies a history of perinatal stress is found, in the small babies it is not. The small babies may well have been insulopenic *in utero*, due to delayed maturation of the beta-cells (Ferguson and Milner, 1970), itself a consequence of a familial tendency for the pancreas to be selectively affected by poor placental nutrition. Six of these 30 babies have gone on to permanent diabetes. Dorchy, Ooms and Loeb (1975) describe a further case that became permanent. The small babies have been shown to have low plasma insulin (Ferguson, 1967), in which respect they are the opposite of the large babies with hyperinsulinism (Baird and Farquhar, 1962) born to diabetic mothers. The non-diabetic small-for-dates baby has normal or high plasma insulin, so the small babies with neonatal diabetes and low insulin have not been produced by placental insufficiency alone.

Management is essentially the same as for any diabetic infant, described in the next section. As all the carbohydrate in the neonate is taken as sugar, it is desirable to start with a minute dose of insulin, for example, one unit, before each feed or every second feed. In giving one unit of insulin a mother may feel more confident that she is being accurate if she takes the insulin up to the third mark and injects down to the second. Kuna and Addy (1979) have successfully located transient neonatal diabetes with chlorpropamide, after first gaining control with insulin.

DIABETES IN INFANCY

Diabetes in the first year is rare, but quite well documented. It is essentially the same as diabetes occurring later in childhood, but poses some problems of its own. It is seldom diagnosed before admission, or even at admission, because polyuria is virtually lost as a symptom and thirst may not be recognized but may be regarded as irritability. The vomiting of ketosis combined with weight loss may suggest gastroenteritis, or the child may be sent to a fever hospital in pre-coma as a case of meningitis. The diagnosis is most likely to be suspected from the first urine test in hospital, and even then the diagnosis may well be, and perhaps should be, 'glycosuria, for investigation' rather than 'diabetes mellitus'.

The particular bug-bear of treatment is the fear of insulin-induced hypoglycaemia. The infant spends much of his day asleep, and even the normal infant may go pale in sleep, so that hypoglycaemia can be missed. The normal child who is beginning mixed feeding is notoriously capricious about his intake of solids, the mother of a diabetic may well be all the more anxious when she knows he should have regular food, and a vicious circle involving an anxious mother and a suspicious child can easily occur. The mother can be reassured that if her baby's blood sugar is low he will be ready to feed but this is not strictly true and the risk of hypoglycaemia, particularly missed hypoglycaemia, is very real. The brain cells of the infant need more energy from sugar than those of an older child and it is believed by many that infantile diabetes leads on to fits and mental defect. This is true, but the prognosis for infant diabetics is not quite as black as it is painted, and is described in detail in Chapter 12.

In the last edition of this book I suggested that the infant diabetic should be on three injections of soluble insulin daily, but in the past year or so my experience of infant diabetes has doubled as we have admitted babies who developed diabetes at two, four and 11 months old respectively. The first of these was treated with two injections of Semitard MC till the age of 11 months, when she was changed to one injection of Retard without loss of control. This led to the other two being put on one injection of Retard as soon as initial control was obtained. As this one injection has so far given satisfactory control I now regard it as 'routine' for infants. It has the added advantage of not turning babies into pin-cushions.

Collection of urine is easier than one might think. Urine bags should not be used as they will eventually break the skin but if the baby is held on the pot on its mother's knee for up to half an hour three or four times a day it is quite easy to obtain specimens. These are likely to be post-prandial due to the workings of the infant bladder but valuable information can still be obtained. Clinistix strips in the night nappies give a fair indication of whether there is a risk of overnight hypoglycaemia, and this can be supplemented by Dextrostix if there is any suggestion that hypoglycaemia may have occurred.

The carbohydrate intake of a baby is based on milk. Milk given to a baby has usually been sweetened to contain 6–7 per cent sugar, so that 150 ml can be taken to contain 10 g of carbohydrate. In the second six months of life the baby will need 50–60 g of carbohydrate from other sources. Ideally, one would like to space the extra carbohydrate equally between the three main feeds, but the desirable may have to give way to the attainable. If the mother worries too much about feeds the baby may go off solids altogether, so I usually tell the mother not to worry if he doesn't take everything at one meal, because it can always be carried forward to the next. One should try to adjust the regime to the baby's natural inclinations, not vice versa, and one should be satisfied that regular habits, whatever they may be, have been established before he leaves hospital. I can think of one exception to this.

It proved almost impossible to get a child of two years to take food in hospital. He was very irritable, steadily lost weight and was in constant ketosis, presumably due to starvation. With heart in mouth I sent him home in this deplorable state. He began to eat as soon as he went home, and within a week he was well stabilized at the cost of several telephone calls.

This case is an example of fitting the regime to the child, although usually any child who gives trouble with feeding will feed better in hospital with a carefree nurse than at home with an anxious mother. It is therefore highly desirable that the mother should live in hospital with the very young diabetic child or there may be trouble when he goes home.

HEIGHT AT ONSET

It has been stated by many observers that diabetic children are taller than average at the onset of the diesease. A few workers have found them to be only of average height. Such apparent differences may not be real. Helen Pond (1970) found that the average height of diabetic children at the onset was on the 60th centile in London, whereas I reported in 1970 that it was on the 45th centile in Glasgow. However, both of us were using the national averages as a standard; the average for normal Glasgow children falls about the 40th centile, and children in the south of England are 3 to 5 cm taller than children in Glasgow. Thus we were in fact agreeing that diabetic children at the onset of their disease were five to ten centiles above the average height *of the local population*, which is the relevant standard. He who gulps down statistics without question will get hooked, sooner or later.

It is very seldom that one can obtain a reliable series of heights for a year or two before diabetes appears. It is therefore marginally justifiable to give the growth chart of a girl *(Figure 9.1)* (referred to on p. 17) who is suspected of being pre-diabetic. It will be seen that in the course of seven years she has proceeded from the 25th to about the 60th centile. Such observations have suggested the involvement of growth hormone, a known insulin antagonist, in the aetiology of diabetes. The clinical experimental evidence on this subject is inconclusive (p. 148) but suggests that any alteration in growth hormone is the result rather than the cause of disordered carbohydrate metabolism.

Since the above was written this girl has reached the age of 13. Her glucose tolerance test (GTT) is now normal (*see* end of Chapter

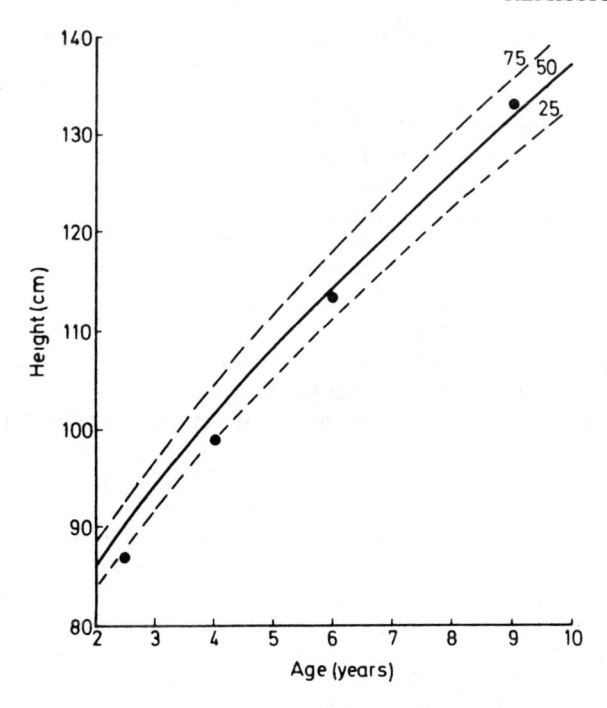

Figure 9.1. This child has been a chemical diabetic for more than seven years, but remains asymptomatic. Her height has increased from below the 25th to above the 50th centile. The 25th, 50th and 75th centiles are shown, and are taken from the Tanner-Whitehouse charts (see text)

1), renal glycosuria is present and her height has returned to the 50th centile.

REMISSION

It has been remarked elsewhere that some diabetic children need more insulin on the fourth or fifth day of treatment to keep them out of ketosis than was needed on the first or second day to abolish ketosis. This is at first sight as surprising as would be the need to increase the flow through an intravenous drip after one had replaced the initial fluid loss. There must be an explanation for this but I do not know what it is. A few days or weeks later the same child may go into remission.

It may seem difficult at the beginning of a remission to decide whether a child is a true diabetic or has simply experienced a transient diabetic state (p. 15) due to stress. In practice the difference is clear-cut. The transient diabetic state passes off in one to three days, more often one than three, whereas the true diabetic will have been on insulin for at least a week before he comes off it.

A complete remission, which implies that the GTT has returned to normal in addition to the patient having given up insulin (Johansen and Ørskov, 1969), is probably rare. One has to say 'probably' as the literature contains little information on GTTs done during this period, but such as have been done are more often abnormal than normal. Remission of a sort is, however, quite common, and may even appear in children who have presented in severe ketoacidosis though it is relatively rare in that group.

Efforts are being made internationally to draw up standards for the definition of 'remission' but so far it remains a period one would rather talk about than define. In checking back on the findings from the Royal Hospital for Sick Children, Glasgow, it was kept in mind that the increased activity of the child on leaving hospital may account for a fall of 20–25 per cent in insulin needs. A fall of less than 33 per cent has therefore been regarded as 'no fall'. The results from 63 consecutive cases are:

No fall in insulin needs	38 cases
Fall of 33–60 per cent	17 cases
Fall of 70–80 per cent	three cases, range of remission four to 20 weeks, average 12 weeks
Completely off insulin	five cases, range of remission three to 12 weeks, average seven weeks

Heavily-built children may have a remission of six months or more, but slim children tend to have shorter remission. This may lead to certain cases being diagnosed as maturity onset type of diabetes in the young ('MODY'), whereas they might be better regarded as juvenile diabetes in some fat children who follow an unusual course in the first few months of their disease. The remission is often abruptly terminated by intercurrent infection, and the parents must always be warned in advance that although a child may have come off insulin entirely he is certain to need it again in the near future. I ask parents to test the urine sugar twice daily during the remission and advise them to start insulin again (two to four units) if two successive urine specimens show the presence of sugar. Such a recurrence may be transient but more often represents the return of manifest diabetes. At this time the child may be very sensitive to insulin, for example, he may show frank hypoglycaemic symptoms on a daily dose of four units of insulin.

There are differing opinions on the management of the child on whom a GTT has not been done but who is regarded as being in 'complete' remission.

(1) Oral hypoglycaemic agents have been given in an attempt to prolong the remission period, but the evidence that they do so is not convincing. It has been mentioned elsewhere that such agents have no demonstrable effect on the GTT in children who are potential diabetics.
(2) Minimal doses of insulin have been persisted with even when the urine is constantly free from sugar, partly in the hope of prolonging the remission and partly to avoid raising false hopes in the child that he has finished with diabetes for good.
(3) My own practice is to take children off insulin if they can do without it. Freedom from the pain of injections for a few weeks seems to me to outweigh the disappointment of starting injections again. The continuation of dieting reminds them that they are still diabetic. This, however, is obviously no more than personal opinion, and each physician is free to make his choice.

What is happing during the remission period? It appears from the work of Johansen and Ørskov (1969) that insulin is being secreted, but the pathology or enzymic activity behind the insulin secretion remains a mystery. It has been suggested by others that children are rather off-colour during the remission period, and are more like their old selves once frank diabetes reappears, and I share this clinical impression. If one questions the mother in as neutral a way as possible: 'Is his general health better or worse since he went back on insulin?' the reply one gets is 'Better' or 'No change'.

During the remission period is insulin keeping the blood sugar down, or is some factor failing to put it up when it should? Weber and Müller-Hess (1972) present further evidence. In the early stages of remission, the rise in insulin in response to oral glucose was slow and never came near to normal levels. Insulin in the children in remission rose to 20 μunit/ml after two hours or more, despite blood glucose levels reading about 22 mmol/l (400 mg/ml); but in normal children insulin rose to 70 μunit/ml after 30 minutes. The GTT may become normal after weight loss in the obese, but there is no related improvement in the insulin response. Weber and Müller-Hess also gave glibenclamide, a sulphonylurea, while performing the GTT. It made no difference to the insulin levels. Its only demonstrable action was to produce a faster decline in the glucose curve in those fat children who had lost weight and in whom the GTT had returned to normal.

The conclusions from this study are that remission is not due to *improved* insulin secretion: that there may be increased peripheral sensitivity to insulin: and that the sulphonylurea effect seems to be extrapancreatic, a view on the action of sulphonylureas which has recently received wider acceptance. These conclusions seem to fit the clinical picture better than the idea that remission is solely the result of a resurgence of insulin secretion.

However, *residual* insulin secretion (rather than *improved* insulin secretion) seems to be important both in the remission period and after it. Pro-insulin is broken down to insulin and C-peptide in a 1:1 ratio. Although much insulin is taken up by the liver and therefore does not reach the systemic circulation C-peptide passes through the liver unchanged and so C-peptide in the peripheral blood is an indicator of the amount of insulin produced by the pancreas. Studies have shown that there is a correlation between vigorous initial therapy to control diabetes, short-lived ketosis at the onset, the presence of remission and the continuing presence of C-peptide even after several years (Ludvigsson and Heding, 1977; Ludvigsson *et al.*, 1977). Grajwer *et al.* (1977) have shown that C-peptide is more commonly to be found in well- rather than poorly-controlled diabetics. If we take C-peptide as an indicator of some residual beta-cell activity, then it is apparent that this is of importance both in remission and in the post-remission period.

GROWTH

The adult height of diabetic children

Almost all available evidence suggests that diabetic children *as a group* are below average height as adults. The first paper written on growth in the insulin era was that of Boyd and Nelson (1928) who found that diabetic children grew better than average. Their method of estimation was open to question, and nobody has agreed with them since. Larsson and Sterky (1962) showed the adult height of males diabetic since childhood to be 5.5 cm below that of the general male population. Sterky (1963) found that diabetic children lagged in growth, particularly boys, but compensated for this to a certain extent by continuing to grow in their late teens. However, the same writer (1967) also found that diabetic children were significantly shorter as adults than their parents, which runs against the present secular trend of children tending to be slightly taller than their parents. The diabetic growth spurt is late, and not as great as in normal children. The diabetics catch up a little in their mid-teens but do not fulfil their adult potential.

In considering these results it must be remembered that children showing a level of control bad enough to result in diabetic dwarfism have been included in the group, so it remains to be decided if *all* diabetic children grow badly or only those in whom control is moderate or poor.

The study of Tattersall and Pyke (1972) on identical twins strongly suggests that nearly all diabetic children fail to attain the height they would have reached had they not been diabetic. A study of twins rules out social, cultural and psychological influences, at least as primary environmental factors inhibiting growth. If such influences appear, they are secondary to the diabetes. The study included 12 identical pairs in whom one member developed diabetes before puberty and the other did not. In only one of these pairs was the diabetic twin equal in height to the other. In the other 11 pairs the diabetic twin was shorter by an average of 5.9 cm, and if only those who had reached adult height were considered the deficit was 7.6 cm. Only 2 per cent of non-diabetic identical twins show a height difference of more than 3.8 cm, so the deficits in the diabetic twins seem definite. These cases were collected from all over the country, so it can be assumed that the level of diabetic control was 'average'.

Growth in childhood

Diabetes in childhood is subject to greater fluctuations than diabetes in adult life, so it can be said that the diabetic state in childhood is unstable. This is not surprising, as childhood itself is not a stable state, but it is relatively stable between the ages of five and 11 years. During that period height is increasing steadily by 5 cm a year and weight by 2.3 kg, rhythms of eating, sleeping and excreting have been established, illness is less alarming and even the psyche can withstand a fair buffeting without showing permanent damage. It is during these years, before the onset of puberty, that insulin needs rise slowly, almost predictably, and diabetes is near to stability.

Several studies have been done on the growth of diabetic children. These studies agree on the fact that diabetic children do not grow as well as normal children, but the results are often set out in a way that makes it difficult to see precisely to what extent the diabetic children do lag, and to compare one's own results with the results from other clinics. The Glasgow figures are therefore offered in a brashly unsophisticated state. Children were studied between the ages of six and ten years, the children studied having been diabetic for at least three years (average 3.7 years) during that period. It was assumed that, if growth was normal, the height would be on the same centile at the end of observation as at the beginning, which may have been expecting a shade much if their initial height had been artificially raised by about 5 centiles due to the pre-diabetic spurt.

Twenty-three boys lagged by 0.2 cm per annum, on average, and 22 girls lagged by 0.1 cm. Beal (1948) who presented her results in a similar way, reported a lag of 0.9 cm per annum. The range involved in the Glasgow figures was considerable, from an annual lag of 2.3 cm in one child to an annual excess of 2.2 cm over expected gain in another. Personal variation is therefore wide.

Growth at puberty

It is agreed that the growth lag in diabetics is most clearly seen at puberty and during the pre-pubertal growth spurt. The Glasgow figures confirm this. Fifteen boys were followed for the three years from their tenth to thirteenth birthdays, the average annual lag being 0.35 cm. Twenty-one girls seemed to do even worse, with an annual lag of 0.8 cm; but the girls have, as it were, more to lose, as normal girls grow more than boys during this age-period, and this will be exaggerated if there is any delay in maturation. The figures are summarized in *Table 9.1*.

TABLE 9.1

Annual growth lag in diabetic children

Age (years)	No.	Sex	Patient-years	Average annual lag (cm)
6–10	23	M	83	0.2
6–10	22	F	84	0.1
10–13	15	M	45	0.35
10–13	21	F	63	0.8

If one adds the Glasgow figures together, the average total lag for diabetic boys is 2.0 cm over the period six to 13 years, and for girls 2.9 cm. Other writers have shown that the tendency to lag persists for a few more years, with some catch-up growth by the diabetics in their late teens when normal children have stopped growing.

Growth and maturation

Diabetics mature late. Does the delay in maturation show itself in childhood and, if it does, can a lag in height be solely attributed to a delay in maturation? A comparison was made at the Royal Hospital for Sick Children between bone-ages (estimated from Tanner and Whitehouse's tables, 1962) of recent and long-standing diabetes. 'Recent' diabetics were a group of 39 children, average age 7.5 years and average duration of diabetes 1.0 years, who showed an average lag in bone-age of 2.2 months. 'Long-standing' diabetics comprised 40 children, average age 10.5 years and average duration of diabetes 5.9 years, who showed an average lag in bone-age of 9.7 months. Linear studies would give information of greater value but, so far as they go, the figures suggest that delay in maturation due to childhood diabetes begins in childhod and is not just a feature of puberty. The point is worth making, as the main factor in maturation in childhood is thyroxin, with the sex hormones assuming importance at puberty. The figures given above are in accord with the evidence that diabetic girls are about one year late in passing through the menarche. Tattersall and Pyke mention two pairs among their identical twins, one of each pair developing diabetes before puberty. The diabetic twins were four years and five years later in the onset of the menarche than their non-diabetic sisters. The normal difference between identical non-diabetic twins is 2.8 *months*, so the differences quoted above become so striking that one must regard them as exceptional.

Bone-age and height-age

If 132 cm is taken as the average height of a boy of nine years, then any boy of that height has a height-age of nine years, whatever his actual age may be. The 40 children mentioned above have been used in a comparison of bone-age and height-age. In 16 of the 40 bone-age and height-age were the same, within 10 percentiles. Bone-age lagged behind height-age in 14 and was ahead in ten. In round terms, bone-age and height-age are the same. This finding suggests that, on the average, a delay in maturation coincides with a lag in height, although this does not necessarily imply that one causes the other.

It must be remembered in assessing such figures in an individual that growth and maturation do not necessarily proceed in parallel, but rather as two flights of stairs which do not always coincide. An extreme example was a diabetic girl who in one year matured by six months and grew by 18 months, the process being exactly reversed the following year. Forecasts of adult height are made from a comparison between bone-age and height-age, and it is thus unsafe to prognosticate about a child's ultimate height until he has been under observation for several years.

Growth and diabetic control

Diabetic control is difficult to define in classic terms, and even if it can be defined it cannot be precisely monitored every day in life. Thus there result some differences of opinion about the relationship between diabetic control and the onset of complications in later life, and the relationship between control and growth in childhood is similarly difficult to assess. About all that can be said is that physicians appear to share the clinical impression that really bad control hastens complications in adults and causes stunting in childhood (*see* p. 256).

Fifty-four children who had been diabetic for at least three years were classified by the amount of sugar found in several overnight urine specimens tested at the clinic. The choice of standard is wilful and unscientific, but probably as reliable as, say, random blood-sugars. Burditt, Caird and Draper (1968) found a good correlation between urine sugars and blood-sugars taken at the same time.

TABLE 9.2

Growth in relation to degree of glycosuria. Patients seen at the RHSC, Glasgow

Amount of sugar in urine	Very high	High	Moderate	Good
Numbers of patients	8	29	13	4
Height range, per annum (cm)	−1.25 to +0.48	−2.10 to +2.20	−2.30 to +1.10	−2.18 to −0.50

In *Table 9.2* the standards for subdividing the sugar levels from 'very high' to 'good' are immaterial, as the point to be demonstrated is that relatively good control of glycosuria does not guarantee good growth. Indeed, the four best controlled in terms of glycosuria all showed a lag in growth, probably a coincidence from the small number, but there is no good evidence that growth varies inversely with glycosuria.

A similar assessment was made of ketosis *(Table 9.3)* and the

TABLE 9.3

Growth in relation to ketosis

Frequency of ketosis	Very frequent	Frequent	Infrequent	Seldom or never
Numbers	3	9	9	33
Height range per annum (cm)	−0.63 to 0	−2.30 to +2.20	−2.10 to +1.10	−2.18 to +0.85

conclusions to be drawn are similar also. Neither high urine sugars nor frequent ketosis correlate strongly with poor growth.

One would expect hepatomegaly (*see* p. 256) to be associated with poor growth. One would also expect poor social circumstances to be related to poor growth, if for no other reason than that normal children in poor circumstances are shorter than those coming from physically better homes. In fact, there does seem to be an association (using an odd parameter) between hepatomegaly and poor social circumstances. As a *jeu d'esprit* I once worked out how often the diabetic children failed to keep their clinic appointments, counting it as a failure only if no attempt had been made to notify the clinic of their impending absence. They may have had no telephone and the nearest public telephone might have been vandalized, or perhaps the parents were not used to writing notes, or perhaps they just forgot appointments or lost their cards, but these excuses themselves are indicative of a rather irregular background, and possibly even a better social index than the number of rooms in the house or the number of persons per room. Be that as it may, the list was headed by three children with more than 65 per cent failures to attend who were in fact the only three children on whom liver biopsies had been done (a practice now abandoned) because of extreme hepatomegaly. Two of these showed very poor growth. The third showed normal growth, despite two admissions for hypoglycaemia and 14 for ketoacidosis in a two-year period. Yet hepatomegaly and poor social circumstances were both present.

The reader by now may be feeling confused. This is right and proper, because it is a very confusing situation, which is summarized in the next paragraph.

It is not denied that there is such a thing as poor diabetic control, but it is difficult to find a simple indicator of it. It we take growth as an indicator of poor control we cannot be certain of finding frequent ketosis, hyperglycaemia or even hepatomegaly in the background.

This statement can be inverted, and it can be said that though marked hepatomegaly is linked with poor growth an occasional child with hepatomegaly may grow well.

Others have claimed that height *is* adversely affected by poor diabetic control. Readers wishing to go further into the controversy will find appropriate references quoted by Jivani and Rayner (1973). We have now come back to the view that 'diabetic control is difficult to define in clinical terms'. Poor control is the outcome of pathological, physiological, psychological and inherited social conditions, all of which have to be assessed in each case.

In a letter, Rayner and Jivani (1973) stressed points they had made in a previous paper (Jivani and Rayner, 1973). They found that growth lag was present in the diabetic child, became most marked at the time of delayed puberty and was not fully compensated for by a relatively poor pubertal spurt. They also mention that, if anything, children with a tendency to hyperglycaemia grow better than the strictly controlled children; and that hyperglycaemia is less dangerous to a child's intellectual and physical development than hypoglycaemia. The Glasgow children were not followed through puberty, but in other respects the Glasgow figures are in accord with those suggestions. Very bad diabetic control may lead to dwarfing, as in the Mauriac syndrome, but bad control and hyperglycaemia are not simply related. Perhaps the most physiologically desirable level of blood sugar in a diabetic is slightly above the normal. It is a point worth considering.

INSULIN REQUIREMENTS

The need for insulin increases as a child grows older. Roughly speaking, he needs about 10 units a day at the age of two, up to 20 units when beginning school at the age of five, and up to 40 units at the age of ten years, but there is considerable individual variation. The amount of insulin needed does not necessarily reflect difficulty in control; a child having about 40 units a day may be well balanced, another child of the same age needing about 20 units a day may show marked fluctuations in his urine charts and clinical state. Chance (1969) mentions a child who had hypoglycaemic attacks on two units a day and was ketotic on 1 unit a day.

Priscilla White (1965) has described stages in the evolution of childhood diabetes in relation to insulin requirements. These stages are:

(1) initial stabilization;

(2) 'perfect' control, using little or no insulin;
(3) 'good' control, using small doses of insulin (10–20 units);
(4) an increase in insulin requirements, often sudden.

Stage (2) is the remission period, which usually lasts less than six months.

Stage (3) represents a period in which the pancreas is producing a little insulin, not enough to control the diabetes completely but presumably enough to supply a little endogenous insulin in time of need, and probably enough to take care of the night hours (when the child is taking no food) in particular. Such children may be satisfactorily controlled on a single morning injection of a medium-acting insulin (including Semitard or Semilente). In theory, others who respond well to exercise during the day might need only a small injection at night, but I have not met this situation. The regime has to be fitted to the child and not vice versa. Stage (3) may last three or four years.

Stage (4) represents 'total diabetes'. This often, but not invariably, coincides with the pre-pubertal growth spurt.

This outline refers, of course, to a child aged four or five years at the onset of diabetes. A girl becoming diabetic at the age of 12 years might find herself very quickly in Stage (4). Furthermore, the evolution of the disease can be altered greatly either by poor care or individual variation in diabetic stability. Nevertheless, this 'programme' is worth bearing in mind, and may be found useful when explaining an increase in insulin requirements to a worried parent. Parents as well as children may 'deny' diabetes and may condone the under-scoring of urine sugar levels by the child, in the mystic hope that low readings in the chart will keep 'total diabetes' at bay. An explanation of what is going to happen just as it begins to happen may nip deceit in the bud.

To state that the requirements rise to about 80 units in the three years before puberty is true of a mythical average, but conceals the fact that in the individual the rise may be dramatic. I have known a girl's requirements to rise from 40 to 100 units in six weeks, and stay at that high level thereafter, so the parents should be warned that this may happen. On the other hand, I saw recently a girl who had serenely passed through her menarche the previous week, still on only 26 units a day. The latter occurrence is rare, the former common. The pre-pubertal rise in insulin requirements also occurs in boys. It is not usually as marked in them as it is in girls, but it may be considerable.

REFERENCES

Baird, J. D. and Farquhar, J. W. (1962). Insulin-secreting capacity in newborn infants of normal and diabetic women. *Lancet*, **I**, 71

Beal, Carolyn K. (1948). Body size and growth rate in children with diabetes mellitus. *J. Pediat.*, **32**, 170

Boyd, J. D. and Nelson, M. V. (1928). Growth studies of children with diabetes mellitus. *Am. J. Dis. Child.*, **35**, 753

Burditt, A. F., Caird, F. I. and Draper, G. J. (1968). The natural history of diabetic retinopathy. *Quart. J. Med.*, **37**, 303

Chance, G. W. (1969). Out-patient management of diabetic children. *Br. med. J.*, **2**, 493

Craig, J. O. (1970). Growth as a measurement of control in the management of diabetic children. *Postgrad. med. J.*, **46**, 607

Dorchy, H., Ooms, H. and Loeb, H. (1975). Permanent neonatal diabetes mellitus: a case report with plasma insulin studies. *Z. Kinderheilk.*, **118**, 271

Ferguson, A. W. and Milner, R. D. G. (1970). Transient neonatal diabetes mellitus in sibs. *Arch. Dis. Childh.*, **45**, 80

Ferguson, I. C. (1967). Neonatal hyperglycaemia: case report with plasma insulin studies. *Arch. Dis. Childh.*, **42**, 509

Grajwer, L. A., Pildes, R. S., Horwitz, D. L. and Rubinstein, Z. H. (1977). Control of juvenile diabetes mellitus and its relationship to endogenous insulin secretion as measured by C-peptide immunoreactivity. *J. Pediat.*, **90**, 42

Hutchison, J. H., Keay, A. J. and Kerr, M. M. (1962). Congenital temporary diabetes mellitus. *Br. med. J.*, **II**, 436

Jivani, S. K. M. and Rayner, P. H. W. (1973). Does control influence the growth of diabetic children? *Arch. Dis. Childh.*, **48**, 109

Johansen, K. and Ørskov, H. (1969). Plasma insulin during remission in juvenile diabetes mellitus. *Br. med. J.*, **I**, 676

Kuna, P. and Addy, D. P. (1979). Transient neonatal diabetes mellitus. *Am. J. Dis. Child*, **133**, 65

Larsson, Y. and Sterky, G. (1962). Long-term prognosis in juvenile diabetes mellitus. *Acta paediat.*, **51**, Suppl. 130

Ludvigsson, J. and Heding, L. G. (1977). C-peptide in juvenile diabetes. *Acta paediat. Scand.*, Suppl. 270, 91

Ludvigsson, J., Heding, L. G., Larsson, Y. and Leander, E. (1977). C-peptide in juvenile diabetics beyond the postinitial remission period. *Acta paediat. Scand.*, **66**, 177

MacDonald, M. J. (1974). Neonatal diabetes. *Lancet*, **I**, 737

Pond, Helen (1970). 'Some aspects of growth in diabetic children. *Postgrad. med. J.*, **46**, 616

Rayner, P. H. W. and Jivani, S. K. M. (1973). Growth in diabetic children. *Lancet*, **II**, 1260

Sterky, G. (1963). Diabetic schoolchildren. *Acta paediat.*, **52**, Suppl. 144

Sterky, G. (1967). Growth pattern in juvenile diabetes. *Acta paediat.*, Suppl. 177, 80

Tanner, J. M. and Whitehouse, R. H. (1962). *Standards for Skeletal Maturity*. Paris; International Children's Centre

Tattersall, R. B. and Pyke, D. A. (1972). Diabetes in identical twins. *Lancet*, **II**, 1120

Weber, B. and Müller-Hess, R. (1972). Plasma insulin response versus clinical course in juvenile diabetics. *Acta paediat. Scand.*, **61**, 257

White, Priscilla (1965). The child with diabetes. *Med. Clin. N. Am.*, **49**, 1065

CHAPTER 10

The Aetiology of Diabetes

> The statements was interesting, but tough.
> Huckleberry Finn

> My wee laddie's wee doggy's the Duke of Argyll's head keeper's
> wee laddie's wee doggy's wee brother.
> (Traditional Scottish claim to kinship with the nobility)

It is well known that diabetes is commoner in some families than in others, but attempts to explain this by simple genetic theory led to complications similar to those in the quotation above. It must now be accepted that diabetes appears as a combination of many factors, hereditary, infective, dietetic and environmental.

HEREDITY

The elucidation of the genetic factor in diabetes is bedevilled by many variables.

(1) Diabetes may appear at any age. Even within the juvenile onset type of diabetes there may be stumbling blocks, for example a father may develop diabetes after his son.
(2) Juvenile onset and maturity onset diabetes are two diseases rather than one. They differ in many ways *(Table 10.1)*. This table alone does not establish that they are different diseases. We know that one disease may act differently at different ages, for example some forms of cancer progress rapidly in the young and may hardly advance at all in the very old.
(3) Diabetes may show a definite genetic pattern when it is linked

with other diseases such as Friedreich's ataxia (*see* Chapter 11). However, this genetic pattern may differ between families with different diseases. For example (a) 'DIDMOAD' (the syndrome of diabetes insipidus, diabetes mellitus, optic atrophy and deafness) appears to be transmitted as a recessive characteristic, but (b) 'MODY' (maturity onset type of diabetes appearing in the young) is transmitted as a dominant characteristic.

(4) Occasional families are found in which the incidence of diabetes is very high, not conforming to other 'rules' of diabetic inheritance.

TABLE 10.1

The differences between juvenile onset and maturity onset types of diabetes

Points of difference	Juvenile onset	Maturity onset
Age	Young	Elderly
Physique	Average	Often obese
Onset	Acute	Gradual
Symptoms	Severe	Mild
Plasma insulin	Eventually absent	May be normal
Ketosis	Ketotic	Non-ketotic
Treatment	Insulin dependent	Diet, oral agents
Stability	Unstable	Stable
Genetic factors	HLA	Present, but different
Islet cell antibodies	Very common	Rare

In addition to this, there may be difficulty in defining diabetes. Should chemical diabetes be classed simply as diabetes? This is sometimes done. Personally, I prefer to regard diabetes as a clinical diagnosis, particularly as a diminished glucose tolerance shown by testing may last a lifetime without frank diabetes appearing, but there is no denying that the two groups, the chemical and the clinical, may overlap.

Juvenile and maturity onset diabetes

It is important at this early stage of discussion to try to clarify the difference between the juvenile and maturity onset types of diabetes. The clinical differences have been mentioned. Differences between their modes of inheritance will now be considered.

The major study by Lestradet, Battistelli and Ledoux (1972) is of great interest. The families of 926 insulin-dependent child diabetics were studied, involving 11 733 persons, i.e. a ratio of one diabetic to 13 relatives. Insulin-dependent diabetes was found in 19.3 per cent of these families, non-insulin-dependent diabetes in 25.2 per cent. As controls the families of 300 non-diabetic children were studied, involving 4 060 persons (again a ratio of 1:13). In this group only 4.3 per cent of families showed insulin-dependent diabetes, but 26.6 per cent, virtually the same as in the study group, showed non-insulin dependent diabetes. Here again we have the impression that genetic factors are very important in the appearance of juvenile onset insulin-dependent diabetes. It should not be assumed from what has been written that maturity onset diabetes is *not* inherited. All that can be assumed is that if it is inherited it is not inherited in the same way as the juvenile onset type. There will be less confusion in the study of the heredity of diabetes if juvenile onset and maturity onset diabetes are regarded as two different diseases.

The recessive gene theory

A concept which for some time held the field was that diabetes was due to a single recessive gene, with emphasis subsequently being laid on its varying penetrance and expressivity in an effort to fit the theory to observed fact. On the recessive gene theory all the offspring of two diabetics should become diabetic, but this does not happen. The older studies do not discriminate between juvenile and maturity onset diabetes, which does not help the paediatrician. When the paediatrician talks of diabetic parents he is really concerned with parents who are diabetic when they consult him, i.e. during the childbearing age. Nor is the paediatrician very interested in whether this couple will have a child likely to become diabetic at the age of 60; he wants to know if they are likely to have a child who will develop juvenile onset diabetes. In a large study Pyke (1968) included 20 couples in whom diabetes had appeared in *one or both* before the age of 40. These 20 couples had borne 57 children of whom seven had become diabetic at the time of the study. There is an old figure (Cooke *et al.*, 1966) which estimates the chance of a child born to *two* diabetic parents as one in four, but this confuses juvenile onset and maturity onset diabetes and so could be an overestimate (by including maturity onset diabetes in the *children*) or an underestimate (by including maturity onset diabetes in the *parents*). Taking Pyke's figures into consideration it appears that the chance of a diabetic child being born to young parents, one or both of whom has diabetes, could be about one in eight, possibly rather worse than one in four if both parents are affected; but there is a lot of guessing on the way to that conclusion.

The child of one diabetic parent

If one parent is diabetic (not one or both, as studied by Pyke), the chance of him or her having a child who will develop diabetes has been calculated as one in 15. This figure is the result of studying occurrence rates, not of applying genetic theory. The words 'will develop' mean no more than they say: the diabetes may not appear until adult life. The risk of anybody developing diabetes in adult life is quite high, and the single diabetic parent can be reassured that 'one in 15' does not indicate an inordinate risk.

Siblings of diabetics

An investigation by the College of General Practitioners showed that 3.0 per cent of the siblings of diabetics were themselves diabetic. On the other hand, studies of identical twins have shown that if one twin becomes diabetic there is a 50:50 chance that the other twin will become diabetic also. The appearance of diabetes in each of a pair of identical twins has been separated by as much as 48 years, which underlines the difficulty of making genetic studies on diabetes and probably explains in part why observed findings are lower than calculated findings.

The inheritance of insulin antagonists

Vallance-Owen (1966) described the finding of a synalbumin insulin antagonist inherited as a dominant in a number of families. Various forms of stress could theoretically convert these 'essential' diabetics into overt diabetics. This theory is itself open to theoretical objections (for example insulin antagonism is not demonstrable in all diabetics) and it has not found universal acceptance in the years

'High-risk' families

Families in which the rate of diabetes is abnormally high do exist but are fortunately uncommon. Elsewhere in this book I have quoted the case of a family in which three children were diabetic by the time the eldest was seven and a half years, and a family tree is appended *(Figure 10.1)*.

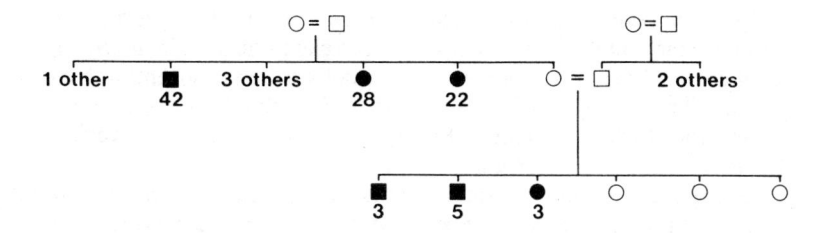

Figure 10.1. A family tree showing an unusually high rate of diabetes. The family is widely scattered and details of all members are not known but it is known that the woman who developed diabetes aged 42 has a diabetic child. In the youngest generation, all three affected children are identical for both haplotypes; as is one of the unaffected brothers, giving him an even chance of becoming diabetic in the future. (Numerals refer to age of onset of diabetes)

Since the first edition of this book this family has been subjected to HLA-typing. The three diabetic children are identical in HLA-typing, and one of the non-diabetic boys is also identical, so he must be considered a one-in-two risk *(Figure 10.1)*. The other two boys show markedly different HLA types.

ENVIRONMENTAL FACTORS

Diabetic mortality

The mortality rate from diabetes dropped by 40 per cent in Britain during and immediately after the Second World War, while rationing was in force (Himsworth, 1949). During the First World War it had dropped by 25 per cent while there was rationing. After the First World War diabetic mortality began to rise and the introduction of insulin in 1922 made no apparent impact on this rise. Admittedly, the period 1918–1922 was too short for a basic rate of rise to be established. Possibly the rise would have been steeper had there been no insulin, but even with insulin the pre-war mortality rate had been reached by 1935. It is true that all diabetics die sooner or later, but one could have expected a flattening of the mortality rate for several years after the introduction of insulin until those whose lives had been prolonged by insulin began to die in their later years. No such flattening occurred.

An explanation for the fall in mortality in wartime is not difficult to propose. Food was short, so there could be no dietary excess and, therefore, no diet-breaking. Unfortunately, it is much more difficult to fit the known facts to the theory. There was *no* fall in the average calories consumed, and attempts to correlate the fall in mortality with either a fall in fat or a rise in carbohydrate consumption have failed. The reason for the fall in mortality during hard times is not clear, and further attempts to find a cause would not even be theorizing, they would be guessing.

The overall rise in diabetic mortality in the years between the two World Wars could be explained by an increase in the prevalence of the disease, with insulin coming just in time to prevent a mortality explosion. As has been seen, it is dangerous to accept 'obvious' theories about diabetes, and it is worth looking at some morbidity figures.

Diabetic morbidity

Pyke (1968) remarks that 'there is a general impression that diabetes is becoming commoner', but points out that the population is ageing and that diagnostic methods are now simpler, so the apparent increase in diabetes may not be a true one. However, the childhood population, though increasing slightly in numbers, is not 'ageing', and in this age-group diagnostic methods are unimportant in the sense that the disease does not have to be sought but obtrudes itself on the consciousness of the physician, and has always done so. It is possible that a few cases of childhood diabetes of very rapid onset may die undiagnosed, but these cases cannot be many and can be assumed to occur in the same proportion to diagnosed cases whether the morbidity is rising or falling. It therefore seems pertinent to show the number of new cases seen each year at the Royal Hospital for Sick Children, Glasgow *(Figure 10.2)*.

It will be seen that there was a fall in morbidity of about 70 per cent during the Second World War. This dramatic fall can be partly

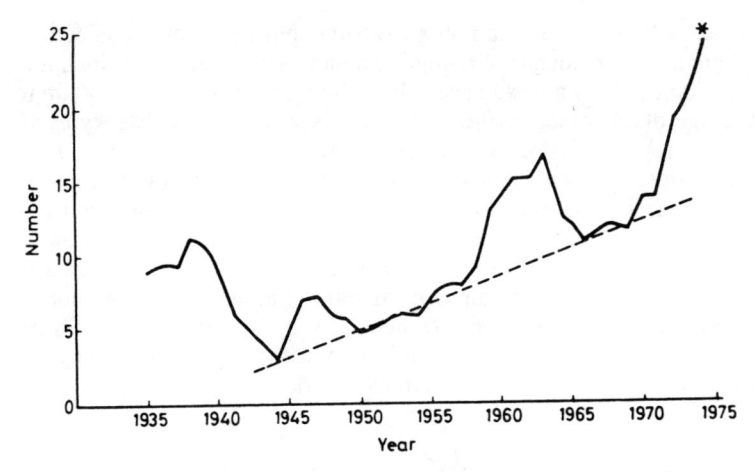

Figure 10.2. Number of new cases of diabetes mellitus seen at the RHSC each year, 1935–1974. More recent figures (Table 10.2 and Figure 10.5) *show a further rise to a new high plateau*

explained by the evacuation of many children from the city during the war, but the evacuation rate was not 70 per cent, nor did evacuation proceed steadily till 1944, as did the drop in morbidity.

After 1944 morbidity rises. It is true that such an increase in morbidity in childhood cannot be correlated directly in time with an increase in adult mortality; if the increased morbidity occurred only in childhood one would expect a gap of 40 or 50 years before it showed as an increase in adult mortality. It seems likely, then, that the figures for childhood are an indicator of a process happening throughout the population and that the 'general impression that diabetes is becoming commoner' is probably correct.

The graph of increasing incidence from the year 1944 has the appearance of being bi-factorial. A dotted line has been inserted (without attempting a statistical fit as the numbers are small) and this line suggests a basic rate of increase on which one small and two large peaks have been superimposed. The basic increase could be due to some genetic or environmental factor which is increasing slowly but constantly in its effect, such as a change in dietary habits or the adoption of a more sedentary life-style (although it is not suggested that these two things have occurred). The peaks could be caused by some other influence which appears and disappears, such as epidemics of infection, a possibility which is attracting considerable attention at present.

It is possible that the recent Glasgow figures represent a peak which will fall again to a rising base-line, but this is only conjecture. There is good evidence of rising incidence in other areas. Calnan and Peckham (1977) now suggest a British incidence of 1.42/1000 up to the age of 16, much higher than figures given before. Sterky et al. (1978) report a Swedish incidence of 1.3/1000 *up to the age of 14*, almost identical with British figures, and they go on to show marked variations between areas and from year to year in Sweden. The fluctuating Glasgow incidence has been discussed, and it can now be said that the rise seen in the 1970s was also noted in Edinburgh and Kirkaldy (i.e. through our central industrial belt) but was not as marked in Aberdeen and Dundee. Mann, Thorogood and Smith (1978) describe space-clustering in Oxfordshire. Deckert (1980) has found no significant recent rise in Denmark.

Seasonal incidence

> In the spring the air being impregnated with the salubrious effluvia of opening flowers, will be more refreshing than the autumnal air loaded with steams of putrefying vegetables, which, unless dispersed by wind frequent at that season, would soon produce fatal effects.
>
> Burton, *Non-naturals*, 1738*

A seasonal incidence in the appearance of juvenile diabetes mellitus has been the subject of comment since the 1920s. The maximal incidence is in the autumn and early winter. Extensive evidence to this effect is at present being collected in the British Diabetic Association study. In the meantime, *Figure 10.3* presents data from King's College Hospital, London, between 1955 and 1968, similar data from the Royal Hospital for Sick Children, Glasgow, for 1948–1968, and additional data from the RHSC for 1969–1974.

The curves resemble each other in two respects. They reach a peak about November, and they are low in the summer months. The use of three-month moving averages obscures some of the more dramatic findings. At King's College Hospital only two of 273 new cases first appeared in June. At the RHSC, in the period 1969–1974 not one of the 105 new cases appeared in June, yet during 1948–1968 there were 15 new cases in June out of a total of 188, i.e. it was an average

* The Non-naturals were Aliment, Air, Rest and Exercise, Sleep and Wakefulness, Repletion and Evacuation, and the Passions and Affections of the Mind. McKenzie (*The History of Health*, 1759) objected to the application of the word 'Non-naturals' to the essentials of life. 'The very sound of the epithet' he wrote, 'is extremely shocking'. He inveighed further against 'this ill-fancied appellation, which arose merely from the jargon of the Peripatetic schools' and finally lapsed into Latin to express the full measure of his indignation. Medicine still has its 'ill-fancied appellations'.

ENVIRONMENTAL FACTORS 217

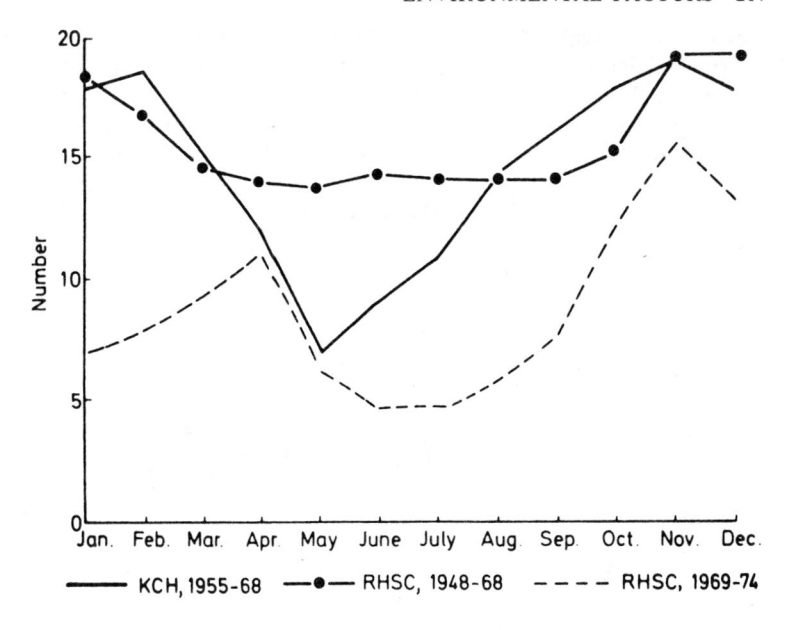

Figure 10.3. Total number of new cases seen each month at KCH and RHSC as three-monthly moving averages. Note the relatively high incidence in the summer months at RHSC in the period 1948–1968

month. In the period 1969–1974 the complete absence of new cases in June was offset by the appearance of 23 in November. It is unwise, however, to become too concerned about minutiae, particularly when unusual findings at one time are found to be commonplace at another, and all that should be derived from the figures so far submitted is that the onset of childhood diabetes is relatively common in the late autumn and early winter. However, the odd little variations mentioned do suggest that there may be some varying influence at work rather than, or as well as, some constant factor such as climate.

In *Figure 10.4*, the two sets of figures from the RHSC have been added together and compared with the King's College Hospital figures, no resort being made to moving averages. This form of presentation is used to coincide with that of Gamble (1974), and the year is shown as beginning on May Day for the same reason, not because of some pagan whim. The very low June figure for King's College Hospital still stands out, but otherwise the graphs coincide fairly well except that RHSC seems to lag by a month or two, possibly because it is 400 miles to the north-west of King's College

218 THE AETIOLOGY OF DIABETES

Hospital and possibly because the RHSC figures refer to the time of the first discharge from hospital and not to the first admission.

Figures obtained from the British Diabetic Association's Register of newly diagnosed diabetic children show a high incidence in the autumn and winter months, with peaks in October and January (Gamble, 1975). At the time of writing, the latest report on the Register was made by Bloom, Hayes and Gamble (1975).

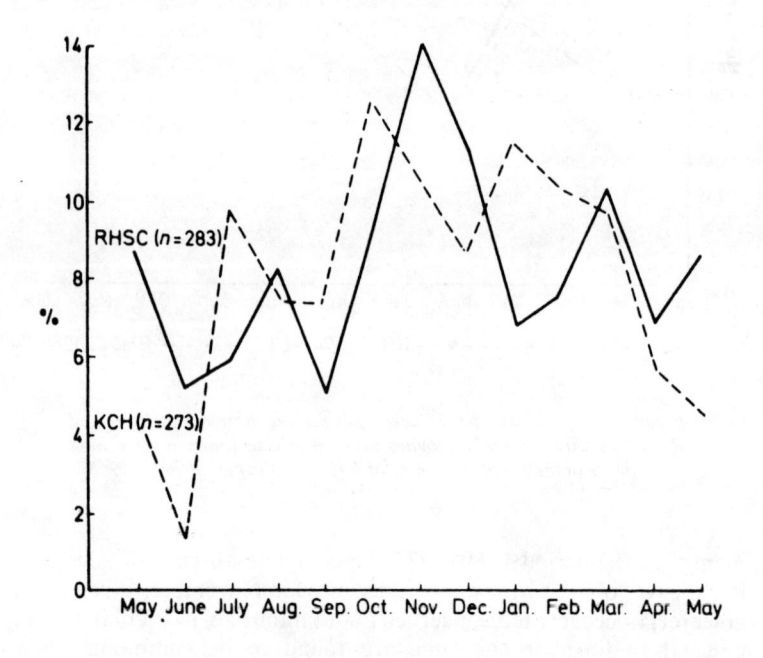

Figure 10.4. Total number of new cases seen each month at KCH and RHSC data as for Figure 10.3, but RHSC figures added together, 1948–1974

The RHSC figures from 1975 are set out in *Table 10.2*. It will be seen from the three-month moving averages that the pattern has reverted to that of 1948–1968, the winter high and summer low being less marked than in 1969–1974. Indeed, the only strikingly low summer month is July. It may be rather surprising to note that when a figure for one particular month is unusually high, that figure is usually isolated. The only sustained high spell is January to March, 1980. It is obviously dangerous to speculate from small numbers and it is better to wait for the next review from the National Register.

TABLE 10.2

Monthly incidence of new cases of diabetes,
January, 1975–July, 1980

Month	Year						Three-month moving average	Year
	1975	1976	1977	1978	1979	Total		1980
Jan	2	1	3	5	4	15	14.3	5
Feb	1	3	3	2	4	13	13.3	7
Mar	2	4	1	2	3	12	12.7	5
Apr	3	1	3	6	0	13	13.3	3
May	5	4	2	3	1	15	12.7	2
Jun	2	4	1	1	2	10	9.7	2
Jul	0	1	0	1	2	4	9.3	1
Aug	2	6	1	4	1	14	10.3	—
Sep	2	0	3	7	1	13	12.3	—
Oct	2	2	2	0	4	10	12.0	—
Nov	3	1	6	2	1	13	12.7	—
Dec	4	3	3	1	4	15	14.3	—
Total	28	30	28	34	27	147	—	(25)

Is infection a precipitating factor?

The role of infection in initiating diabetes in childhood will be considered under two headings, general and specific.

General considerations

The seasonal incidence of the onset of diabetes appears to be well established. The reasons for this incidence are not so clear. Earlier explanations have included the suggestions that it could be due to the nervous stress of returning to school, the relative inactivity during school hours, the shortness of daylight cutting down exercise or some climatological effect of cold or warmth. It now seems that Burton, with his 'steams of putrefying vegetables' may be as near the mark as any, if such steams are to be taken as symbolic of infection.

Gamble has found that the ages of maximal incidence are five and 11 years, the ages at which children in Britain either begin at school or move to a different school. This draws particular attention to nervous stress and infection as possible precipitants, but hardly diminishes the possibility that other factors (for example exercise and climate) may play important roles. It could still be that the really important precipitating cause, constant throughout childhood, is (say) lack of exercise, with infection only supervening to supply little peaks of incidence at five and 11 years. One must not jump to the conclusion that infection is the sole precipitant of childhood diabetes, or even the most important precipitant. This point is, I think, worth labouring, lest the present interest in the infection theory should slip into uncritical acceptance.

Gamble has also shown that children who begin school before the age of five (for example by attending nursery school) develop diabetes at an earlier age than those who start school later. By combining this fact with the age at which diabetes actually appears the concept emerges that it may take a year or two of repeated infections before diabetes finally manifests itself. Gamble raises the possibility that a combination of viruses may produce diabetes in the individual, and that the age of onset may vary with that combination.

At the run-of-the mill clinical level many physicians must have felt that certain cases of diabetes were brought on by infection. Little 'outbreaks' of diabetes occur. Six new diabetics were admitted to the RHSC, Glasgow in the first fortnight of October, 1974, nearly a quarter of the total for that year. Two sisters developed diabetes within a week of each other, immediately after 'measles'. Other clinicians have had like experiences, and the obvious explanation is infection acting in a specific way on insulin balance. One must resist the temptation to generalize from a few cases.

Specific evidence

There is a sizeable body of pathological evidence, reviewed by Doniach (1974), suggesting that infection may cause juvenile diabetes. Doniach's material included nine juvenile diabetics who had died untreated in the period 1907–1930, the bulk of such material obviously dating from the pre-insulin era. Seven of the nine showed reduction in the number of islets, which may show atrophy or hypertrophy, and in the beta-cells. The average weight of the pancreas was less than half of the normal for the age. The presence of inflammatory cells (lymphocytes, macrophages and a few polymorphs) has been described by Gepts (1965) but insulitis was not prominent in Doniach's series. Plasma cells were not obvious, which is against an immunological reaction without ruling it out entirely. Gepts' work is often quoted, but has not been universally confirmed. However, where insulitis has been recorded it has always been associated with a very acute history, so it is possible that insulitis, which is rare, is the result of direct infection.

Experimental evidence from animals seems stronger than pathological evidence from humans in incriminating viruses as potential precipitating agents of diabetes. Taylor (1974) provides a valuable introduction to the subject. A variant strain of the encephalomyocarditis virus has a specific effect on the islets of mice, producing insulin deficiency diabetes. Coxsackie B3 virus often produces pancreatitis in mice but affects the acinar more than the islet tissue, unless a particular strain of mice (CD1) is used. In that strain insulitis occurs, which hints at the importance of genetic factors. The same strain of mice inoculated with Coxsackie B4 show marked insulitis. The blood sugar tends to fall for about five days, suggesting the release of insulin from degenerating beta-cells, and then rises in the next two weeks to diabetic levels. The infiltration in the islets of these mice is lymphocytic in type.

This work involves two important principles.

(1) It is only a special strain of virus (M strain of EMC virus or B4 of Coxsackie) which will cause diabetes in mice.
(2) These viruses will only cause diabetes in special strains of mice, bred to be unduly susceptible to diabetes. We can inquire further into how far these principles operate in man. A study in 1969 showed antibodies to Coxsackie B4 in 65 per cent of diabetics and 41 per cent on non-diabetics and a further study of an older age-group (Gamble, Taylor and Cumming, 1973) raised the figures to 87 per cent and 65 per cent, very significant differences, though the question 'significant of what?' remains to be answered as controls and diabetics were not matched geographically. On the other hand, levels of antibodies to Coxsackie B1, B2, B3 and B5 showed no difference between diabetics and controls, so B4 stands suspect provided it invades a suitable host. That Coxsackie B4 *can* cause diabetes in man has recently been shown by Yoon *et al.* (1979) who isolated the virus from the pancreas of a boy who had died at the onset of diabetes, grew the virus in culture, injected it into a susceptible strain of mice who developed diabetes, and then found viral antigens in the necrosed B-cells of the mice.

The work done on Coxsackie B4 should not blind us to the fact that other viruses may be involved and indeed some have been implicated on less direct evidence.

(1) Diabetes may appear shortly after mumps (McCrae, 1963) or an increased incidence may be noted a year or two after an epidemic (McLaren, 1977; Sultz et al., 1975). Diabetes, even with ketoacidosis, may be a transient phenomenon during mumps, but mumps is a common disease and the association with diabetes may not be very strong.
(2) Oli and Nwokolo (1979), observing a small outbreak of diabetes after an epidemic of *infectious hepatitis* found that in about half the cases the diabetes was transient.
(3) *Coxsackie B2* seems to have precipitated one case of diabetes (Wilson et al., 1977).
(4) The rate of diabetes has been shown to be very high in survivors of congenital rubella (Menser, Forrest and Bramsby, 1978), of particular interest as there is a long interval between insult and the development of diabetes. It is worth dwelling for a moment on the possible gap that might exist between the original insult and the appearance of diabetes. Steel, Gray and Clarke (1979) found that 27 per cent of babies born to mothers who *subsequently* developed insulin-dependent diabetes were above the 90th centile for weight, arguing that the diabetic state in the mother may have been smouldering for a long time before it appeared.
(5) Ward, Galloway and Auchterlonie (1979) reported a case of diabetes appearing at the age of 13 months in a child with congenital *cytomegalovirus* infection.
(6) Pancreatitis has been reported with *infectious mononucleosis* (Burgess, Kirkpatrick and Menser, 1974).

It seems probable that infection is a precipitant of at least some cases of juvenile diabetes in man. What is known about the second principle mentioned above, the susceptibility of the host? This is discussed in the next section.

Susceptibility of the host: the HLA system

The HLA system may not be the only factor in determining if a child is susceptible to diabetes, even though the volume of recent literature gives that impression, but it is certainly a foot in the door to aetiology. The one thing certain about the HLA system is that whatever is written here will be out of date by the time it is printed.

It was first noted that certain alleles situated on chromosome 6 (HLA—A1, A2, B8, B15, B18, B40 and CW3) were about twice as common in insulin-dependent diabetes as in the general population (Cudworth and Woodrow, 1974, 1975; Nerup et al., 1974). It has since been realized that these alleles are linked to DW3 and DW4, these two latter factors being even more closely related to diabetes. The most recent arrival on the stage, a very promising newcomer, is a rare genetic type, BfF1, which so far has the closest relationship of all with diabetes mellitus. Raum et al. (1979) have detected it in 22.6 per cent of patients with insulin-dependent diabetes, but in only 1.9 per cent of the general population.

There is evidence that when two antigens are present in the same haplotype (B8 and B15, and probably B8 and B40) the possibility of diabetes appearing is increased still further. This does not apply to a double dose of the one high-risk antigen (for example, B8, B8 or B15, B15). It must be stressed that the simple possession of these factors does not imply that the carrier will develop diabetes. Indeed, the majority of people with B8 do *not* develop diabetes, but the *percentage* of people with B8 is higher among insulin-dependent diabetics.

It is desirable to say a word about haplotypes. A haplotype is that part of the genotype obtained from one parent only. The parent will transmit one of his or her two haplotypes to the child. The haplotype carries a number of HLA factors, not a single factor. If we simplify this by taking one letter to represent a haplotype carrying a number of factors, and if we represent one parent as AB and the other as CD, a child could be AC, AD, BC, or BD. AC and AD are identical for one haplotype, but if two children both are AC they are identical for two haplotypes, 'identical' meaning 'identical within the limits of our present knowledge'. What are the clinical implications of these statements? If two siblings have two identical haplotypes and one of them is diabetic, the chance of the other child developing insulin-dependent diabetes is one in two, the same as for identical twins. If a number of children in one family have diabetes they will probably each have two identical haplotypes, and will certainly develop diabetes closer to each other in time than if they had one identical haplotype (*see* p. 203, High-risk families). Furthermore, heaping Pelion on Ossa (which takes more effort than it is worth), a second child with two identical haplotypes is more likely to develop diabetes *in winter* than if he had one. These observations serve to show that quite recent theories on the inheritance of diabetes have been simplistic in the extreme.

It is probable that diabetic heredity depends on groups of antigens rather than single antigens and it is possible that certain groups of high-risk antigens may be inherited together as an autosomal recessive (Rubinstein, Suciu-Foca and Nicholson, 1977). This theory is still under discussion as it may be that two high-risk antigens acting on a single locus (over-dominance) can mimic recessive inheritance. The concept of gene-complexes is gaining ground (Bertrams et al., 1979).

In contrast to high-risk factors there are low-risk factors, for example B7 and DW2, which appear *less* often in diabetics than in the general population. To that extent they appear to be 'protective' against diabetes.

High-risk HLA antigens are associated with signs of autoimmunity, most simply the appearance, usually transient, of islet-cell antibodies (ICA or PICA). These ICA are present in 85 per cent of juvenile onset diabetics within a week of the first diagnosis of the disease but 16 years later in only 10 per cent, and the early and transient nature of their appearance has led in the past to underestimation of their presence. Thyroid, gastric and adrenal antibodies are also more common in juvenile diabetics than in the general population, implying that such diabetics have inherited a widespread defect in autoimmune mechanisms. It is thought that the 10 per cent who retain their ICA may form a rather different group as they have a later age of onset of diabetes and are predominantly female in a ratio of nearly 2:1. Autoimmune diseases such as hypothyroidism, Addison's disease and pernicious anaemia later in life are more common in diabetics than in the general population.

The HLA system in relation to infection

Are the ICA the cause of an attack on the islet cells or the result of it? Do T-lymphocytes lose their controlling influence over K-lymphocytes or do they themselves run wild, destroying islet cells? There is not yet agreement on the answers to those questions and until there is the carnage among the B-cells must remain hidden under the smoke of battle. At the end of the day the B-cells lie in ruins, a few viruses slink around, the lymphocytes dust themselves down and a troop of the ICA marches off into the blood stream. The high-risk HLA factors appear to have altered the normal response to viral infection into autoimmunity. A more learned discussion of this process is given by Farquhar (1979).

Summary

There is no doubt that infection and the HLA antigens play important roles in the aetiology of juvenile onset diabetes, but it cannot be assumed that they are the only cause. The last word on the subject may fairly go to Dodge and Laurence (1979) who have described for the first time congenital absence of the Islets of Langerhans in two siblings.

LOOKING FOR DIABETES

It could be argued that, while seeking for the cause of diabetes, we have so far only been looking at the tip of the iceberg. No mention has been made of the many 'normal' people at present walking the earth with latent or chemical diabetes, and it is possible that if they were brought into the discussion further light might be shed on the aetiology of diabetes. An adult with maturity onset diabetes may have sugar in the urine for months or years before he develops symptoms, but a child will only show sugar for days or weeks before becoming ill. Screening an adult population every year or two would reveal many cases of diabetes before symptoms had appeared. Screening a childhood population would have to be done every week or two for a like result to be obtained.

Screening all children for clinical diabetes or chemical diabetes is a useless exercise, but screening of potential diabetics for chemical diabetes is more realistic. At the research level it is fair to convert the term 'potential' diabetes into 'possible high risk' of diabetes, and various high-risk groups have been studied—obese children, siblings of diabetics and children with symptoms suggesting hypoglycaemic episodes (including those with symptomatic hypoglycaemia as neonates). Such screening will ultimately only prove justifiable if the results indicate that the eventual appearance of diabetes can be delayed or averted.

A large group of papers dealing with various aspects of screening in childhood was published in 1973 in *Metabolism*, vol. 22, pp. 209–420. Those daunted by such a reference will be glad to know that the results were summarized by Rosenbloom, Drash and Guthrie (1972, before the detailed reports appeared). Various high-risk groups were studied. Two hundred children with chemical diabetes were found. Of these, 11 per cent had developed insulin-dependent diabetes during a follow-up of one to 17 years. This is an impressive figure, but the 89 per cent who did not develop diabetes are also impressive in their own way, as they had been specially selected for screening because they were considered to be at special risk of developing diabetes. Thus screening gives valuable information about groups, but not about individuals. A child with an abnormal glucose tolerance test may revert to normal, stay much as he was or proceed to overt diabetes, and there is no obvious way of forecasting which course he will follow. If one could make such a forecast one would be nearer to the justification of screening, but full justification would only come if the information obtained were sufficient to avert diabetes. Until that day comes, screening is of some academic but no clinical value.

Screening can be done in many ways. The glucose tolerance test may be modified by giving cortisone before it. One can estimate the growth hormone response to intravenous glucose, tolbutamide or glucagon, or one can estimate the free fatty acid response to oral or intravenous glucose. Morphological studies may be made of the blood vessels, or one can study the normal haemoglobin component AL_cHbA_1 which is raised in diabetes, though not in chemical diabetes. None of these methods is of certain value in making a prognosis for the individual child.

Reports have been collected (Rosenbloom et al.) of 33 children considered at risk in whom attempts were made to delay the appearance of diabetes by giving sulphonylureas (for example tolbutamide). Follow-up ranging from two months to five years showed that carbohydrate intolerance improved in 19, was unchanged in two and was worse in 11. No worker could distinguish drug effect from natural history, so there seems little hope that treatment with the sulphonylureas will prove preventive.

Obesity is a rather different matter (Bloom, 1971). There is a theoretically effective method of treating obesity and curing obesity is in itself desirable, whether or not that prevents the appearance of diabetes. There is a higher percentage of obesity in adult diabetics than there is in the normal population. Obese non-diabetic adults have insulin levels which are above normal, which may also be the case in obese diabetics. This seems to represent an effort by insulin to maintain normoglycaemia, an effort which is hampered by the relative insensitivity of muscle and fat cells to the action of insulin, and suggests that the rational treatment is to reduce the mass of fat rather than give more insulin. It should be remembered, however, that under the age of 30 obesity is no more common in diabetics than it is in the normal population, and to put a fat child on a diet in order to prevent the appearance of diabetes is to make several unwarranted assumptions.

Chiumello et al. (1969) found no relationship between obesity and abnormal GTTs except in children with a strong family history of diabetes. The findings of Court et al. (1971) were in almost direct opposition. Twenty-seven of 46 obese children had abnormal GTTs, but no relationship was found between impaired glucose tolerance and a family history of diabetes. Drash (1973) studied 18 grossly obese adolescents, all of whom showed hyperinsulinism in response to glucose, glucagon or arginine. Seven of these, who had lower peaks of insulin response than the others, also showed some impairment of the GTT. Weight loss was achieved by diet in hospital, but attempts to maintain this on an outpatient basis were not successful, an experience all too common in the treatment of obesity. Nevertheless in a follow-up extending to three years no case of overt diabetes had appeared. One can sense some of the pent-up irritation that always accompanies attempts to treat obesity in Drash's comment that the only satisfactory approach to obesity is prevention, and that parents should realize that 'the maintenance of normal body weight is as important as immunizations and the treatment of infectious diseases'. So far, however, no clear-cut connection has been demonstrated between childhood obesity and juvenile diabetes.

It appears, then, that screening tests for childhood diabetes based on carbohydrate tolerance, even in children particularly at risk, are unlikely to yield much of value. The GTT cannot be taken as a completely reliable guide to the future, and too much worry about a doubtful result might cause unnecessary anxiety for years. I have never been asked by a parent to carry out such a screening test on the sibling of a diabetic, but if I were I would only do so if I thought parental anxiety was already so great that testing could only allay rather than increase that anxiety. Otherwise I would say that such screening tests are not reliable. It is also possible to envisage a situation where a screening test might generate not only anxiety but guilt. Suppose that an obese sibling with an abnormal GTT failed to lose weight (which is likely) and then did develop diabetes, would not a feeling of guilt be added to the other anxieties of the disease? I do not know, but see little point in taking the chance. It seems to me that the only clinical value of a screening test is to allay gross familial anxiety, and that it cannot give adequate warning of impending diabetes. A screening test should be regarded as no more than a tool in research. In clinical practice, let sleeping dogs lie.

Diabetes in developing countries

It may be that what has just been written about the aetiology of diabetes does not apply in some of the developing countries. The number of diabetics with first degree relatives who are also diabetic has been quoted as 21.2 per cent in Britain, but in Malaysia it is 0.5 per cent and in Bangladesh 0.2 per cent. Perhaps much of this difference lies in difficulty in case-finding, but even so the difference is so striking that one must suspect that the hereditary factor is low in the two latter countries. Oli *et al.* (1980) raise another possible point of difference when they point out that islet cell antibodies appear to

228 THE AETIOLOGY OF DIABETES

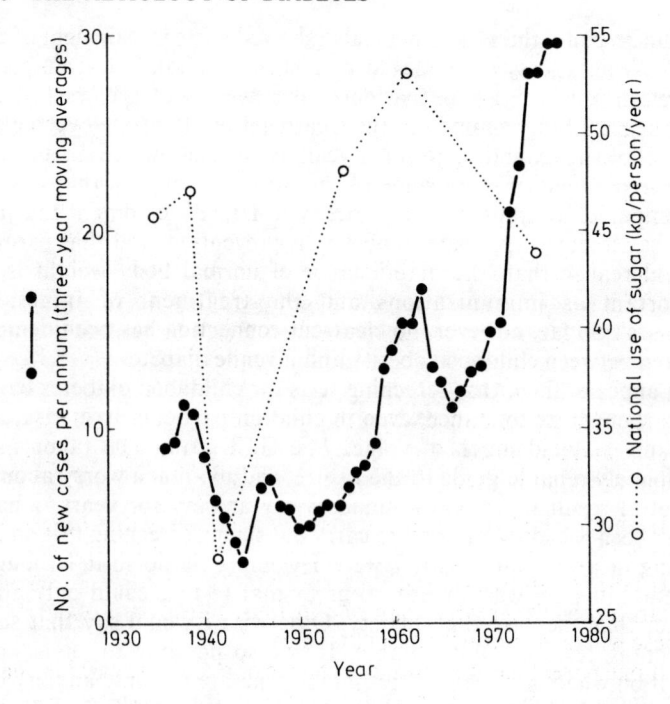

Figure 10.5. The national sugar intake compared with the occurrence of childhood diabetes in the RHSC, Glasgow. (Although a little British sugar comes from sugar beet, virtually all is imported and the National Use is derived from the imported tonnage, thus covering loose sugar and that used in jams, candies, and other manufactured products.) The graphs 'fit' until the late 1960s, but thereafter diverge markedly, a nice example of 'proof by association' coming unstuck

be much less common in juvenile-onset Nigerian diabetics than in whites. Apart from the family history, the incidence of diabetes seems to vary from nation to nation. It is rare among the Eskimo, extremely common in certain Red Indian tribes now living a 'civilized' life. It appears that the more advanced a civilization the more diabetes there is, possibly an extension of the observation already made that diabetes is less common in time of war. Commercially purified sugar has been blamed by some as causing diabetes. That it does not seem to do so in *juvenile* diabetics in the Glasgow area is shown by *Figure 10.5*. Diabetes has been described as a 'thrifty genotype', lying hidden in times of starvation and want and thus interfering not at all with the survival of a race under pressure, but becoming manifest when the survival of the race seems assured*. It certainly appears to be true that diabetic morbidity rises when the living conditions of immigrant or subject races are improved. This might be due to a more liberal diet, to a fall in physical exertion, to exposure to new infections or to other unidentified factors. Whatever the cause, it appears to be a fact.

Counselling

If ever HLA-typing becomes generalized it will be possible to state more accurately the risk of a child becoming diabetic. At present, however, we must still rely on observed occurrence rates, slowly being revised by disentangling juvenile onset from maturity onset diabetes, and the conclusions that can be drawn from them. Approximations are summarized below.

(1) If an identical twin has diabetes the chances of the other twin developing diabetes are one in two.
(2) If both parents have diabetes, the chances of a child developing it are probably greater than one in four, but a bare majority of these will have maturity onset diabetes.
(3) If one parent has diabetes, the chance of a diabetic child is one in 15, including maturity onset diabetes. This forecast may be a little optimistic.
(4) If a child has diabetes and does not qualify under (1)–(3) above, the chance of a sibling developing it is one in 33, but if a sibling can be shown by HLA-typing to carry two haplotypes identical with the proband the chance is as high as one in two.

Provided he is sure that his questioner understands what has been said about rates of probability a counsellor has no moral right to offer advice. If two diabetic adults want to marry, that is their own business. If they ask me if they *should* marry, then it becomes my business. There is really very little bar to diabetics marrying. Diabetes is not a fatal disease, like cystic fibrosis; the chances of it being transmitted are not very high; and it may not appear until relatively late in life.

Counselling may become a matter of personality assessment. In a recent letter to *Balance*, the journal of the British Diabetic

---

* I cannot resist dragging in at this point the case of a certain strain of diabetic fat mice, referred to by Pyke. The homozygous mice are so fat and such noted trencher-mice that in times of abundance they become too fat to copulate, leaving it to the slimmer heterozygous mice to perpetuate the race. The analogy is obscure, but possibly a principle is involved somewhere.

Association, a diabetic mother described the guilt she felt when her son developed diabetes at the age of 12. I do not suggest that one could identify such a mother at a single interview but, having read that letter, I think one might include the question 'What would you feel like if you *did* have a child with diabetes?', to give one the opportunity to quell guilt feelings before they arise, or at least to give the subject an initial airing. It is consoling to remember, in this difficult situation, that the couple will probably do what they feel like doing, whatever I may say. If a couple who already have a diabetic child decide they do not want another child they may not be very fond of children anyway.

Can diabetes be prevented?

The possibility of preventing diabetes is the subject of a review by Farquhar (1979). The situation can be summarized thus:

(1) HLA-screening may show siblings at special risk of diabetes.
(2) Inoculation of these siblings, or indeed all the siblings, against viruses (Coxsackie B4 and such as may be identified in the future) might prevent future diabetes.
(3) Poor control of diabetic pregnancy in the past may have allowed insulin antibodies from the mother and/or the overstimulated B-cells to produce an auto-aggressive response in the fetal B-cells, heralding possible diabetes in the future. Purified porcine insulins might help here.

Such a programme might be costly, but when one considers the cost of being diabetic for life it might well turn out to be economic in the long run. The possibility of preventing even a few cases is a new ray of light that, ten years ago, few would ever have expected to see.

REFERENCES

Bertrams, J., Baur, M. F., Gruneklee, D. and Gries, F. A. (1979). Association of BfFl, HLA–B18 and insulin-dependent diabetes mellitus. *Lancet*, **2,** 98

Bloom, A. (1971). Obesity and diabetes. *Postgrad. med. J.*, **47,** 430

Bloom, A., Hayes, T. M. and Gamble, D. R. (1975). Register of newly diagnosed diabetic children. *Br. med. J.*, **3,** 580

Burgess, J. A., Kirkpatrick, K. L. and Menser, M. A. (1974). Fulminant onset of diabetes mellitus during an attack of infectious mononucleosis. *Med. J. Aust*, **2,** 706

Calnan, M. and Peckham, C. S. (1977). Incidence of insulin-dependent diabetes in the first sixteen years of life. *Lancet*, **1,** 589

REFERENCES

Chiumello, G., Guercio, M. J. D., Carnelutti, M. and Bidone, G. (1969). Relationship between obesity, clinical diabetes and beta-pancreatic function in children. *Diabetes*, **18**, 238

Cooke, A. M., Fitzgerald, M. G., Malins, J. and Pyke, D. A. (1966). Diabetes in children of diabetic couples. *Br. med. J.*, **II**, 674

Court, J. M., Dunlop, M., Leonard, I. and Leonard, R. F. (1971). Five-hour oral glucose tolerance test in obese children. *Arch. Dis. Child.*, **46**, 791

Cudworth, A. G. and Woodrow, J. C. (1974). HL-A antigens and diabetes mellitus. *Lancet*, **II**, 1153

Cudworth, A. G. and Woodrow, J. C. (1975). Evidence for HL-A linked genes in juvenile diabetes mellitus. *Br. med. J.*, **3**, 133

Cudworth, A. G. and Feldenstein, H. (1978). HLA genetic heterogeneity in diabetes mellitus. *Med. Bull.*, **34**, 285

Deckert, T. (1979). Childhood diabetes and diet in Scotland (in discussion). *Pediat. adolesc. Endocr.*, **7**, 26

Dodge, J. A. and Laurence, K. M. (1977). Congenital absence of islets of Langerhans. *Arch. Dis. Childh.*, **52**, 411

Doniach, I. (1974). Post-mortem histology of the islets of Langerhans in juvenile diabetes mellitus. *Postgrad. med. J.*, **50**, 544

Drash, A. (1973). Relationship between diabetes and obesity in the child. *Metabolism*, **22**, 337

Farquhar, J. W. (1979). Juvenile diabetes mellitus: possibility of prevention. *Arch. Dis. Childh.*, **54**, 569 (gives 134 references)

Gamble, D. R. (1974). Epidemiological and virological observations on juvenile diabetes. *Postgrad. med. J.*, **50**, 538

Gamble, D. R. (1975). Diabetes mellitus: viral and epidemiological studies. *Proc. R. Soc. Med.*, **68**, 256

Gamble, D. R., Taylor, K. W. and Cumming, H. (1973). Viral antibodies in diabetes mellitus. *Br. med. J.*, **3**, 627

Ganda, O. P. and Soeldner, J. S. (1977). Genetic, acquired and related factors in the etiology of diabetes mellitus. *Arch. intern. Med.*, **137**, 461

Gepts, W. (1965). Pathologic anatomy of the pancreas in juvenile diabetes mellitus. *Diabetes*, **14**, 619

Himsworth, H. P. (1949). The syndrome of diabetes mellitus and its causes. *Lancet*, **I**, 465

Lestradet, H., Battistelli, J. and Ledoux, M. (1972). L'hérédité dans le diabète infantile. *Diabète*, **20**, 17 (Abstracted in *Novodok*, 72–1360)

McCrae, W. M. (1963). Diabetes mellitus following mumps. *Lancet*, **I**, 1300

McLaren, N. K. (1977). Viral and immunological bases of beta-cell failure in insulin-dependent diabetes. *Am. J. Dis. Child.*, **131**, 1149

Mann, J. I., Thorogood, M. and Smith, P. G. (1978). Space clustering of juvenile-onset diabetes. *Lancet*, **1**, 1369

Menser, M. A., Forrest, J. M. and Bransby, R. D. (1978). Rubella infection and diabetes mellitus. *Lancet*, **1**, 57

Nerup, J., Platz, P., Andersen, O. O., Christy, M., Lyngsoe, J., Poulsen, J. E., Ryder, L. P., Nielsen, L. S., Thomsen, M. and Svejgaard, A. (1974). HL-A antigens and diabetes mellitus. *Lancet*, **ii**, 864

Oli, J. M., Bottazzo, G. F. and Doniach, D. (1980). Islet-cell antibodies in Nigerian diabetics. *Lancet*, **1**, 1090

Oli, J. M. and Nwokolo, C. (1979). Diabetes after infectious hepatitis: a follow-up study. *Br. med. J.*, **1**, 926 (see also Correction, *ibid.*, p. 1324)

Pyke, D. A. (1968). In *Clinical Diabetes and its Biochemical Basis.* p. 210. Ed. Oakley, W. G., Pyke, D. A. and Taylor, K. W. Oxford; Blackwell

Raum, D., Alper, C. A., Stein, R. and Gabbay, K. H. (1979). Genetic marker for insulin-dependent diabetes mellitus. *Lancet,* **1,** 1208

Rosenbloom, A. L., Drash, A. and Guthrie, R. (1972). Chemical diabetes in childhood: report of a conference. *Diabetes,* **21,** 45

Rubinstein, P., Suciu-Foca, N. and Nicholson, J. F. (1977). Genetics of juvenile diabetes mellitus: a recessive gene closely linked to HLA D and with 50 per cent penetrance. *New Engl. J. Med.,* **297,** 1036

Steel, J. M., Gray, R. S. and Clarke, B. F. (1979). Obstetric history of diabetics: its relevance to the aetiology of diabetes. *Br. med. J.,* **1,** 1303

Sterky, G., Holmgren, G., Gustavson, K. H., Larsson, Y., Lundmark, K. M., Nilsson, K. O., Samuelson, G., Thalme, B. and Wall, S. (1978). The incidence of diabetes in Swedish children, 1970–1975. *Acta paediat. Scand.,* **67,** 139

Sultz, H. A., Hart, B. A., Zielezny, M. and Schlesinger, E. R. (1975). Is mumps virus an etiologic factor in juvenile diabetes mellitus? *J. Pediat.,* **86,** 654

Taylor, K. W. (1974). Viruses in experimental and human diabetes. *Postgrad. med. J.,* **50,** 546

Vallance-Owen, J. (1966). The inheritance of essential diabetes mellitus from studies of the synalbumin insulin antagonist. *Diabetologia,* **2,** 248

Ward, K. P., Galloway, W. H. and Auchterlonie, I. A. (1979). Congenital cytomegalovirus infection and diabetes. *Lancet,* **1,** 497

Wilson, C., Connolly, J. H. and Thomson, D. (1977). Coxsackie B2 virus infection and acute-onset diabetes in a child. *Br. med. J.,* **1,** 1008

Yoon, J-W., Austin, M., Onodera, T. and Notkins, A. L. (1979). Virus-induced diabetes mellitus. *New Engl. J. Med.,* **300,** 1173

CHAPTER 11

Diabetes Associated with Other Diseases

> They lard their lean books with the fat of others' work.
> Burton, *Anatomy of Melancholy*.

Diabetes may appear in association with another disease either because the pancreas has been directly affected (pancreatic diabetes) or because there is a genetic link with another disease. This genetic link may be direct, or it may represent no more than a shared tendency to autoimmune disease.

PANCREATIC DIABETES

'Pancreatic diabetes' is a term used for those cases of diabetes which follow destruction or removal of all elements of the pancreas, in whole or in part. Patients who have survived pancreatectomy need relatively little insulin, often less than 40 units in the day, which emphasizes the importance of insulin antagonism in juvenile diabetes, as many juvenile diabetics need more insulin than that. However, despite the low dose of insulin, many of the post-pancreatectomy patients have unstable diabetes, which underlines the fact that those on high doses of insulin are not necessarily the least stable.

Ketosis may occur in pancreatic diabetes, though it is reputedly less common than in juvenile diabetes mellitus. Complications are believed to be less common in pancreatic diabetes but it is difficult to be certain of this as post-pancreatectomy patients as a rule do not live long. Whether they are less common is largely immaterial, as they certainly may occur.

Pancreatic diabetes may be classified as follows.

Cystic fibrosis (CF)

Rosan, Schwachman and Kulczycki (1962) describe ten children with cystic fibrosis who went on to develop diabetes. The survival time after the appearance of diabetes might be as little as a month or two, but several were still alive six or seven years after the diagnosis of diabetes. My own experience has been more limited and less fortunate. Of three patients known to me, two died within months of the appearance of diabetes. The third was last heard of still alive after several years, having gone through a secretarial course and taken up a job in an office.

These children are difficult to treat. Lung infection encourages loss of diabetic control, and loss of diabetic control encourages lung infection. While the lung infection is severe, ketosis is common, but while the lung infection is under reasonable control there may be heavy persistent glycosuria without ketosis. There is a failure of absorption of protein and fat in cystic fibrosis and the intake of carbohydrate must therefore be high. I have the clinical impression that these children seem brighter and healthier when on a high carbohydrate, high insulin regime.

The reason for the appearance of diabetes in cystic fibrosis seems cut and dried, the crushing of islet tissue by progressive fibrosis in the pancreas. It is not now certain that this explanation is correct. Although it is known that there is a degree of insulinopenia (short of frank diabetes) in about 40 per cent of patients with CF, the islet tissue has appeared histologically normal. There has also been demonstrated in children with CF *and in their parents* a factor which interferes with the transport of sugar, which could affect either the entero-insular axis or the pancreatic cells themselves. The parents of CF children excrete less insulin than normal controls (Goodchild and Brown, 1972). This evidence is enough to rock the boat, but not enough to exclude pancreatic fibrosis as the eventual cause of the diabetes, and Kjellman and Larsson (1975) hold to the view that fibrosis is the important clinical factor.

Pancreatectomy

In childhood, partial pancreatectomy is most likely to be done to eradicate an insulinoma leaving too little pancreas behind for adequate insulin production. Kim, Johnson and MacMillan (1973) describe an infant with hyperplasia of the islets who still suffered hypoglycaemic attacks even after removal of 85 per cent of the pancreas. Total pancreatectomy was therefore carried out and the child was maintained on insulin but, after appearing to do well, the child developed hyperosmolar non-ketotic coma and subsequently died.

Haemochromatosis

Excess iron deposits in the body are found in haemochromatosis, particularly in liver, heart and pancreas. It exists in two main forms, idiopathic and acquired, the latter being due either to repeated blood transfusions or to an excessive intake of iron.

Idiopathic haemochromatosis has a familial element, has been associated with malnutrition and alcoholism and is essentially a disease of middle age. It has been recorded in a boy of 13 years, but really does not come within the scope of this book. Walsh, Malins and Bloom (1978) reinforce the opinion that the diabetes of the idiopathic form may not be due to secondary islet destruction but to a genetic link between the two diseases.

Acquired haemochromatosis could well occur in those children who receive repeated transfusions for such disorders as erythrogenesis imperfecta, but in fact the interference with organ function which is seen in the idiopathic type is uncommon, so diabetes is relatively rare. Haemochromatosis due to excess iron ingestion has been reported among primitive peoples using iron cooking pots, but is little more than a medical curiosity.

Ketosis is relatively uncommon. Oakley (1968) reports only four episodes of ketosis in 13 patients, but found that all patients needed insulin and a moderate degree of insulin resistance was common. This provides another example of stable diabetes in the presence of a need for moderately high insulin dosage.

Chronic pancreatitis

This is a rare cause of diabetes, particularly so in children, though its onset in adult life has been traced back to childhood. It is more likely to be detected by finding glycosuria while investigating steatorrhoea, or by noticing calcification in the pancreas in an x-ray of the abdomen, rather than by any symptomatic manifestation. The bile duct and pancreatic duct enter the ampulla of Väter together; infection of the bile duct may lead to chronic pancreatitis, and calculus formation may aggravate it. The implication, however, is that chronic pancreatitis is essentially a disease of adult life.

Hereditary pancreatitis manifesting itself in childhood appears to be relatively common in the USA, but not in the UK. Sibert (1975) found it in only one of nine cases. In four of these nine the cause of pancreatitis was not apparent; the others followed viral infection or trauma.

Exceptional circumstances may exist in East Africa, where chronic pancreatitis with calcification is relatively common and most of those who have it die before the age of 45. This argues an onset at a relatively early age, but even in East Africa one would not expect to see it in childhood. As might be expected, malnutrition and alcohol have been suggested as aetiological factors.

DIABETES AND THE DUCTLESS GLANDS

The relationship between diabetes and the ductless glands is twofold.

(1) Diabetes may be secondary to a disease in a ductless gland, for example a pituitary adenoma or a phaeochromocytoma.
(2) Diabetes and a disorder of a ductless gland may coexist from a common cause, a tendency to develop autoimmunity.

The first group of disorders is described here.

The pituitary

Diabetes mellitus is found in about 10–15 per cent of cases of *acromegaly*, a disease which is associated with a high level of growth hormone, an insulin antagonist. Circulating insulin levels are normal, but inadequate in the circumstances, and the acromegalic often needs a high dose of insulin. It is true that acromegaly is a disease of adult life, but its omission here would have looked more peculiar than its inclusion. The childhood equivalent of acromegaly is pituitary gigantism, but I do not know of a case combining this disorder and diabetes.

The adrenal

Although a *phaeochromocytoma* may arise wherever there is chromaffin tissue, for example in the sympathetic chain, it is classically a tumour of the adrenal and is therefore included here. The tumour produces catecholamines and results in hypertension usually, but not always, paroxysmal, with which glycosuria may be associated. It may also produce attacks of low-grade fever, headache, tachycardia and malaise, and if the blood pressure is not measured an erroneous diagnosis of primary diabetes mellitus (or even 'virus infection, unspecified' in the absence of urine-testing) may be made.

Correct diagnosis is essential, as the logical treatment of the glucosuria is not by insulin but by removal of the tumour.

Cushing's syndrome is produced by overactivity of the adrenal cortex (either from hyperplasia, adenoma or adenocarcinoma), associated with an overproduction of glucocorticoids which may produce diabetes mellitus in two forms. These two forms are more easily understood if an underlying tendency to diabetes is present in some but not in others. In those with this tendency, Cushing's syndrome may push them over the brink into frank clinical diabetes mellitus. In those without the tendency diabetes may be manifest only as hyperglycaemia, glycosuria and pruritus, with little or no thirst, polyuria or ketosis. Whatever the underlying cause, the two different forms exist.

The thyroid

Thyrotoxicosis produces an abnormal glucose tolerance curve rather than overt diabetes. Thyroxine appears to speed the absorption of sugar from the gut, with a sharp rise in the blood sugar at half an hour or an hour, but not thereafter. As would be expected, an intravenous GTT is normal in thyrotoxicosis. Diabetes has been reported to occur in some women, who were obese but otherwise normal, and who had taken thyroid unnecessarily in an effort to slim, but this does not apply in childhood.

DIABETES AS AN AUTOIMMUNE DISEASE

The concept of juvenile diabetes mellitus as an autoimmune disease resulted originally more from its association with other autoimmune diseases than from direct proof of the autoimmune nature of diabetes. Antibodies to gastric parietal cells and thyroid cytoplasm in the serum of juvenile diabetics are twice as common as in the serum of controls. These antibodies are fairly common (in about 7 per cent) of the population as a whole. Antibodies to intrinsic factor and adrenal cortex are very rare, but both are found in diabetics much more often than in controls.

Islet cell antibodies have now been convincingly demonstrated in the sera of almost 50 per cent of juvenile diabetics of recent onset (Lendrum, Walker and Gamble 1975), and many of those scored as negative were in fact doubtfully positive. These antibodies are very rare in adult diabetics even when they are insulin-dependent, so the antibodies may be present for only a short period. Their detection in children does, however, strengthen the impression that autoimmunity is of importance in precipitating diabetes in some children. Further evidence is supplied by Bottazzo, Florin-Christensen and Doniach (1974) and MacCuish et al. (1974).

The type of insulitis which is found in some juvenile diabetics, a perivascular cuffing, is also reminiscent of autoimmune disease. A similar lesion may be found in adrenalitis and thyroiditis, but is never seen in adult diabetics. Insulin-dependent diabetics show inhibition of lymphocyte migration, but elderly diabetics do not.

It is not suggested that all cases of diabetes have an autoimmune basis, only that some cases of the juvenile type probably have it. This subject has been discussed in the previous chapter on aetiology.

COELIAC DISEASE AND DIABETES

The clinical association between coeliac disease and diabetes mellitus was reported as an oddity by Walker-Smith and Grigor (1969) in a letter to the *Lancet*. This provoked a considerable correspondence suggesting that the association was not as uncommon as might be supposed, although it was necessary to differentiate between coeliac disease and non-coeliac steatorrhoea.

Hooft, Devos and van Damme (1969) have investigated gastrointestinal function in 19 *unselected* diabetics. Thirteen showed some evidence of malabsorption, although the majority of these did not have diarrhoea. Steatorrhoea might or might not be present. Of the six jejunal biopsies performed, four were normal and two showed 'flattened villi'. There was thus evidence that malabsorption and steatorrhoea were unexpectedly common in juvenile diabetes, but almost always clinically silent.

Visakorpi (1969), writing from Finland, stated that in his experience 4 per cent of all coeliacs and 10 per cent of those diagnosed after the age of two years developed diabetes. He quoted five cases, in which diabetes appeared anything from one month to eight years after coeliac disease was diagnosed. Although coeliac disease diagnosed before the age of one year may be followed by diabetes, the impression gained from the literature is that it is the coeliac of relatively late onset who is most likely to develop diabetes. This is certainly true of the three coeliac diabetics who have recently passed through the clinic at the Royal Hospital for Sick Children, Glasgow. In one of Visakorpi's cases diabetes preceded coeliac disease. This is unusual, but is enough to suggest that when malabsorption and diabetes occur together one should not be regarded as a complication of the other, which in turn suggests that there may be a common immunological link. This link may well be the HLA-B8 antigen which is present in 80 per cent of children with coeliac disease (McNeish, Nelson and Mackintosh, 1973) and in 54 per cent of juvenile diabetics (Cudworth and Woodrow, 1974).

Children with coeliac disease and diabetes combined present no great theoretical problem. Two of our three cases have done well. The only deviation from the routine treatment of diabetes is that gluten must be excluded from the diet. The customary generous supply of carbohydrate is given and two of our patients have seemed perfectly happy and under no particular strain. The growth spurt which follows treatment of the coeliac disease appears to be uninhibited by the presence of diabetes (*Figure 11.1*).

This boy began treatment for both diseases at the age of five and a half years, when his height was on the 10th centile. It had reached the 50th centile by the age of seven years and remained there till he was 12. There was a slight falling off at 13 years, when his bone-age was 11.8 years.

One of our three patients did badly. She had coeliac disease and unstable diabetes which was difficult to control even in hospital. In addition she was mentally retarded, had urinary incontinence (which made urine testing capricious), and she lived in poor social circumstances. It is perhaps not surprising that she died in her teens with her liver full of glycogen, her case finally being reported by Manderson *et al.* (1968). The main adverse factors here were that neither her diabetes nor her coeliac disease were adequately controlled. If a similar child fails to thrive in a good home environment the original diagnosis of coeliac disease may be wrong. Steatorrhoea plus *partial* villous atrophy do not add up to a safe diagnosis of coeliac disease.

A summary can be given at this point:

(1) Many juvenile diabetics show malabsorption, either clinically or subclinically.

(2) Diabetics may have steatorrhoea without having coeliac disease.
(3) There is, however, a link between diabetes and coeliac disease.
(4) A child with coeliac disease and diabetes at the same time should do well, in a good home.

A combination of coeliac disease, diabetes mellitus and hyperthyroidism in the same patient has been reported by Chambers (1975). A familial syndrome of diabetes mellitus, IgA deficiency, malabsorption and the HLA haplotype A2, B8 and DW3 has been described (Van Thiel *et al.*, 1977). This leads on to the next section.

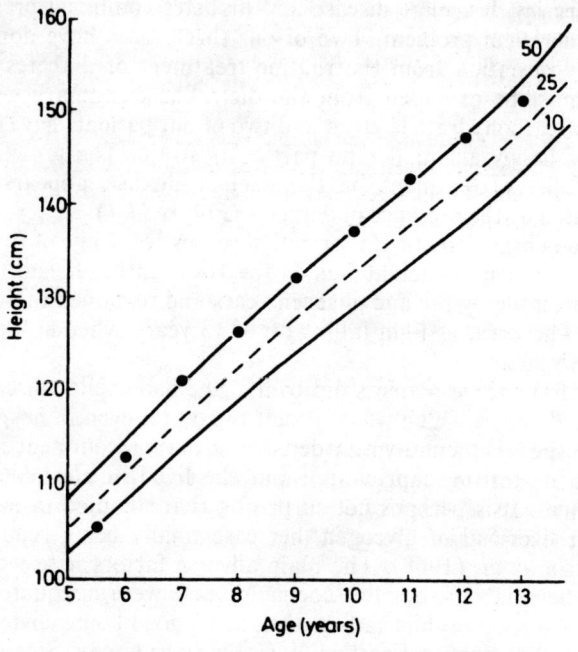

Figure 11.1. Growth of a boy in whom diabetes mellitus and coeliac disease were diagnosed almost simultaneously at the age of five and a half years, the late onset of coeliac disease being the rule when it is associated with diabetes. Diabetes does not prevent the growth spurt which occurs when coeliac disease is treated, but apparently declares itself in the pre-pubertal lag in height, which in this boy falls well below the 50th centile. The 10th, 25th and 50th centiles are shown, and are taken from the Tanner–Whitehouse charts

THYROIDITIS AND DIABETES

In 1972, Green and Winter described 21 patients with thyroiditis, four of whom went on to develop diabetes mellitus within three years of the onset of thyroiditis. Some time later, another had developed diabetes and two more had abnormal GTTs. On the other hand, thyroiditis may appear *after* diabetes, as can be seen from the following case-history.

A girl, born in 1967, developed diabetes mellitus at the age of 15 months. She came to Glasgow from England in 1970, having a daily injection of Lente insulin. Her mother had diabetes and sarcoidosis, her maternal grandmother had Hashimoto's disease and her paternal grandfather had thyrotoxicosis. She was therefore subjected to a battery of ten tests for immunofluorescent antibodies, all results being negative. Height and weight were on the 50th centile.

In the last few weeks of 1971 she had six hypoglycaemic attacks, having had only one in her life before. The majority of these were in the small hours, and the attacks stopped after adjusting her diet and substituting some of her Lente insulin with Semilente. During 1972 she gained a lot of weight and by 1973 it was realized that while her height was still on the 50th centile her weight had reached the 97th. She was also becoming lethargic. Investigation showed definite hypothyroidism (PBI 1.3 ng per cent, T4 undetectable, TSH greatly elevated at 290 nunits/ml). Her bone-age was at the 25th centile but there was no epiphyseal dysgenesis.

The ten tests for antibodies were repeated, and now gave strong positives against gastric parietal cells and thyroid microsomes and a weak response to the rheumatoid factor. One year later, on treatment with thyroxin, her height is still on the 50th centile and her bone age on the 25th, but her weight has fallen to between the 75th and 90th and she is very bright and active.

There are two interesting points in this story. First, it is very tempting to relate the sudden appearance of hypo attacks to the onset of hypothyroidism*. Lack of circulating thyroxin could have led to a delay in the absorption of sugar from the bowel, a feature which was held in check by altering her insulin and carbohydrate intake. Secondly, there is the appearance of immunofluorescent antibodies in the serum some years after the onset of diabetes, so there can be no doubt that the diabetes preceded the thyroiditis.

That thyroid antibodies are more common in diabetes than in controls has already been mentioned. That the connection between clinical diabetes and clinical thyroiditis is not particularly uncommon is implied in the work of Green and Winter (1972). That the

---

* Priscilla White remarks that a second remission should make one suspect the onset of hypothyroidism.

paediatrician should keep in mind the possibility of thyroiditis appearing in a diabetic child is therefore obvious.

DIABETES IN RELATION TO OTHER DISEASES

Diabetes may coexist with certain other diseases, either in numbers which suggest the association is not the result of chance, or in families where a genetic link seems obvious. Such associations will now be discussed.

Optic atrophy

The connection between juvenile diabetes mellitus (JDM) and optic atrophy (OA) was discussed by Rose et al. (1966) in a very helpful review. The association between the two diseases has been recognized for over 100 years, but at first the optic atrophy was regarded as a complication of diabetes. Later, it was thought that optic atrophy seemed to be no more common in diabetics than in controls, and their appearance in the one patient was regarded as fortuitous. Recently, diabetes and optic atrophy have been found to run together in certain families, which suggests that there is indeed an aetiological link between the two.

Rose and his colleagues looked for cases of diabetes combined with optic atrophy in special schools and in organizations for the blind. They found seven and decided that this must be near to the total for England and Wales. They found 39 other reported cases, making 46 in all, many of which were associated with other diseases as well, for example diabetes insipidus (DI), Refsum's disease, Friedreich's ataxia, Alstrom's syndrome and the Laurence–Biedl syndrome, and several of these were deaf. They can be tabulated thus:

```
JDM+OA        :13
JDM+OA+deafness:12
JDM+OA+Friedreich's ataxia:10 (9 female)
JDM+OA+DI:5
JDM+OA+Refsum's syndrome:2
JDM+OA+Alstrom's syndrome:3
JDM+OA+Laurence–Biedl syndrome (including DI):1
```

Diabetes and optic atrophy, with or without deafness

The onset of the diabetes mellitus is early (average 7.5 years, range three to 15 years), that of the optic atrophy somewhat later (average 10.8 years, range four to 24 years), and the deafness, if present, usually appears subsequent to both of them. In five cases optic atrophy preceded diabetes mellitus.

In one family, one child was an ament with a goitre, two others in the same family had epilepsy, and two aunts had goitres. Other defects of the nervous system, such as ataxia and neurogenic bladders, have been reported. A recent description of the DIDMOAD syndrome (diabetes insipidus, diabetes mellitus, optic atrophy and deafness) is given by Richardson and Hamilton (1977).

Diabetes, optic atrophy and Friedreich's ataxia

The recurring statement that diabetes mellitus occurs in 20 per cent of cases of Friedreich's ataxia derives from Thorén's (1962) report of nine cases of diabetes, to which he added one case with an abnormal intravenous GTT, in a total of 50 cases of Friedreich's ataxia examined. Thorén regarded this result as falsely low as the mean age of the non-diabetics was 20.5 years, and the mean age of the onset of diabetes in the affected patients was 21.9 years (range eight to 41 years, which just qualifies the association for paediatric consideration). Diabetes occurred long after the ataxia, at a time when the patients were no longer able to walk. All showed cardiac myopathy. The clinical picture of diabetes in Friedreich's ataxia is typical of juvenile onset diabetes, i.e. it is ketosis-prone and insulin-dependent, and post-mortem examination shows a small pancreas with reduced islet tissue.

Of the ten cases mentioned above, where diabetes and Friedreich's ataxia are combined with optic atrophy, the age of onset of diabetes is available in five, the average being 18 years (range 15–21). The age of onset of the optic atrophy is recorded in only three, occurring one to four years after the diabetes.

The combination of *diabetes insipidus* with Friedreich's ataxia has been reported. Though very rare, it is a diagnostic hazard.

The coexistence of diabetes mellitus and insipidus *without* optic atrophy has long been recognized (Raiti, Plotkin and Newns, 1963: Stoppoloni, Pierantoni and Pacelli, 1969) but may be a difficult diagnosis to make, in which case certain tests are available.

A boy suspected of having both diseases was admitted for hormone investigation to the Western Infirmary, Glasgow (Dr J. J. Brown). He was allowed free intake of water and food for 24 hours, during which time he passed 7580 ml of urine with a urinary antidiuretic hormone (ADH) of 0.88 ng/hour (normal 2.5–17 ng/hour). Water deprivation, aimed at producing a weight loss of 4 per cent was carried out for 18 hours, by which time he had lost 4.3 per cent of his weight. His basal ADH was 3.3 pg/ml; after 12 hours of deprivation it was 4.0 pg/ml and after 18 hours 3.2 pg/ml (normal 4–9 pg/ml). The results were low and showed no increase during the period of water deprivation. The urinary osmolality was 113 mmol/kg at the start, 235 mmol/kg after 13½ hours and 312 mmol/kg after 18 hours. The plasma osmolality after 18 hours was 291 mmol/kg, indicating a failure to concentrate urine to an osmolality significantly greater than that of the plasma during the test. These observations confirm the suspicion of ADH deficiency.

At the simple clinical level, a well-controlled diabetic in hospital who is passing in the region of five litres of urine in the day with only slight glycosuria can be assumed to have diabetes insipidus and a trial with pitressin is indicated. Treatment with pitressin can be maintained and does not appear to alter the control of the diabetes mellitus.

The coincidence of diabetes mellitus and insipidus may be fortuitous or may be due to pituitary dysfunction, but when optic atrophy is also present a genetic link seems probable. Either form of diabetes may appear first.

Refsum's syndrome and others

Refsum originally named his syndrome heredopathia atactica polyneuritiformis, which is as good a way as any of ensuring that a syndrome will be linked with one's own name! It is a hereditary syndrome involving atypical retinitis pigmentosa, polyneuritis and ataxia and has been described in association with diabetes mellitus and optic atrophy in childhood. The diabetes appears first.

Alstrom's syndrome and the Laurence–Biedl syndrome resemble Refsum's syndrome in certain ways, but only Refsum's syndrome shows ataxia and polyneuritis, only the Laurence–Biedl syndrome shows polydactyly and mental defect, and Alstrom's syndrome shows none of these four features, but does show obesity. All may show atypical retinitis pigmentosa, deafness and hypogonadism. All have been associated in a few patients with concurrent diabetes mellitus and optic atrophy.

DIABETES AND OTHER CONDITIONS

Prader–Willi syndrome

The literature on this syndrome was recently reviewed by Ridler, Garrod and Berg (1971). A good description is given by Hoefnagel, Costello and Hatoum (1967). The syndrome presents at birth an infant with hypotonia, cyanotic attacks, a small mandible, a poor cry, poor movements, a small penis and an empty scrotum. Obesity appears in the first or second year, and is accompanied by hyperphagia, a small head, small stature and small hands and feet. A GTT may be abnormal. In adolescence diabetes may appear. The diabetes shows no weight loss or ketosis and is not helped by insulin, but responds well to oral hypoglycaemic agents. The IQ is in the range 20–90. Juul and Dupont (1967) collected 46 cases, of which five were frankly diabetic and ten showed chemical diabetes. Two of the five diabetics had developed diabetes by the time they were 12 years old.

At present I have one case under observation, but he has not yet reached the 'diabetic' age.

Acquired lipoatrophic diabetes

The original description of this condition was given by Laurence in 1946, and little has been added since. It may occur in childhood and is more common in females. There is widespread loss of body fat. If diabetes supervenes it is insulin-resistant and non-ketotic. Enlargement of the liver, which may go on to cirrhosis, is a striking feature. Hyperlipidaemia and greatly raised triglycerides are found, so that xanthomas on the skin are common.

Occasional cases have been seen in which the lipoatrophy involves single dermatomes, and a neural basis for the lipatrophy has been proposed. However, hypothalamic dysfunction involving the pituitary seems a more likely basis. Releasing factors for corticotrophin and follicle stimulating hormone are high in the plasma of patients with lipoatrophic diabetes, but how they could be involved in its causation is obscure. In short, the metabolic basis of this syndrome is unexplained.

Dunnigan et al. (1974) described a familial form of lipoatrophic diabetes in which the face was unaffected and the liver normal in size. Dunnigan's paper gives a helpful review of the lipoatrophies and lipodystrophies.

Klinefelter's syndrome and Turner's syndrome

Facts may be classified into two types, 'Oh?' facts and 'Let-me-at-it!' facts. In the former category, it seems to me, is the fact that a family history of diabetes is often found in association with Klinefelter's syndrome (Nielsen, 1966) and Turner's syndrome (Menzinger, Fallucca and Andreani, 1966). Chthonic clinicians are likely to be unmoved by this revelation, but deeper thinkers may be intrigued by the link between diabetes and the sex chromosomes, as opposed to the autosomes. Nielsen found abnormal GTTs in six of ten patients with Klinefelter's syndrome, but did not report overt diabetes.

Others

Farquhar (1979) lists further rare associations with diabetes, i.e. ataxia telangiectasia, glucose 6-PD deficiency, Type I glycogen storage disease, Huntington's chorea, hyperlipoproteinaemias, isolated growth hormone deficiency, leucoderma, muscular dystrophy, myotonic dystrophy, pineal hyperplasia, acute intermittent porphyria and the syndromes of Cockayne, Schmidt and Werner.

REFERENCES

Bottazzo, G. F., Florin-Christensen, A. and Doniach, D. (1974). Islet cell antibodies in diabetes mellitus and autoimmune polyendocrine deficiencies. *Lancet*, **II**, 1279

Chambers, T. L. (1975). Coexistent coeliac disease, diabetes mellitus and hypothyroidism. *Arch. Dis. Childh.*, **50**, 162

Cudworth, A. G. and Woodrow, J. C. (1974). HL-A antigens and diabetes mellitus. *Lancet*, **II**, 1153

Dunnigan, M. G., Cochrane, M. A., Kelly, A. and Scott, J. W. (1974). Familial lipoatrophic diabetes with dominant transmission. *Quart. J. Med.*, **43**, 33

Farquhar, J. W. (1979). Juvenile diabetes mellitus: possibility of prevention. *Arch. Dis. Childh.*, **54**, 569

Goodchild, M. C. and Brown, G. A. (1972). Insulin excretion in cystic fibrosis. *Arch. Dis. Childh.*, **47**, 152

Green, O. C. and Winter, R. J. (1972). Spring meeting of the pediatric Societies, Washington: abstracted in *Year-book of Pediatrics* (1973), p. 273

Hoefnagel, D., Costello, P. J. and Hatoum, K. (1967). Prader–Willi syndrome. *J. Ment. Defic. Res.*, **11**, 1

Hooft, C., Devos, E. and van Damme, J. (1969). Coeliac disease in a diabetic child. *Lancet*, **II**, 161

Juul, J. and Dupont, Annalise (1967). Prader–Willi syndrome. *J. ment. Defic. Res.*, **11**, 12

Kim, C. B., Johnson, W. W. and MacMillan, D. R. (1973). Hyperglycaemic non-ketotic coma in a postpancreatectomy diabetic infant. *Am. J. Dis. Child.*, **125**, 755

REFERENCES

Kjellman, N-I. M. and Larsson, Y, (1975). Insulin release in cystic fibrosis. *Arch. Dis. Childh.*, **50**, 205
Lendrum, R., Walker, G. and Gamble, D. R. (1975). Islet cell antibodies in juvenile diabetes mellitus of recent onset. *Lancet*, **I**, 880
MacCuish, A. C., Barnes, E. W., Irvine, W. J. and Duncan, L. J. P. (1974). Antibodies to pancreatic islet cells in insulin-dependent diabetics with co-existent auto-immune disease. *Lancet*, **II**, 1529
McNeish, A. S., Nelson, R. and Mackintosh, P. (1973). HL-A1 and 8 in childhood coeliac disease. *Lancet*, **I**, 668
Manderson, W. G., McKiddie, M. T., Manners, D. J. and Stark, J. R. (1968). Liver glycogen accumulation in unstable diabetes. *Diabetes*, **17**, 13
Menzinger, G., Fallucca, F. and Andreani, D. (1966). Gonadal dysgenesis and diabetes. *Lancet*, **I**, 1269
Nielsen, J. (1966). Diabetes mellitus in parents of patients with Klinefelter's syndrome. *Lancet*, **I**, 1376 (and **II**, 748)
Oakley, W. G. (1968). Pancreatic diabetes and haemochromatosis. In *Clinical Diabetes and its Biochemical Basis*, p. 675. Ed. Oakley, W. G., Pyke, D. A. and Talyor, K. W. Oxford; Blackwell
Raiti, S., Plotkin, S. and Newns, G. H. (1963). Diabetes mellitus and insipidus in two sisters. *Br. med. J.*, **II**, 1625
Richardson, Joyce E. and Hamilton, W. (1977). Diabetes insipidus, diabetes mellitus, optic atrophy and deafness: three cases of DIDMOAD syndrome. *Arch. Dis. Childh.*, **52**, 796
Ridler, M. A. C., Garrod, O. and Berg, J. M. (1971). A case of Prader–Willi syndrome in a girl with a small extra chromosome. *Acta paediat. Scand.*, **60**, 222
Rosan, R. C., Schwachman, H. and Kulczychi, L. L. (1962). Diabetes mellitus and cystic fibrosis of the pancreas. *Am. J. Dis. Child.*, **104**, 625
Rose, F. C., Fraser, G. R., Friedman, A. I. and Kohner, E. M. (1966). The association of juvenile diabetes mellitus and optic atrophy: clinical and genetical aspects. *Quart. J. Med.*, **35**, 385 (This paper gives references to some of the rarer syndromes mentioned above)
Sibert, J. R. (1975). Pancreatitis in children: a study in the North of England. *Arch. Dis. Childh.*, **50**, 443
Stoppoloni, G., Pierantoni, G. and Pacelli, V. (1969). Two children with diabetes insipidus and diabetes mellitus. *Lancet*, **II**, 1425
Thorén, C. (1962). Diabetes mellitus in Friedreich's ataxia. *Acta paediat.*, **51**, Suppl. 135, 239
Van Thiel, D. H., Smith, W. I., Rabin, B. S., Fisher, S. E. and Lester, R. (1977). A syndrome of immunoglobulin A deficiency, diabetes mellitus, malabsorption and a common HLA haplotype. *Ann. int. Med.*, **86**, 10
Visakorpi, J. K. (1969). Diabetes and coeliac disease. *Lancet*, **II**, 1192
Walker-Smith, J. A. and Grigor, W. (1969). Coeliac disease in a diabetic child. *Lancet*, **I**, 1021
Walsh, C. H., Malins, J. M. and Bloom, S. R. (1978). Diabetes mellitus in idiopathic haemochromatosis. *Br. med. J.*, **2**, 1267

CHAPTER 12

Complications

The complications of diabetes in childhood will be discussed under three main headings:

(1) Complications occurring at the time of, or near to the first admission: these are ketoacidosis, coma, hypoglycaemia, skin lesions, oedema, neuropathy and pneumomediastinum.
(2) Complications occurring later in childhood:
    (a) Common—hepatomegaly, poor growth, fat atrophy and hypertrophy, neuropathy, joint contractures.
    (b) Uncommon—CNS damage, eye disorders, nephropathy.
(3) The prognosis for childhood diabetics in adult life. The actual complications of adult life will not be discussed in detail.

It used to be tacitly accepted that one did not have to worry very much about diabetic complications occurring in childhood but new sophisticated techniques (for example fluorescein angiography) suggest that there is no room for complacency. Lawrence and Locke pointed out in 1963 that proteinuria and neuropathy may occur in childhood, possibilities which are often overlooked.

EARLY COMPLICATIONS

Ketoacidosis and coma are discussed in Chapters 7 and 8.

Hypoglycaemia is discussed on p. 126

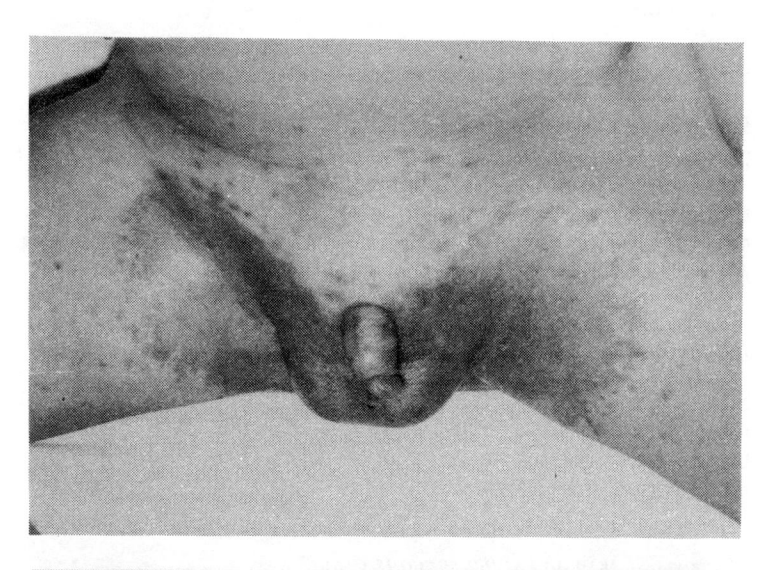

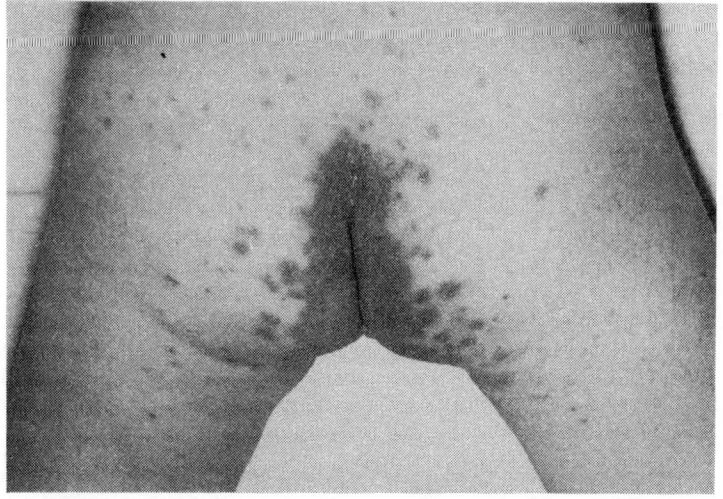

Figure 12.1. Perineal candidiasis (thrush) at the onset of diabetes. It is true that thrush may appear in the absence of diabetes, particularly in the napkin-wearing age-group, but this little boy had no problem till diabetes appeared. Involvement of the depths of the flexures and the presence of spotty lesions round the periphery suggest thrush rather than ammoniacal dermatitis

Skin lesions

Moniliasis

Pruritus is not common in childhood diabetes but moniliasis is, particularly in the perineal region. If there is a perineal rash in a diabetic one should always consider the use of local nystatin as a therapeutic trial, even although monilia has not been identified in scrapings. The perineal rash is not confined to females, as *Figure 12.1* shows.

Erythema at injection sites

Some children show a transient localized erythema at the sites of insulin injection for a month or two after insulin therapy has been begun. This does not imply infection, is harmless, and calls for no modification in treatment.

Necrosis of skin and subcutaneous tissue

Necrobiosis lipoidica diabeticorum (Bauer *et al.*, 1964) is a skin condition which may occur in diabetics or pre-diabetics, and occasionally in non-diabetics. It is most marked around the front of the legs. A purplish discoloration slowly spreads and develops a central pale area which becomes atrophic and may ulcerate. It is of interest in that 18 per cent of cases have been reported to occur before the diabetes, and indeed the average time interval is over three years. The condition has occurred in childhood.

The condition about to be described represents a more superficial necrosis.

> A girl of 12 years was admitted with a one-week history of thirst and polyuria, mild enough to have escaped the notice of the parents except on one occasion when they had been out on a family walk. She had been ambulant but lethargic the day before admission, went to bed early and was found in deep coma next morning. At admission, she was moderately ketotic but had a blood sugar of 180 mmol/l (3240 mg per cent).* The details of treatment do not concern us here. Briefly, she responded well to routine small doses of insulin given hourly, was talking sensibly after 48 hours, and has made a complete recovery in all respects except for her skin lesions. These are shown in *Figure 12.2*. They presented as flat reddish erythematous areas, but within about six hours looked much as in the illustration. A scab formed and the lesions appeared to be healing

---

* This child has been seen since *Figure 1.1* was drawn up.

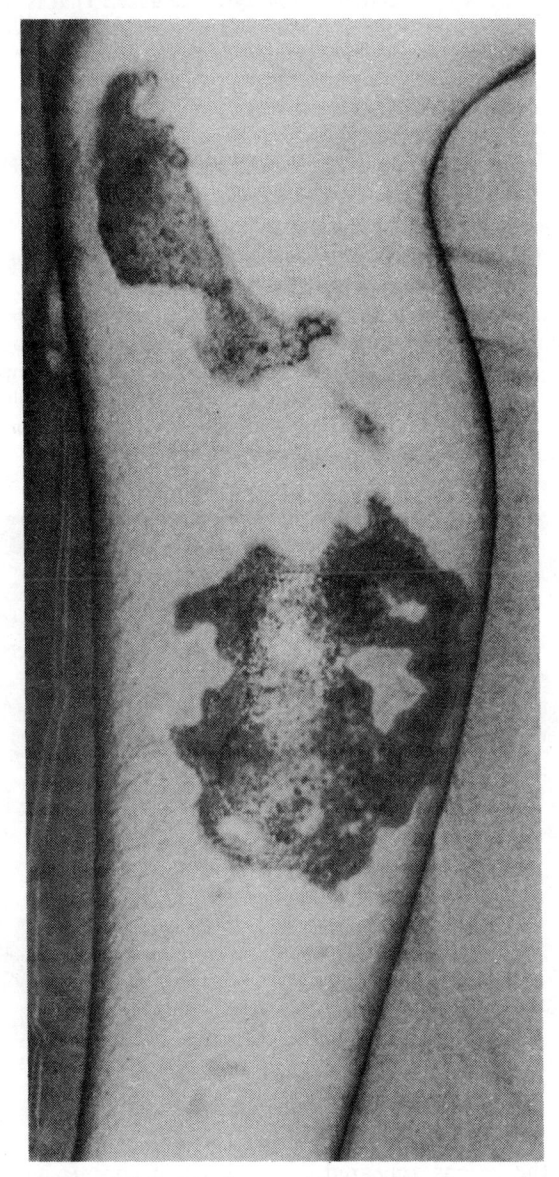

Figure 12.2. Lesion of very rapid onset during deep coma

well, but a month after discharge a thick scab was still present with obvious underlying infection, but no systemic upset. That is the position as I write. Our pleasure at her recovery, which at first seemed very unlikely, has been marred by the fact that permanent scarring of the legs seems certain.

A similar case was under the care of Dr Isabel Ferguson at the Southern General Hospital, Glasgow.

A boy of nine and a half years had also had thirst and polyuria for a week. At the time of admission he was semicomatose and showed marked discoloration at the pressure points. These areas very quickly proceeded to bed-sores *(Figure 12.3)*. His blood sugar at the time of admission was 138 mmol/l (2480 mg per cent) and the pH of the blood was 6.92. He also responded well, but to larger and less frequent doses of insulin than were given in the first case. His skin lesions healed uneventfully. Another complication noted at the time of admission was a drop-foot on the right. This will be discussed below, in the section on neuropathy.

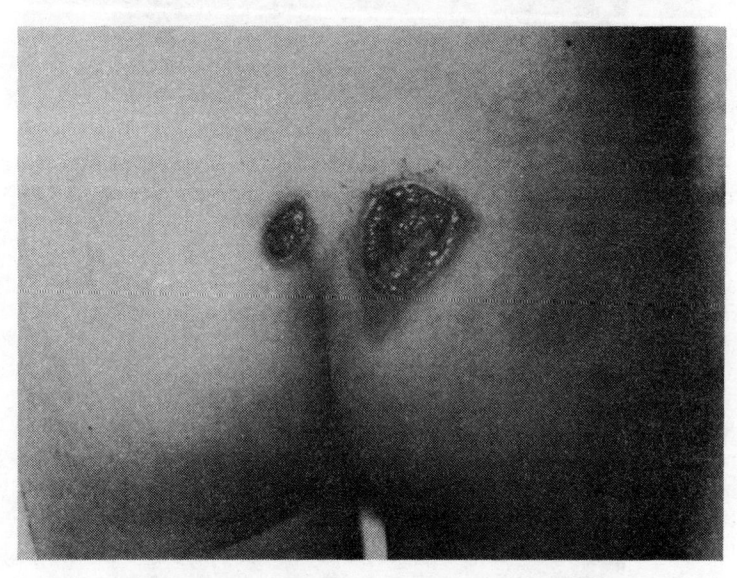

Figure 12.3. Bedsores of very acute onset in new diabetic

One striking feature which the cases have in common is the speed at which the lesions appeared. Neither set of parents had realized there was anything there, yet within 24 hours gross changes were apparent, despite all efforts to ease pressure. The second striking feature held in common was the gross hyperglycaemia. The third is the short history, with the disease apparently running a mild course until sudden deterioration in the day before admission. Biopsies were not done on the lesions and their aetiology remains unexplained, but it is desirable to record that such lesions may appear, apparently in rather exceptional circumstances.

Oedema

I was about to write that oedema in diabetes is a well-known entity, but I doubt if it is. It was described in 1928 by Leifer, who even then commented that it was more common than reports would suggest.

Oedema is associated with an improvement of control in diabetes. I have seen it during the first admission, and also during the re-stabilization of badly controlled patients. Rosenbloom and Giordano (1977) have found oedema to be one sign of overtreatment which is not necessarily a contradiction of what has just been written, because in overtreatment there may be a rapidly fluctuating state between too much and too little insulin action. The diagnosis is easy if one remembers the circumstances in which it occurs, and if one finds no abnormality in the urine, blood or cardiovascular system *(Figure 12.4)*.

One's first impression is that the oedema appears to be due to an 'overshoot' in the correction of fluid loss. Dunnigan (1976) suggests that there may be a carbohydrate-linked electrolyte imbalance. Clinically, the condition seems to blend with the idiopathic oedema of adult females. Dunnigan has found that this latter condition, often found in association with a family history of diabetes, responded better to controlling the carbohydrate intake and giving an antidiabetic drug than it did to diuretics. A further clinical link is that diabetic oedema is more common in girls than boys and is also more persistent in girls, who may show this benign oedema for weeks or months, whereas in boys it may disappear after a few days. Diabetic oedema occurs after a period of relative carbohydrate starvation due to insulin lack, and the sex incidence suggests that a hormonal factor is also involved.

Neuropathy

Reske-Nielsen *et al.* (1970) studied nine patients at the onset of juvenile diabetes mellitus, three of them under the age of 20. One patient was asymptomatic, seven had a history going back three

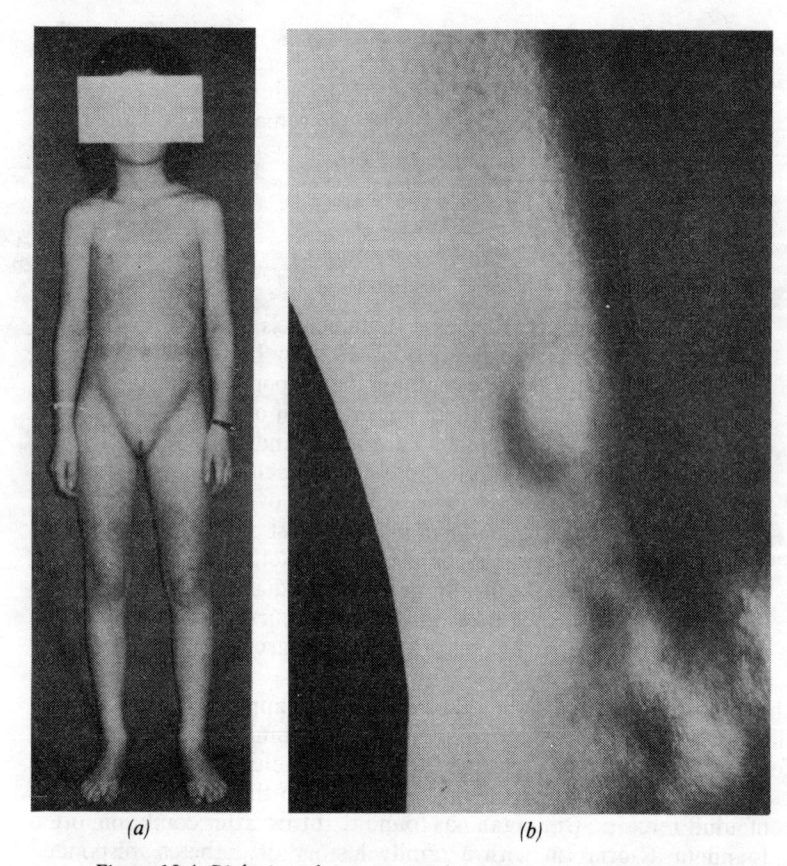

Figure 12.4. Diabetic oedema may not be obvious, and is apparent in (a) only as the mark made by clothing at the waist; but (b), taken of the same girl at the same time, shows that oedema may be obvious if one specifically looks for it (photographs by courtesy of Dr M. G. Dunnigan and Dr A. Ford, Stobhill General Hospital, Glasgow)

to ten weeks and one had a history of 26 weeks. Biopsies on leg muscles were performed. The end-plates were described as 'bizarre' and the terminal expansions were unusual in various ways, but at the same time regenerative changes were also noted. In addition to these findings the mean conduction velocity in the nerves was 45.9 m/second (normal 50.8 m/second) and vibration sense was also impaired. Simple clinical tests showed no abnormal neuromuscular signs. Three biopsies were repeated three to five weeks after the blood sugar had been restored to normal, but diabetic signs were still present.

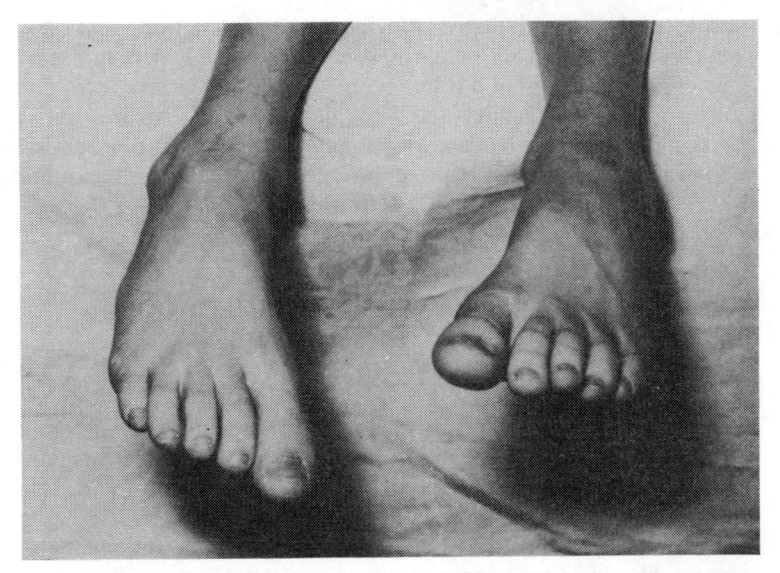

Figure 12.5. Same boy as in Figure 12.3, showing right drop-foot

Against this background one can consider the case of the boy with the drop-foot, described above in *Figure 12.3*. Biopsy was not done in his case but electromyography was, and the report read, in part, as follows. 'There is a neurogenic disturbance affecting the muscles which appears to be more marked in the peripheral muscles. The total study would appear to support a neuropathic process although this is not affecting to any severe extent the major nerve trunks, but presumably the active process is involving the very fine nerve terminals within the muscles.' The drop-foot took six months to recover, but eventually did so. It is worth repeating that neuropathy in diabetic children is commoner than is generally realized.

Autonomic neuropathy does not seem to have attracted much attention in childhood, but has certainly been noted in young adults. There are many tests of autonomic function of which the heart-rate response when changing position from standing to lying appears to be both simple and reliable (Ewing, *et al.*, 1978).

Pneumomediastinum

When I first encountered pneumomediastinum in diabetic ketoacidosis I did not know what it was. I heard an odd kind of pericarditic squeak, and the radiologist provided the explanation next day. Pneumomediastinum is thought to be caused by the hyperventilation of severe ketoacidosis, and it has been described by Grieve, Bird and Collyer (1969) and Zahler and Skoglund (1978). It is rare, but is mentioned here as it has escaped many textbooks. The prognosis is good. Seldom can one remove the cause of pneumomediastinum as quickly as one can in diabetic ketoacidosis.

LATER COMPLICATIONS IN CHILDHOOD

Hepatomegaly and dwarfism

Hepatomegaly and dwarfism in diabetes were most often found together when the only type of insulin available was soluble (regular) insulin. If one goes back to 1938 one finds a description by Marble et al. of 60 diabetic children with enlarged livers, 30 of them being dwarfs with frequent attacks of alternating ketosis and hypoglycaemia. The liver size decreased in 47 of the 60 when they were changed to a daily injection of depot insulin (protamine zinc, the only longer-lasting insulin then available). When one comes to think of it, it is illogical to treat a condition characterized by rapid fluctuations in blood sugar with the very type of insulin, soluble insulin, best calculated itself to produce rapid swings in blood sugar. Yet the idea that a child who is unstable on one injection of a depot insulin should automatically be changed to soluble died hard. Two injections of a medium acting insulin are to be preferred.

Hepatomegaly may be associated with other abnormal signs. The syndrome of hepatomegaly, dwarfism, obesity and hypogonadism in the diabetic child was described by Mauriac and now bears his name. An account of this syndrome, amounting to a monograph, was given by Wagner, White and Bogan in 1942. Hepatomegaly was very common. In a group of diabetic children, enlargement of the liver by 1 cm or more below the costal margin was found in 51 per cent of boys and 53 per cent of girls (controls, 17 and 15 per cent respectively). Enlargement of 3 cm or more was found in 15 per cent of boys and 17 per cent of girls (controls 8.6 and 2.6 per cent respectively). As no child was more than 20 per cent below his expected height, the shorter patients (8.3 per cent of the total) were referred to as 'pseudodwarfs' rather than 'dwarfs'. However, the stunting in this group was considerable. The age of maximal retardation was 15 years, at which time the average lag in height was 8.8 in (22 cm). If one can imagine the average adult male having a height of 4 ft 11 in instead of 5 ft 8 in one can get some idea of the degree of retardation. It approaches science fiction.

Cases of Mauriac's syndrome have recently been described by Mandell and Berenberg (1974) and Lee and Bode (1977) but the full-blown syndrome is now rarely seen. Hepatomegaly, however, remains common. Just how common is it? This is not an easy question to answer, partly because there may be error in clinical assessment and partly because it may be difficult to decide on a standard of hepatomegaly.

A house officer may write 'Liver not palpable' when in fact the liver is considerably enlarged. This happens because the diabetic liver is usually soft and difficult to feel. For my part, I must confess that if I concentrate hard enough I can feel a liver edge that is not there, and recently I decided that a 4 cm liver was probably a muscle ridge*. I am not trying to make myself out a fool. I am just insinuating that a clinician who does not doubt his ability to assess liver size correctly any time he cares to try may be deluding himself. I prefer to temper a clinical judgement with objective evidence.

Standards of liver size from x-ray measurements were laid down by Deligeorgis *et al.* (1970, 1973), and I am glad to say that they did not find a good correlation between their clinical and x-ray assessments either. These papers prompted us to x-ray our own patients for liver size, using the same technique, as nearly as possible to their thirteenth birthdays. The x-ray estimations were carried out by Dr Elizabeth Sweet, and we suggest that this measurement should be used in future as it does give a reasonably precise figure and a standard of comparison between different observers.

Forty children were x-rayed for liver height within two weeks of their thirteenth birthday. The results are shown in *Figure 12.6*.

Liver height correlates with total height which has a virtually symmetrical distribution curve, so the pronounced tail in the figure suggests that a liver height of over 20 cm is definitely abnormal at this age. Even excluding those with a liver height of over 20 cm the average liver height was 17.6 cm, about 1.5 cm higher than the figure which can be deduced approximately from the scattergram given by Deligeorgis *et al.* While admitting that Greek figures cannot be applied to British children, the suspicion remains that the

---

* A word on the *scratching test* for liver size may be of help. The bell of the stethoscope is placed on the abdomen just above and to the right of the umbilicus. A fingernail scratches the skin briskly with a side-to-side movement while at the same time moving from the ribs down over the abdomen in a curve which keeps it at a constant distance from the stethoscope. When the scratching finger leaves the liver edge the noise in the stethoscope becomes suddenly louder.

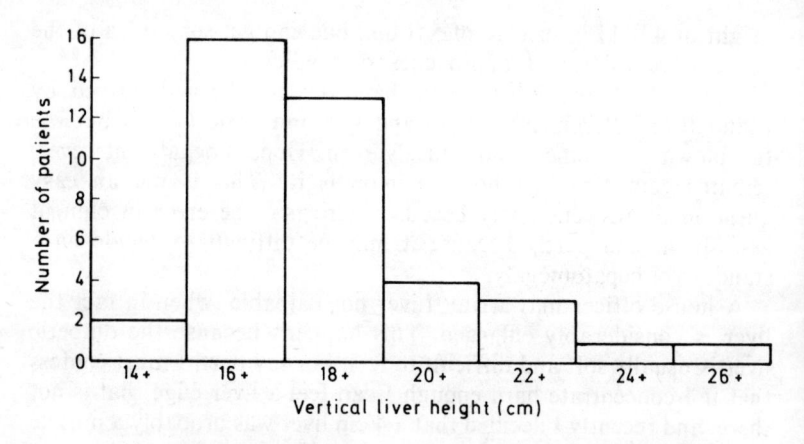

Figure 12.6. Vertical liver height (x-ray measurement) in 40 diabetic children aged 13 years. Liver height is known to correlate with patient height so one would expect this histogram to show an almost symmetrical Gaussian distribution, which it certainly does not. The assumption is that many diabetic children have abnormally large livers but it is difficult to be sure in the individual case unless the enlargement is gross

majority of diabetic children may have some hepatic enlargement, albeit mild in most cases.

The eight children with the largest livers had unsatisfactory backgrounds, the parents being unable to benefit from the clinic for social or emotional reasons. These children also grew poorly. *Figure 12.7* shows that even if their height at 13 years was average they had in fact declined from a higher level, and indeed nearly all showed a falling-off in height from early in their diabetic careers. There was no clear relationship between hepatomegaly and the duration of diabetes and, although the children with hepatomegaly had an insignificantly greater delay in bone-age than those with smaller livers (11.7 years against 12.0 years at a calendar age of 13 years) this delay was insufficient to account for stunting in height.

Why is the liver big?

In the early days of insulin it was thought that hepatomegaly was due to fatty infiltration, but it is now known to be due to the deposition of glycogen. The accumulation of glycogen in the livers of unstable diabetics was discussed by Manderson *et al.* (1968). The amount of glycogen may be as great as in glycogen storage disease, but in

Growth in children with hepatomegaly (diagrammatic)

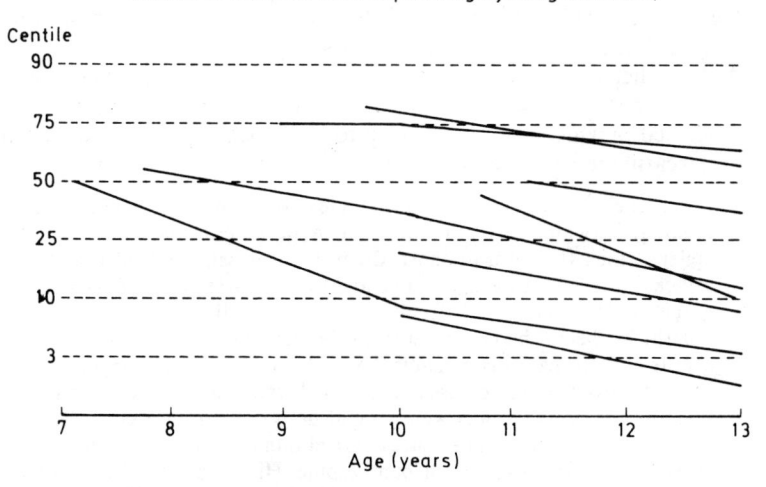

Figure 12.7. Height in relation to hepatomegaly. These eight children were found to have definite hepatomegaly at the age of 13 years. The unbroken lines represent their percentile status for height during their diabetic lives and indicate that all has not been well from an early stage. Even the two children who are above the 50th centile were originally on or above the 75th and one child, on the 50th centile when contracting diabetes at the age of seven, had fallen to the 3rd centile at the age of 13. When one remembers that liver height correlates with patient height and when one notes that five of these children are far below average height the degree of hepatomegaly becomes all the more striking

diabetes the chain length of the glycogen is normal. It appears to be in a very stable form as the blood sugar does not rise after the infusion of glucagon, which may account for the frequent hypoglycaemic attacks which accompany hepatomegaly. It may be that unstable diabetes leads to excess glycogen in the liver and resultant hypo attacks, rather than unstable diabetes with frequent hypo attacks leading to hepatomegaly, though the latter is the more popular theory. There is fairly general agreement in the literature that hepatomegaly results from over-eating in the presence of relative insulin deficiency. However, Asherov et al. (1979) describe a case in which hepatomegaly was the result of the patient deliberately taking extra insulin and they hold the view that hepatomegaly is a sign of overtreatment; which coincides with earlier opinions (Middleton and Hockaday, 1965; Rosenbloom and Giordano, 1977). My own view, taking the history of the syndrome over the last 50 years or so into account, is that hepatomegaly is the result of overtreatment particularly if it is irregular due to too much soluble (regular) insulin being used. So far, so good; but Pavy described diabetic hepatomegaly in 1885, long before the insulin era, so there may be more causes than one. To illustrate this a case will be described in which the relationship to the type of insulin used and to overtreatment is not clear.

At the age of seven months, Gerald developed pneumococcal meningitis, which left him retarded, hyperkinetic and epileptic. His epilepsy took the form of short absences, drop seizures and grand mal attacks. In 1965, at the age of two and three-quarter years, he developed diabetes. He was very difficult to control in all respects. Within 18 months his height had dropped from the 25th to a point below the 10th centile and his liver was palpable 7.5 cm below the costal margin. Biopsy showed gross glycogen excess in the liver. Hypo attacks mixed freely with fits, and his drop seizures were so bad he was wearing a crash helmet. However, these particular seizures were eliminated by nitrazepam and his other seizures improved on carbamazepine. His behaviour also improved when he was put on dexamphetamine after he had been threatened with expulsion from his occupational centre because of one-man riots. Indeed at this period neighbours with a movie camera would take Gerald into the country and set the camera rolling, because he could be guaranteed to produce a forest fire and a couple of floods every Saturday afternoon. His height in 1971 was just above the third centile, and his liver had not decreased in size. He was then put on two daily injections, and by 1974 his height was above the 50th centile, his behaviour was much better, and his liver was barely palpable, though x-ray in 1975 showed it to be just over the upper limit of normal (20.5 cm). His growth spurt was accompanied by rapid maturation, and by the age of 12½ years his voice had broken and he had the makings of a moustache. I have not seen such a spurt in height and maturation in a diabetic before and the history of previous intracranial pathology makes one careful about attributing the spurt to Rapitard. On the other hand, the decrease in liver size does seem definitely attributable to the twice-daily injections. The change to two injections was delayed as it was thought that one injection of a depot insulin was all that we could expect to be carried out regularly in his special circumstances, but we were wrong. I regret to say that Gerald is now in the hands of the police for lifting up the skirts of little girls. I think he must be regarded as an exceptional case.

Hypertrophy and atrophy of fat

Areas of *fat hypertrophy* ('fatty tumours') occur at an injection site which has been used too often, although some children seem almost immune and others are very susceptible. These lumps can be of considerable importance to the teenage girl from a cosmetic point of view, but they are of even greater importance in their effect on diabetic control. The absorption of insulin from such areas is irregular and may cause anomalous control which varies from day to day. This may occur whatever previous instruction the mother has had. The areas become partially anaesthetized, the child wants to use them and 'He just won't let me give it anywhere else' is the mother's usual defence. She has to be supported through this minor crisis, and when new areas are brought into play the fall in insulin requirements can be surprising. The mother should be warned of the increased possibility of hypo attacks when the change is first made. A fatty tumour resolves over the years if it is left to itself.

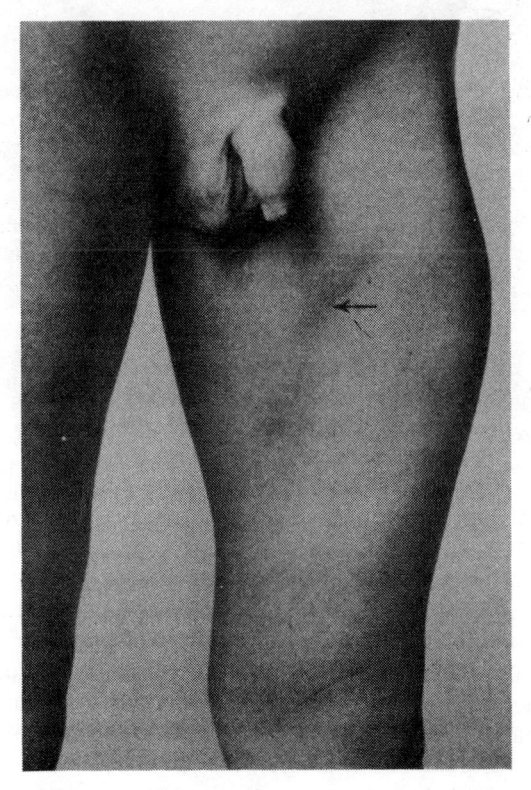

Figure 12.8. Shows fat hypertrophy of outer thigh, and Y-shaped fat atrophy of inner thigh, the latter at a site never used for injections

Fat atrophy is a phenomenon which is as yet unexplained. It may be present at the same time as fat hypertrophy. In childhood boys are

262 COMPLICATIONS

affected as often as girls, from puberty it is more common in girls. Various causes have been suggested, usually involving the local action of insulin or its impurities, but the phenomenon may be seen at a site where no injection has ever been given *(Figures 12.8 and 12.9)*. The subject has recently been reviewed by Teuscher (1974). It is common. The fat disappears without an exudative reaction or appreciable fibrosis. This is not due to an immunochemical reaction between fat and insulin, nor is it related to the pH of the insulin, to

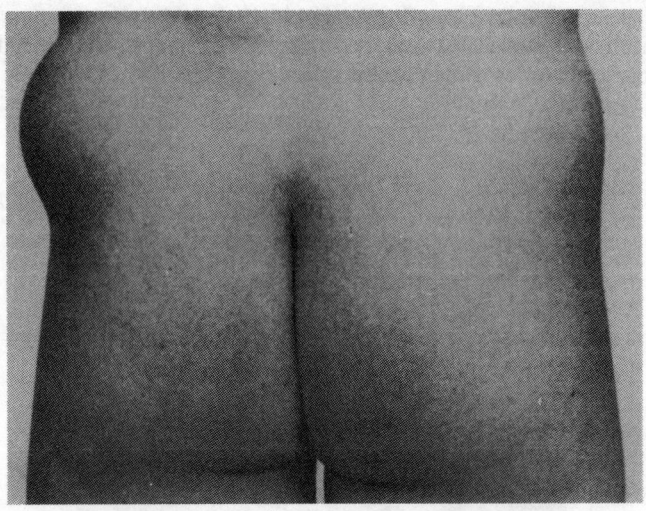

Figure 12.9. Same boy as in Figure 12.2. In a pre-disposed child, fatty tumours may appear at any site used

preservatives, to local trauma or to alcohol in the syringe. It is not related to circulating insulin antibodies and skin tests to various insulins are negative. It appears after three to six months of treatment and subsides after two to three years. Teuscher found that Monocomponent insulin, the purest form of insulin then made, and free from pro-insulin, arginyl insulin etc., did not produce lipoatrophy, so it may be the impurities which cause the trouble. Pork insulins may be less likely than beef insulins to produce atrophy. The recommended treatment is to inject the daily dose or doses of insulin around the edges of the lesion, gradually working towards the centre, and success has been claimed with a variety of insulins when using this method. Unfortunately, I have had difficulty in getting children to sustain this form of treatment, as such injections seem to hurt more.

Joint contractures

In 1976 Grgic *et al.* described contractures of the finger joints found in 28 per cent of 229 diabetics under the age of 18 years, the little finger being most commonly affected. The contractures correlated with the duration of the disease but could appear as early as one year after onset. Multiple contractures were associated with short stature. Major joints were involved in a few. The condition can be detected by asking the patient to place his hand palm down on a table with the fingers slightly spread; it is then viewed from the side. The abnormalities are confined to the connective tissue, the bone appearing normal on x-ray. The cause of the changes is not yet clear. I can confirm that these changes can be found if one looks for them *(Figure 12.10)*.

Robertson, Earnshaw and Campbell (1979) describe similar changes (not Dupuytren's contracture) and their surgical treatment in later life.

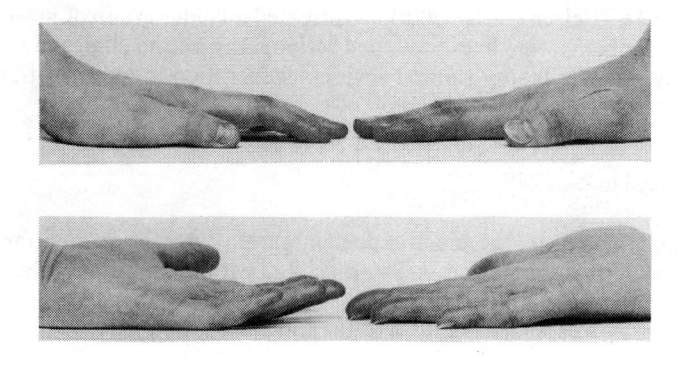

Figure 12.10. Diabetic joint contractures (patient on left, control on right). The patient is a girl of 12 years who has been diabetic for five years. Control is poor and she has had several recent readmissions for recurrent ketoacidosis. These are 'Stage 2' changes, 'Stage 1' involving one finger only. The abnormality in this girl was asymmetrical, only the ring and little fingers being involved in the other hand

Neuropathy

The occurrence of neuropathy in the early days of diabetes has been discussed above. There may be a persisting neuropathy throughout childhood, but the clinician may well underestimate the incidence as neuropathy is demonstrable by laboratory tests before it is recognized clinically.

Nerve conduction tests are not carried out as a routine at the RHSC, Glasgow. One of our patients was admitted to another hospital, where delay in nerve conduction in the legs was demonstrated. This was surprising, as she was the star of her school netball team.

Eeg-Olofsson and Perersen (1966) examined a group of children aged eight to 15 years and found pathological delay in conduction in the ulnar nerve in 2 per cent and in the perineal in 9 per cent. Abnormal findings were related to the interlinked triad of age, duration of the disease and poor control. Abnormal electroencephalograms were found in 35 per cent (and in 13 per cent of controls), which finding was not related to the triad but to the frequency of hypoglycaemic coma. The findings of Gamstorp et al. (1966), who also encountered difficulty in separating the effects of duration and poor control (as control deteriorates with the duration of the disease), were essentially similar.

Reske-Nielsen et al. (1968) investigated an older group of juvenile onset diabetics who had developed retinopathy but no clinical neuropathy. Muscle biopsy showed severe degeneration in terminal fibres and end-organs.

Damage to the CNS

Abnormalities in the electroencephalogram have been mentioned above. They are not necessarily associated with seizures, but seizures are relatively common in the child who develops diabetes before the age of two years *(see below)* and mental retardation may sometimes occur.

Eeg-Olofsson (1977) discusses neurological disturbances and EEG findings associated with hypoglycaemia and favours the idea that there may be a *genetic* 'diabetic encephalopathy' with individual sensitivity to hypoglycaemia varying on a genetic basis. If it is decided that a diabetic child is having seizures independently of hypoglycaemia the drug of choice is probably carbamazepine. The phenytoins interfere with insulin production and usage and may cause ketosis.

Timperley et al. (1974) describe six cases who, in the course of diabetic ketoacidosis, developed cerebral intravascular coagulation which was thought to be the cause of death. Perhaps suprisingly, cerebrovascular lesions do not appear as clinical sequelae, at least as far as my experience goes.

Eye disorders

Transient disorders of vision may be present in hypoglycaemic attacks, during severe dehydration or during marked hyperglycaemia, and a poorly controlled child may complain of variations in vision without being acutely ill, but such disorders seem too transient to be properly classed as complications.

Cataracts are known to occur in childhood diabetes, and indeed if they occur at all they are likely to occur early in the disease. Danowski (1957) reports their presence in 1 per cent of diabetic children between the ages of 12 and 15 years, and my own impression is that they are very rare. Earlier writers have reported a higher incidence which may mean that the overall management of child diabetics has been improving since then, but this is not certain. Both progression and regression of cataracts have been reported during periods of good control, so the part played by good control in the prevention or treatment of cataracts is doubtful. Bilginturan, Jackson and Ide (1977) have recently discussed transitory cataracts and lens opacities from the biochemical aspect.

Retinopathy must first be defined. Hardin *et al.* (1956) describe nine grades. The earliest signs are venous dilatation (Grade 1) and a few punctate haemorrhages or capillary aneurysms (Grade 2). 'Diagnostic' diabetic proliferative retinopathy is Grade 9. If Grades 1 and 2 were excluded, the time required for the appearance of retinopathy was 13 years. After this basic period of 13 years the duration of the disease did not seem to be important in the progressive retinal deterioration, but the level of diabetic control did seem important. Pond and Oakley (1968) mentioned retinopathy in six of 134 children under the age of 16, but all six showed only the changes of Grades 1 and 2 so their findings are consistent with those of Hardin *et al.* The technique of fluorescein angiography (Toussaint *et al.*, 1976; Dorchy *et al.*, 1977) has, by showing small fluorescein leaks as the first signs of retinopathy, virtually doubled the diagnosis rate of retinopathy in childhood; but the condition is potentially reversible with improved control. Joos and Johnston (1957) discuss 44 children diagnosed as diabetic before the age of 15 years, and followed for an average of 14 years. Of the 44, 18 had developed retinopathy, and retinopathy was present in all those who had complications of any kind, which implies that retinopathy precedes other angiopathic complications, a view which is generally held. They also related retinopathy to poor control, but Knowles *et al.* (1965) introduced the puberty factor, pointing out that those who developed diabetes around puberty developed retinopathy five years earlier in the disease than those who had developed diabetes as young children.

Suggestions have been made that the appearance of retinopathy may be related to certain HLA types and immune complexes but this matter is still under debate.

In summary, diabetic retinopathy in childhood appears only as mild vascular changes, and even those are rare. The appearance of retinopathy in later life is linked with, if not entirely dependent on, the level of control and the deleterious influence of puberty.

Nephropathy

Like retinopathy, nephropathy has to be defined. Microangiopathy has been assessed by kidney biopsy and claims to have demonstrated focal basement capillary membrane thickening even before diabetes appeared have been made. Doubt has been cast on the specificity of these changes, if they indeed exist. Fox *et al.* (1977) have shown that, in rats with streptozocin-induced diabetes, the appearance of capillary basement membrane thickening was associated with high blood glucose.

If one considers only the more definite signs of kidney damage, there is very little evidence pointing to nephropathy in childhood. Balodimos, Legg and Bradley (1971) describe a boy of nine years who died in one of many attacks of ketoacidosis, death being due to cerebral oedema. Glycogen nephrosis was present, and in addition many glomeruli showed diffuse mesangial thickening. The findings stop short of the classic Kimmelstiel–Wilson type of glomerulosclerosis.

The presenting sign of nephropathy in a diabetic who is being kept under supervision is persistent proteinuria. Nephritis, pyelonephritis, and other causes of albuminuria have to be excluded. One isolated finding of protein is not likely to be significant. Pond found evidence of diabetic glomerulosclerosis in four out of 12 with persistent proteinuria in her 134 children examined under the age of 16. Although the urine of the Glasgow children is tested for albumin at each visit to the clinic, I have not found persistent proteinuria to be a problem, probably because they are referred to an adult hospital on their thirteenth birthday. It is worth noting that only one of the four with nephropathy referred to by Pond had retinopathy, which belies the belief that retinopathy always comes first.

THE PROGNOSIS FOR CHILDHOOD DIABETICS IN ADULT LIFE

Life expectancy and the significance of puberty

Pyke, Oakley and Taylor (1968), using figures from the Joslin Clinic, state that a child diabetic at the age of ten years can expect to live for a further 44.3 years. The expectancy for a normal ten-year-old is 61.5 years, so the diabetic child has a life expectancy which is 73 per cent of normal. This percentage figure is in fact marginally better than is found for diabetics of later onset, so the idea that a child diabetic is plunging towards an early grave whereas a man who gets diabetes in middle age will come close to his allotted span is false.

In discussing prognosis with parents I point out that the *average* life expectancy for a diabetic child is 75 per cent of normal but I go on to stress that this is only an average which includes neglected and neglectful diabetics and that good control can result in a life of normal length. This is meant to be encouraging, while at the same time stressing the need for taking every care in management.

Puberty is a dangerous time for the childhood diabetic, and it seems to be at that time rather than in earlier childhood that the basis of serious complications is laid down. Larsson, Sterky and Christiansson (1962) followed children for varying periods up to 19 years. Of 24 children who had developed the disease under the age of six years, three were dead; of 20 with the onset between the ages of six and ten, four were dead; of 15 with the onset between 11 and 15, seven were dead; and the length of follow-up was the same for all groups. They also took notice of the signs of angiopathy (essentially retinopathy and nephropathy) and found no correlation between the duration of diabetes and angiopathy, those in the 11–15 years group being much more likely to get it than those in the 0–5 years group. This difference might be simply the effect of chronological age, but in fact no correlation was found between chronological age and angiopathy, except for vascular calcification. The impression given is that angiopathy, or the clinical manifestations of angiopathy, is related to puberty rather than to the age at which a child develops diabetes.

Larsson, Sterky and Christiansson see the dangers of puberty as an argument for the paediatrician retaining control of his patient up to the age of 16 years, presumably because they think it unfair to present adult physicians with new cases at their most unstable, though this is not actually said. I would not go as far as this myself. The lesson I take from the figures is that the paediatrician may have a period of several years in which little serious may be happening, during which he should be concentrating on promoting in the child an attitude to his diabetes which is honest, accepting and responsible.

The prognosis for the very young diabetic

The long-term prognosis for children who develop diabetes before the age of two years is of particular interest and sheds light on the prognosis for children as a whole. Imerslund (1960) reported on 134 such children who had attended the Joslin Clinic between 1922 and 1956. One must bear in mind that a study going back to 1922 will cover the earliest days of insulin, and that the rate of complications will be relatively high. Of the 134, 20 were dead and 25 were lost to follow-up. Imerslund's results may be summarized as follows.

(1) *Deaths.* Seven of the 20 dead had died before the age of five years. Coma and infections were the commonest causes of death, but there had been no death from coma since 1948, nor from infection since 1954. Antibiotics, the fall in the prevalence of tuberculosis and improved intravenous therapy have reduced the death rate considerably.
(2) *Height.* The females had attained normal adult height. The males were 7 cm below the average. This sex difference is striking and is in accord with the findings of other writers in children with diabetes of later onset. Pond (1971) thinks that inability to adhere to diet is commoner in the growth-retarded group, but it seems likely that the sex hormones also play a part.
(3) *Intelligence.* Five were 'feeble-minded', and two of these were also epileptic. On the other hand, one had a PhD. The remainder were within the normal range of intelligence. Intelligence is normal in children with diabetes of later onset.
(4) *Epilepsy.* Epilepsy alone, without mental defect, was found in seven. Mental retardation and epilepsy are two striking complications which are mainly confined to children with diabetes of very early onset and which are presumably due to frequent *undetected* hypoglycaemia. The significance of these serious complications is lost if one considers life-expectancy alone.
(5) *Retinitis* was the first 'adult' complication to appear and was present in 10 per cent of the ten to 14 year age group. The severity of the retinopathy was not fully discussed. Retinopathy in some form was present in all by the age of 30–40 years, but retinitis proliferans in only 16.7 per cent.
(6) *Proteinuria and neuropathy* were not found before the age of 18

years, but investigations have become more sophisticated since Imerslund wrote her paper and there is evidence now (*see above*) that involvement of the kidneys and nerves may occur earlier in childhood.

(7) *Hypertension* appeared first at the age of 25 years, although 30 per cent had shown calcified arteries in the 20–24 years age group. This finding again reflects the early days of insulin.

These results refer to an exceptional age group. Three further studies should be mentioned to give an impression of the prognosis for children who develop diabetes later.

Children developing diabetes before the age of ten

Pyke, Oakley and Taylor (1968) report on the fate of 110 children who developed diabetes before the age of ten, and who were reviewed after at least 15 years of diabetes. Deaths were excluded, but were few.

Retinopathy was present in 64, but only five of these were seriously affected. Sixteen showed lens opacities, 13 of those in association with retinopathy.

Persistent proteinuria was found in 31, but in only seven of these was there further evidence of renal damage.

Hypertension was found in four cases. Absent arterial pulsation at the foot was also found in four.

In all, only nine patients were seriously affected, five by retinopathy and four by renal damage.

Children developing diabetes before the age of 15

White (1960) gives a review of childhood diabetics after at least 30 years of their disease. She reported on 478 patients who had developed diabetes before the age of 15 (not just in the ten to 15 years age group).

Thirty years on, 90 per cent of the patients showed retinopathy, but proliferative retinopathy was present in only 30 per cent and blindness in 8 per cent.

Persistent proteinuria was present in 42 per cent.

Fifty-six (12 per cent) had died, 29 from heart disease, 17 from renal failure.

It should be noted that this report again takes us back to the 1920s, and that the series includes puberty-onset cases, so there is reason to hope that the prognosis for the child diabetic is now better than these figures suggest. Further discussion of the complications of adult life is beyond the scope of this small book, but can be pursued in a textbook on diabetes in adults.

Death in childhood diabetes

Imerslund's report on deaths of very young diabetics is given above. In a recent review, Smith and Hudson (1976) comment that the Registrar General's returns show that the death rate from diabetes in England and Wales in children under 15 years has run for many years at about 25 per annum. This conveys little information and they therefore summarize ten deaths occurring in their own practice over a period of 25 years. The major factor contributing to death in childhood is a profound metabolic disturbance. At the Royal Hospital for Sick Children, Glasgow, where the diabetic population is about the same size, there have been eight deaths in the past 16 years. One died within three hours of admission of hyperosmolar coma, one was admitted moribund from another hospital, one died of dysentery in a fever hospital and two who had severe cystic fibrosis had developed diabetes almost as a terminal phenomenon, the essential cause of death being cystic fibrosis. Two died of cerebral oedema, probably because of being given too much hypotonic fluid too early, but one has the clinical impression that there may be patient-to-patient variation in susceptibility to cerebral oedema as I have once seen it occur when even retrospectively there seemed to be no flaw in management.

REFERENCES

Asherov, J., Mimouni, M., Varsano, I., Lubin, E. and Baron, Z. (1979). Hepatomegaly due to self-induced hyperinsulinism. *Arch. Dis. Childh.*, **54,** 148

Balodimos, M. C., Legg, M.A. and Bradley, R. F. (1971). Diabetic glomerulosclerosis in children. *Diabetes*, **20,** 622

Bauer, Marjorie F., Hirsch, P., Bullock, W. K. and Abul-Haj, S. K. (1964). Necrobiosis lipoidica diabeticorum. *Arch. Dermatol.*, **90,** 558

Bilginturan, A. N., Jackson, A. L. and Ide, C. H. (1977). Transitory cataracts in children with diabetes mellitus. *Pediatrics*, **60,** 106

Danowski, T. S. (1957). *Diabetes mellitus, with Emphasis on Children and Young Adults.* p. 433 Williams and Wilkins; Baltimore

Deligeorgis, D., Yannakos, D., Panayotou, P. and Doxiadis, S. (1970). The normal borders of the liver in infancy and childhood; clinical and x-ray study. *Arch. Dis. Childh.*, **45,** 702

REFERENCES

Deligeorgis, D., Yannakos, D. and Doxiadis, S. (1973). Normal size of liver in infancy and childhood: x-ray study. *Arch. Dis. Childh.*, **48**, 790

Dorchy, H., Toussaint, D., Devroede, M. and Ernould, C. (1977). Angiofluorescein studies in infantile diabetic retinopathy. *Acta paediat. Belg.*, **30**, 59

Dunnigan. M. G. (1976). Personal communication

Eeg-Olofsson, O. (1977). Hypoglycaemia and neurological disturbances in children with diabetes mellitus. *Acta paediat. Scand.*, Suppl. 270, 91

Eeg-Olofsson, O. and Perersen, I (1966). Childhood diabetic neuropathy. A clinical and neurophysiological study. *Acta paediat.*, **55**, 163

Ewing, D. J., Campbell, I. W., Murray, A., Neilson, J. M. M. and Clarke, B. F. (1978). Immediate heart-rate response to standing: simple test for autonomic neuropathy in diabetes. *Br. med. J.*, **1**, 145

Fox, C. J., Darby, S. C., Ireland, J. T. and Sönksen, P. H. (1977). Blood glucose control and glomerular capillary basement membrane thickening in experimental diabetes. *Br. med. J.*, **2**, 605

Gamstorp, I., Shelbourne, S. A., Engleson, G., Redondo, D. and Traisman, H. S. (1966). Peripheral neuropathy in juvenile diabetes. *Diabetes*, **15**, 411

Grgic, A., Rosenbloom, A. L., Weber, F. T., Giordano, B., Malone, J. I. and Shuster, J. J. (1976). Joint contractures—common manifestation of childhood diabetes. *J. Pediat.*, **88**, 584

Grieve, N. W. T., Bird, D. R. H. and Collyer, A. J. (1969). Pneumomediastinum and diabetic hyperpnoea. *Br. med. J.*, **I**, 186

Hardin, R. C., Jackson, R. L., Johnston, T. L. and Kelly, H. G. (1956). The development of diabetic retinopathy. Effect of duration and control of diabetes. *Diabetes*, **5**, 397

Imerslund, Olga (1960). The prognosis in diabetes with onset before the age of two. *Acta paediat.*, **49**, 243

Joos, T. H. and Johnston, J. A. (1957). A long-term evaluation of the juvenile diabetic. *J. Pediat.*, **50**, 133

Knowles, H. C., Guest, G. M., Lampe, J., Kessler, M. and Skillman, T. G. (1965). The course of juvenile diabetes treated with unmeasured diet. *Diabetes*, **14**, 239

Larsson, Y., Sterky, G. and Christiansson, G. (1962). Long-term prognosis in juvenile diabetes mellitus. *Acta paediat.*, **51**, Suppl. 130

Lawrence, D. G. and Locke, S. (1963). Neuropathy in children with diabetes mellitus. *Br. med. J.*, **1**, 784

Lee, R. G. L. and Bode, H. H. (1977). Stunted growth and hepatomegaly in diabetes mellitus. *J. Pediat.*, **91**, 82

Leifer, A. (1928). A case of insulin edema. *J. Am. med. Ass.*, **90**, 610

Mandell, F. and Berenberg, W. (1974). The Mauriac syndrome. *Am. J. Dis. Child.*, **127**, 900

Manderson, W. G., McKiddie, M. T., Manners, D. J. and Stark, J. R. (1968). Liver glycogen accumulation in unstable diabetes. *Diabetes*, **17**, 13

Marble, A., White, P., Bogan, I. K. and Smith, R. M. (1938). Enlargement of the liver in diabetic children. *Arch. int. Med.*, **62**, 740

Middeton, G. M. and Hockaday, T. D. R. (1965). Glycogen-laden hepatomegaly in diabetes. *Diabetologia*, **1**, 116

Pavy, F. W. (1885). Introductory address to the discussion on the clinical aspect of glycosuria. *Lancet*, 1085

Pond, Helen (1971). Diabetes mellitus. In *Recent Advances in Paediatrics*. p. 317. Ed. D. Gairdner and D. Hull. London; J. and A. Churchill

Pond, Helen and Oakley, W. G. (1968). Diabetes in children. In *Clinical Diabetes and its Biochemical Basis*. Ed. W. G. Oakley, D. A. Pyke, and K. W. Taylor. Oxford; Blackwell

Pyke, D. A., Oakley, W. G. and Taylor, K. W. (1968). The prognosis of diabetes. *Ibid*
Reske-Nielsen, E., Gregersen, G., Harmsen, A. and Lundbaek, K. (1970). Morphological abnormalities of the terminal neuromuscular apparatus in recent juvenile diabetes. *Diabetologia*, **6**, 104
Robertson, J. R., Earnshaw, P. M. and Campbell, I. W. (1979). Tenolysis in juvenile cheiroarthropathy. *Br. med. J.*, **2**, 971
Rosenbloom, A. L. and Giordano, B. (1977). Chronic overtreatment with insulin in children and adolescents. *Am. J. Dis. Child.*, **131**, 881
Smith, C. S. and Hudson, F. P. (1976). Mortality in juvenile diabetes mellitus over 25 years. *Arch. Dis. Childh.*, **51**, 297
Teuscher, A. (1974). The treatment of insulin lipo-atrophy with Monocomponent insulin. *Diabetologia*, **10**, 211
Timperley, W. R., Preston, F. E. and Ward, J. D. (1974). Cerebral intravascular coagulation in diabetic ketoacidosis. *Lancet*, **1**, 952
Toussaint, D., Quaetert, M., Dorchy, H. and Loeb, H. (1976). Early diagnosis of retinopathy in juvenile diabetes by fluorescein angiography. *Acta paediat. Belg.*, **29**, 177
Wagner, R., White, P. and Bogan, I. K. (1942). Diabetic dwarfism. *Am. J. Dis. Child.*, **63**, 667
White, P. (1960). Childhood diabetes. Its course, and influence on the second and third generations. *Diabetes*, **9**, 345
Zahler, M. C. and Skoglund, R. R. (1978). Pneumomediastinum associated with diabetic ketoacidosis. *J. Pediat.*, **93**, 529

CHAPTER 13

Food for the Diabetic

For the past 30 years Western nutritionists have shown a growing antipathy towards dietary fat. Their views have been enshrined in the report of the McGovern Committee, *Dietary Goals for the United States* (1977). These views have been widely (but not universally) accepted in other countries and in general endorsed by the American Diabetic Association (1979), though this report does say that there is no absolute proof that a high-carbohydrate, low-fat diet will work as planned. The over-all aim of the dietary recommendations is to lower blood cholesterol levels and thus prevent late vascular degeneration, of particular importance to diabetics. It is argued that, while the total fat should be reduced, the poly-unsaturated fraction should be increased. Dietary fibre should also be increased to flatten the absorption curve of carbohydrate. Cholesterol should be largely avoided.

The British paediatrician will see at once that these recommendations will call for a considerable alteration in the eating habits of British children, for reasons which will be discussed later. He may also muse about breast milk, the natural food for babies, remembering that 50 per cent of the calories of breast milk come from fat. It is now preached that 30–35 per cent of our calories should come from fat. Both breast milk and cow's milk are also high in cholesterol. A 10 lb baby gets about 110 mg daily, as opposed to a recommended adult intake of 300 mg daily. Should nature hang her head in shame at having provided so poorly for her infants or have nutritionists made unwarranted assumptions?

There has as yet been no prospective study to support current theories and such retrospective studies as claim to do so have either been criticized on grounds of methodology or contradicted by rival results (Mann, 1977; McMichael, 1977). Still clearly to be heard are the voices of those who believe that cholesterol deposits in major vessels are not the cause of disease but part of the healing process (Kaunitz, 1977). On the other hand we must remember that White (1933) described severe vascular changes in child diabetics in the early days of insulin treatment so child diabetics are potentially at risk.

The real point at issue is not what is desirable but what is feasible, particularly when dealing with children. Various aspects of the problem will now be discussed in greater detail.

CALORIES

A calorie count may be taken as the starting-point for calculating a strict diabetic diet, or the calories obtained from a loosely-controlled diet may be counted by dietary recall. Both methods will produce inaccurate facts, but in a field where it is impossible to obtain an accurate impression.

A formula often used for children is a daily intake of 1000 cal plus 100 × age in years, which would give a ten-year-old child 2000 cal. If one begins from a required number of calories it is easy to work out the relative amounts of protein (P), fat (F) and carbohydrate (CHO) needed. The old recommended ratio was 20P:40F:40CHO (as calories) but opinion has now swung to a ratio of 15:35:50 in keeping with the present distrust of fat and the high cost of protein. Many clinics in North America and Europe use this method and prescribe exchanges for all three main dietary constituents but the custom in Britain is to prescribe a known amount of CHO (e.g. 100 g plus 10 × age in years) and allow the protein and fat to be free.

Both these systems can be subject to modification. The stricter method may allow extra CHO to be given at times of increased work. The 'limited CHO' method may be accompanied by advice rather than rules on the amount and type of fat and protein to be given.

When I first worked in a diabetic clinic 'Lawrence Lines' were in fashion. If given in the customary ratio of two CHO exchanges to one protein-and-fat exchange the final ratio was 16P:42F:42CHO. An increase in CHO would automatically lower the fat, but would also lower the protein to levels perhaps too low for a growing child. I formed the impression that such strict dietary control was more suited to a motivated adult than to an unmotivated child and I have gone over to 'limited CHO', accepting the attendant risks of a high fat intake. Birkbeck, Truswell and Thomas (1976), using a strict diet for child diabetics in Western Canada, calculated that they were giving a diet balanced 20:32:48, whereas British laissez-faire results in a 14:44:42 intake (not, in fact, very different from the original Lawrence Lines). To push the point to the extreme, one could say that on the one hand we have the strict dieters driving their patients into rebellion by impossible demands and on the other we have the indolent loose dieters spinelessly trying to keep their patients happy while negligently calling down upon them all the complications of the later diabetic life. The following sections are aimed at getting the best of both worlds.

CARBOHYDRATES

Carbohydrates are not the villains they once were. Several studies have shown that the carbohydrate (CHO) intake can be increased considerably, particularly if sustained exercise is being undertaken as at a diabetic camp, without a corresponding increase in urinary sugar. Even the Indian diabetic, who is taking a very high CHO diet without very much exercise, seems to need no more insulin than his Western counterpart. This presumably means that in the past protein and fat have been used as ancillary sources of energy and that extra CHO will prevent this. It is, therefore, far from certain that a rise in CHO intake should be accompanied by a rise in the insulin prescribed. One should wait and see.

There remains a relative prohibition on CHO being given as sugar on the grounds that it causes too rapid a swing in the blood sugar. There is, however, one occasion on which the use of sugar can be justified, and that is immediately before strenuous exercise. This gives one the excuse to allow the child a measured amount of ordinary sweets (candies) and if this results in a sudden increase in the amount of strenuous exercise which the child takes, so much the better.

Starch used to be starch, and that was that. Now there is evidence (Akerblom, 1979) that all starches do not have the same glycaemic effect. The blood sugar appears to rise less sharply after bread than potatoes, possibly because wet cooking (boiling potatoes) bursts the starch granules more than dry cooking (baking bread). This could be one of the many variables, and a minor one at that, which result in day-to-day variations in the blood sugar level. If we assume that all starches behave in the same way we are working from an inaccurate fact.

Akerblom *et al.* (1972) have also observed that fructose raises the blood sugar rather less than starch. But all fruits are not the same. Apples and pears have a high fructose:glucose ratio, bananas have not. Many years ago a mother told me that bananas always gave her son glycosuria whereas other fruits did not. She was a faddist who always referred to her son as a 'man-child' and I dismissed this as another of her daft notions. She was probably right. It is too late to apologize now. 'One piece of fruit equals another piece of fruit' is another inaccurate fact.

SWEETENERS AND DIABETIC PRODUCTS

A wide range of diabetic products are available, but their use is seldom to be recommended. The squashes and low-calorie drinks may be used freely, but most other products such as biscuits, chocolate and tinned fruit do contain some CHO and therefore must be counted in the diet. Each packet or container will have the CHO content clearly marked on it. Sorbitol is often used in diabetic products and this will be discussed below.

Saccharin is many times sweeter than sugar, but is not oxidized in the body to supply energy. It is used to replace sugar in reducing diets and is also of value to diabetics. It is supplied in tablet form only but can be dissolved in hot water to give a liquid sweetener. Saccharin should always be added *after* cooking to avoid a strong 'after-taste'. Saccharin has been suspected as a possible cause of bladder cancer but the connection has been debated and it is still available in Britain, where it is the cheapest of the sweeteners.

Saxin is a trade name for the sodium salt of saccharin. It is more soluble than saccharin, has less after-taste and is supplied in the form of tablets and solution. The solution is convenient for use in preparing food as well as in drinks, and can be added to the milk that is going to be poured over cornflakes. Cornflakes without a sweetener are unacceptable to many. Several proprietary sweeteners containing sodium saccharin are available, including liquid Saxin and Hermesetas.

Sorbitol is a hexahydric alcohol obtained by the reduction of glucose. It is only 60 per cent as sweet as sucrose but the sweetness is very similar to sucrose, with little after-taste. Furthermore, it can be used in the same way as sugar, i.e. it can be boiled and used in all forms of cooking and baking. These features have made it popular, particularly with the manufacturers of diabetic products, but it has disadvantages. These are:

(1) More than 15 g taken in a day may cause diarrhoea.
(2) It is oxidized in the body to supply energy, and Vaaler, Hanssen and Aagenaes (1980) have shown that meals containing sucrose

or sorbitol in equal amounts have almost exactly the same effect on the blood sugar.
(3) It costs a lot.

If we accept Vaaler's findings, sucrose is better than sorbitol, because it costs less. There is general agreement that if sorbitol is given it must be counted as carbohydrate. Logically, I should allow the diabetic children to put a scraping of cheaper, non-diabetic jam on their bread if they want it, and in fact I am tentatively beginning to do so.

Grapefruit skin contains a very strong sweetener which is at present under investigation.

LIPIDS

As has been mentioned, the present belief is that the diabetic diet should be low in fats, and that those fats should contain a high proportion of the polyunsaturated forms. It has been suggested that the ratio of saturated, monounsaturated and polyunsaturated fats should be 1:1:1, and when we remember that the present British intake is more like 5:4:1 it will be realized that there is justification in taking a fairly close look at the fats in our diet.

Neutral fats account for 98 per cent of the lipid intake. They are composed of triglycerides, i.e. glycerol in combination with three variable fatty acids. These fatty acids may be saturated (e.g. stearic), monounsaturated (e.g. oleic) or polyunsaturated (e.g. linoleic, linolenic).

Polyunsaturated fats are 'essential' as they cannot be synthesized in the human body. They are needed in prostaglandin metabolism and in the developing brain and for normal skin metabolism. In addition, it has been shown that a fat intake relatively high in polyunsaturates tends to lower the blood cholesterol, which indeed is why polyunsaturates are recommended, but animal experiments suggest that this may simply be the result of piling the cholesterol into the liver, which might do more harm than good.

The normal diet also includes, in small quantities:

(1) phospholipids, fatty acids in combination with nitrogen and phosphoric acid;
(2) cerebrosides, fatty acids combined with a nitrogenous substance and a sugar;
(3) sterols, which may exist free or form esters with fatty acids, for example cholesterol, which one should remember is essential as a precursor of steroid hormones.

TABLE 13.1

The percentage of fat, polyunsaturated fat and cholesterol in various fatty substances and oils

	Total fat	Polyunsaturated	Cholesterol
'Vegetable fat'	100	7	0
Sunflower oil	99.9	63	0
Soya-bean oil	99.9	60	0
Corn oil	99.9	56	0
Cotton-seed oil	99.9	50	0
Peanut oil	99.9	29	0
Palm oil	99.9	9	0
Olive oil	99.9	8	0
Butter	81	4	0.28
Margarine	81	14	0
'Flora'	80	55	0
Lard	99	10	0.1

There is a widespread belief among the intelligent but not fully informed that all vegetable oils are good, and animal fats bad. *Table 13.1* may go some way towards clearing this up. It will be seen that what is sold as unspecified 'vegetable fat' is low in polyunsaturated fat, and is in fact no better in this respect than lard. Certain British cooking fats come under this heading. The first four oils in the table all contain a high percentage of polyunsaturated fats, but the next three show a falling-off. By far the greatest fat fraction in olive oil is monounsaturated (oleic acid) and some believe that the monounsaturated fats are physiologically closer to the saturated than the polyunsaturated fats. Several branded vegetable cooking oils available in Britain do not state what oil or oils are being used, and this is because the content may vary from batch to batch depending on which oil is available on the world market at a good price. Some cooking oils based on corn oil are a 'good buy', but there is no guarantee that a vegetable cooking oil will be low in polyunsaturates unless the proportion of oils used is clearly stated on the label. Any margarine is better than butter as regards polyunsaturates, but only one or two (for example Flora, Outline) are much better. Again, one has to read the label.

The tired executive in his jet may fondly believe he is doing his arteries a good turn by adding 'non-dairy creamer' to his coffee. True, he may minutely reduce his cholesterol but coconut oil, on which the creamer is based, is 97 per cent saturated fat. Peanut oil, which must be in many cooking oils, seems to be more atherogenic than butter when given to monkeys.

Animal fats do not come off quite so badly as one might think. This is shown in *Table 13.2*. One should not become too excited about the high *percentage* of polyunsaturates in a haddock as the *total* fat content is low. On the other hand, one is entitled to look askance at the low figure for beef, where the total fat content is high. As for the mackerel, I just do not know. I *do* know that around our shores the total fat content of mackerel-meat is 5 per cent in February and 20 per cent in August, so if we eat an August mackerel we are presumably doing well for our daily intake of polyunsaturates. But does the ratio of the fats stay constant through the seasons and, if not, which mackerel figures have got into the table? There must be a lot of inaccurate facts in food tables.

TABLE 13.2

The percentage of total lipids of saturated, monounsaturated and polyunsaturated fats in various foodstuffs, and the cholesterol content as mg per 100g

	Saturated	Mono-unsaturated	Poly-unsaturated	Cholesterol
Haddock	29.6	20.9	45.3	60
Herring	22.3	55.8	19.6	70
Mackerel	27.0	41.3	27.1	80
Canned salmon	27.5	42.6	26.3	90
Turkey	36.5	26.9	29.5	80 dark meat, 50 light meat
Chicken	35.1	47.6	14.9	110 dark meat, 70 light meat
Beef	44.9	49.3	4.3	

Note: The totals for the three fats do not add up to 100 because 'other lipids' are excluded

PROTEIN

The only source of pure natural protein is white of egg. Otherwise, when one gives protein one gives fat. A high P : F ratio (calculated as calories) is best obtained from vegetable sources, particularly the pulses (*see Table 13.3*) though certain white fish are also good.

The figures in the table are often only approximate, particularly

TABLE 13.3

Distribution of protein, fat and carbohydrate in various foods, shown as calories per 100g

	Protein	Fat	CHO	Remarks
Fresh peas	27	4	68	This group is moderately
Tinned haricot beans	24	4	76	high in protein, low in fat
Dried lentils	103	9	237	
Roasted ground nuts	104	390	94	
Potatoes	8	1	76	
Carrot	4	2	36	Turnip similar
Cabbage	6	1	23	Cauliflower similar
Lettuce	5	2	11	
White bread	34	18	208	This group has butter, margarine
Wholemeal bread	38	32	192	or milk added at table, which upsets
Cornflakes	32	6	320	the favourable P : F ratio
Oatmeal porridge	11	5	46	
Milk	13	33	20	
Butter	2	729	2	
Egg	51	104	2	
Cheddar cheese	100	290	8	
Cod	66	3	0	Haddock and plaice similar
Herring	76	60	0	Halibut similar
Trout	77	19	0	
Tinned salmon	88	86	0	
Tinned sardines	103	243	0	Extra oil removed. Tunny similar
Roast chicken	81	113	0	
Lean roast beef	77	117	0	
Grilled steak	68	225	0	
Roast lamb	90	208	0	
Lamb chops, grilled	96	315	0	
Pork chops, grilled	57	288	0	
Bacon, grilled	100	495	0	

for the animal sources where the amount of fat is variable. The mackerel is a striking example, but even in Britain the amount of carcase fat in beef and lamb varies from region to region and from breed to breed. To talk about the fat content of bacon is almost farcical, the variations being obvious to the naked eye.

The *amount* of each food taken in the diet should also be remembered. One need not exclude bacon and butter from the diet on the basis of their high fat content, because they are taken in relatively small quantities. I think food tables are best used as a guide to what a child has been eating so that any excesses can be curbed. I do not think one should sit down with pages of food tables and construct a diet which the wretched child is supposed to take.

FIBRE

Dietary fibre has aroused much recent interest. Helpful reviews are to be found in a *Lancet* editorial (1977) and a paper by Saperstein and Spiller (1978). Readings for fibre in food tables usually refer to crude fibre and exclude pectins, gums and mucilages. The most approved fibre at present is guar, a gum.

The use of guar was first advocated as possibly preventing atheroma, ischaemic heart disease, diverticulitis and colonic neoplasm. It was then observed that meals containing guar appeared to limit the post-prandial rise of blood sugar in diabetics, making it a desirable additive to the diabetic diet. Another school of thought believes that any lowering of blood sugar so obtained may be of little therapeutic value. Furthermore, guar is not palatable and it tends to produce excess wind in the colon.

Karela is a small gourd which is eaten in the East and the Caribbean and which can be obtained in cities such as Glasgow either fresh or tinned. It has been shown to reduce glycosuria when eaten by diabetics, but this appears to be due to interference with the urine tests, the blood sugars being unaffected. It should therefore be remembered as a possible source of false negative urine tests in overseas patients (Gaskin, 1979).

Bran can be used in the diet, either as a breakfast cereal or mixed with other food, but there are few children who like it (though some do) and its effect in diabetes is less than that of guar. It is right to remember that fibre is a constituent of a balanced diet, but I do not think a paediatrician need feel guilty if he does not have all his patients on guar.

NATIONAL FEEDING HABITS

A comparison of eating habits in Britain and some other European countries is given in *Table 13.4*.

TABLE 13.4

Supplies of certain foods in certain EEC countries, 1974–5 (kg/person/year)

	UK	France	West Germany	Italy
Milk	145	65	59	56
Meat	74	97	89	65
Potatoes	99	95	92	37
Fruit	48	79	116	108
Refined sugar	46	38	36	29
Visible fats	22	24	25	23
Wheat	64	70	47	129

(From the Ministry of Agriculture, Fisheries and Food, 1976)

It will be seen at once that Britain is at a disadvantage in constructing an 'ideal' diet for a diabetic child, while still conforming to national custom. We take a great deal of milk and 50 per cent of the calories of milk come from fat, which gets us off on the wrong foot. On the other hand, other Europeans eat more cheese than we do. We take an average amount of potatoes but our vegetable intake is low. We take little fruit. To be thoroughly parochial, the Scottish intake of fruit and vegetables is well below the low British average.

Our consumption of meat is above that of Italy, but well below that of France and West Germany. In addition, the British take the highest percentage of lamb, which contains more fat than beef.

The disadvantages show most clearly in the snacks. Milk is often taken and the favourite solid in this part of the country is potato crisps ('chips' in the USA). Fifty-five per cent of the calories of crisps come from fat. The league is headed at 67 per cent by peanuts ('ground nuts'). Obviously we should be using more fruit, biscuits, etc.

SOCIAL EATING

Meals are more than 'nosh-ups'. They should be times when the family is sitting round a table, enjoying their food, talking and looking at each other's faces. They are the only occasions on which natural, easy, intra-family communication is likely to take place. Playing with children is similar, but it lacks the eye-to-eye contact of meal-times, and play may be too competitive for relaxation. Certainly, there can be rows at meal-times, but ideally there are not.

The diabetic child wants to eat the same as the rest of the family, and our reasons for instructing otherwise must be very strong. Unusual diets may be acceptable to adults and indeed welcomed by hypochondriacs, but they are not for children. It is usually easy for the family to make minor adjustments (for example refraining from sugared cakes) to fit in with the diabetic child. There should be no unnecessary strife around the table. 'Eat up your nice cabbage' is bad enough, 'Eat up your nice guar' is worse. To be too strict with diet is to risk creating a child who is rebellious not just at table but in every aspect of his diabetic life. That is a disaster. It will produce a much more prolonged upset of his diabetic control than will some slight laxity when fitting the eating habits of the diabetic to those of the rest of the family.

Many children, diabetic or not, are difficult with their food. If there is a problem at meal-times, the main thing is to keep regular the quickly available source of energy, carbohydrate. Day-to-day variations in protein and fat are not so important. What he takes in a week has more meaning than what he takes in a day.

SUGGESTED ADJUSTMENTS TO DIET

Various aspects of the diabetic diet have been discussed. The time has come to say what I do in practice. The principles I work on are:

(1) A regular intake of carbohydrate should be prescribed, divided into three main meals and three snacks.
(2) There is probably enough evidence to suggest that fats, particularly saturated fats, should be given in reduced amounts, but there is not enough evidence to justify this if the child objects strongly.

The resultant advice given to mothers works out something like this:

(1) A margarine high in polyunsaturated fats should be used instead of butter, but if the child still demands butter he is allowed it.
(2) Milk should be kept to one pint (540 ml) per day, but if the child is not a meat-eater the milk allowance can be increased.
(3) Meat should be grilled where possible, to minimize the fat content.
(4) Crisps should not be given more than three times a week, eggs should be limited to four or five a week, and cheese should be regarded as a savoury rather than a free food when he is hungry. Crisps may be difficult to limit as it is quite common for a Scottish child to eat two packets a day.
(5) White fish and poultry should be taken more often.
(6) 'Fish and chips', though dietetically unsound because of the frying, can be given once a week as a treat, as it would be unwise to forbid it altogether—in Glasgow, at any rate. Corn oil should be used in the frying.
(7) The use of flour to thicken mince and sauces is not forbidden, as long as the amount used is known and counted as CHO. The amount may be so low as to be negligible.
(8) Fruit should be used more often.
(9) Sweets, chocolates or candy can be taken before strenuous exercise in amounts sufficient to prevent hypoglycaemia.
(10) Ordinary jams and marmalade can be used if spread thinly, and counted as 5 g of CHO.
(11) The prescribed CHO can be raised if he is hungry.

These comments are given as suggestions, not rules, and are open to negotiation.

REFERENCES

Akerblom, H. K., Siltanen, I. and Kallio, A. (1972). Does dietary fructose affect the control of diabetes in children? *Acta med. Scand.*, Suppl. 542, 195

Akerblom, H. K. (1979). An appraisal of the glycaemic effect of some dietary carbohydrates in insulin-dependent diabetics. In *Nutrition and the diabetic child. Paediat. adolesc. Endocr.*, **7,** 69.

American Diabetic Association (Committee Report) (1979). Principles of nutrition and dietary recommendations for individuals with diabetes mellitus. *Diabetes*, **28,** 1027

Birkbeck, J. A., Truswell, A. S. and Thomas, B. J. (1976). Current practice in dietary management of diabetic children. *Arch. Dis. Childh.*, **51,** 467

Gaskin, R. St. C. (1979). Karela and tests for glycosuria. *Lancet*, **1,** 986

Kaunitz, H. (1977). Repair function of cholesterol versus the lipid theory of arteriosclerosis. *Chemistry and industry*, Sept. 17

Lancet (editorial) (1977). Dietary fibre, **2,** 337

McMichael, J. (1977). Dietetic factors in coronary disease. *Eur. J. Cardiol.*, **5/6,** 447
Mann, G. V. (1977) Diet-Heart: end of an era. *New Engl. J. Med*, **297,** 644
Saperstein, S. and Spiller, G. A. (1978) Dietary fiber. *Am. J. Dis. Child.*, **132,** 657
Vaaler, S., Hanssen, K. F. and Aagenaes, O. (1979) Influence of two types of sweetness on the blood glucose after breakfast in young juvenile diabetics. In *Nutrition and the diabetic child. Pediat. adolesc. Endocr.* **7,** 132. Basel; Karger
Weil, W. B. (1979). National dietary goals. *Am. J. Dis. Child.*, **133,** 368
White, P. (1933). *Diabetes in Childhood and Adolescence*, p. 178. London; Henry Kimpton

CHAPTER 14

Notes on Diabetic Diet

Fiona House
(Chief Dietitian, Royal Hospital for Sick Children, Glasgow)

It is assumed that the reader

(1) knows the broad principles of dietetics,
(2) will be using a limited carbohydrate diet,
(3) knows the total amount of carbohydrate to be given in the day (p. 23), and
(4) has decided on the initial distribution of carbohydrate between the meals and snacks.

This section will discuss some special situations which may confront the diabetic. A few recipes will be given. A list of carbohydrate exchanges and a short bibliography are appended for reference.

SOME SPECIAL SITUATIONS

School meals

The problem with the normal school meal as far as the diabetic is concerned is the pudding. This usually consists of a dish high in concentrated carbohydrate which was thought to be impossible to include in a diabetic diet. However, closer examination of the size of the dish and the ingredients per portion have led us to allow our patients to take the normal school pudding and to count this as 30 g

CHO. Allowing the children to take the pudding has the great advantage of making them the same as their peers.

The main course at the meal is less of a problem. Meat dishes such as stew or mince can be allowed freely, the thickening of the gravy being ignored. The potatoes are easily counted. Six chips, one small roast or boiled potato and one scoop of mashed potato all contain 10 g of CHO. In practice most primary schoolchildren are given one scoop of potatoes giving them a total of 40 g at lunchtime including the pudding whereas secondary schoolchildren get two scoops of potatoes giving them a total of 50 g CHO.

Pastry is used a lot at school meals and is more difficult to judge because the CHO content depends on the type of pastry, but a rough guide would be that a 2-inch square is one portion. Breadcrumbs on fried fish count as half a portion. Two fish fingers count as one portion.

The introduction of the choice of menu system to more schools makes it much easier for the older diabetic to choose a suitable meal. The menu often includes fresh fruit, biscuits and cheese, jelly, ice cream and soup all of which the diabetic could judge fairly accurately for CHO content.

Packed lunches are popular with some children but if they are not suitable and the child or parent does not want to allow an ordinary school meal it is possible to have a special school meal provided. Methods for arranging this vary from area to area but generally a letter and a diet sheet from a doctor or dietitian to the Area Community Medicine Specialist is required. He in turn will inform the Area School Meals Organizer.

Eating out

Most hotels offer a wide enough selection of foods on their menu to allow a diabetic to choose a meal to comply with his diet. The following are foods commonly found on the menu:

Tomato juice	Free	
Fruit juice	Small glass	10 g CHO
Melon	Free	
Consommé	Free	
Cream soup	Small bowl	10 g CHO
Fish in sauce	Leave the sauce	

Fish in batter	Leave the batter	
Fish in crumbs	Small fish	10 g CHO
Omelettes	Free	
Salads	Free Leave the mayonnaise dressing	
Roast meats, chops, steaks	Free	
Made-up dishes, e.g. rissottos	Avoid	
Vegetables	Free Except peas, corn, baked beans, potatoes	
Corn	45 g (1½ oz) (2 dessert spoons)	10 g CHO
Peas	4 tablespoons	10 g CHO
Potatoes	4–5 chips	10 g CHO
	1 small roast or boiled	10 g CHO
	1 scoop mashed	10 g CHO
Fresh fruit	1 piece	10 g CHO
Ice cream	1 scoop or 1 small block	10 g CHO
Biscuits and cheese	2 plain biscuits	10 g CHO

After weighing 10 g CHO portions over a period of time the diabetic or his mother should be able to judge the portions by eye. Extra can be left on the plate. When in doubt about what a dish contains ask the waiter to explain.

One ounce weighs 28.35 g and one fluid ounce measures 28.41 ml. In this and subsequent sections one ounce is taken to weigh 30 g and one fluid ounce to measure 30 ml.

Indian and Chinese meals are much more popular now and there is no reason why the diabetic should not enjoy these also. We have included some recipes to try at home, but when eating out or buying a 'carry out' the important thing to be able to do is to recognize an exchange of cooked rice. It does not matter whether it is plain or fried rice, the CHO content is the same. I normally recommend people to weigh 15 g dry rice and cook it so that they can see what a portion looks like but as a rough guide two pudding spoons of cooked rice give 10 g CHO.

Curries are no problem for the diabetic since the ingredients are normally 'free', the exception being the split pea curries, for example, dhal—a kind of concentrated lentil soup which should be counted as such—20 g CHO for a small portion.

One small chapati (the size of your hand) is 10 g CHO and a restaurant portion of pokeras should be counted as 20 g CHO.

Most Chinese dishes consist mainly of protein and free vegetables. The only dish likely to cause a problem is the 'sweet and sour' one which will count because of the batter on the food and the chutney in the sauce. Try the recipe in the book and then you will be able to judge amounts better when you eat out.

Since both Indian and Chinese desserts tend to be very sweet it would perhaps be better to keep to ice cream.

Parties

Most children's parties take place in the afternoon and so the mid-afternoon snack can be given as party fare. An extra 10 g carbohydrate should also be given at this time to cover excitement and extra exercise. Advice to give mothers is as follows.

Going to parties

(1) Take diabetic squash with you.
(2) Tell the hostess in advance and help her to arrange suitable foods for your child. She may appreicate your taking diabetic jelly to the party.
(3) At the party watch your child and help him to choose his CHO allowance.
(4) Make sure he actually eats it.
(5) Watch the child carefully until his next meal in case of a 'hypo'.

Giving parties

(1) Provide diabetic squash for everyone—they will never know the difference and it makes your child the same as everyone else.
(2) Make all your sandwiches up to 10 g or 20 g CHO portions—they can be open sandwiches or rolls with the centre removed and then filled.

(3) Make diabetic jelly for everyone—½ litre (1 pint) squash+15 g (½ oz) gelatine to set. Serve with cream (which has no carbohydrate content) instead of evaporated milk.
(4) Buy your ice cream in bulk, for example ½ gallon tub, and serve it with 60 g (2 oz) potato scoop so that every serving is a portion.
(5) Give out packets of crisps instead of putting them into bowls.
(6) If your child is old enough, decide in advance what he will take as his CHO allowance.

Picnics

(1) Always take the total amount of carbohydrate your child will require for the period you will be away. This will include snacks.
(2) Take plenty of free foods as 'fillers', for example, salad, vegetables, cold meats, hard-boiled eggs, cheese. Flasks of tea, coffee, Oxo, Bovril are very useful.
(3) Carry extra carbohydrate to cover extra exercise.
(4) If you are taking sandwiches or bread for more than one meal it is often easier and safer to label them.
(5) Weight for weight rolls have the same amount of CHO as bread but they are often easier to deal with on picnics. Take the dough out of the centre of the roll and then weigh it. This usually halves the weight of the roll and leaves more space for the filling. Double-decker sandwiches are another way of making the carbohydrate allowance go further. Take three slices of bread and put filling between them.
(6) Extra cold meat, cheese, salad etc. can be carried in plastic airtight containers
(7) Yoghurts, crisps, fruit and ice cream can all be used as part of the picnic.

Illness

If a child is unable, through illness, to take his usual food, the carbohydrate part of the diet must be in another form. Examples of liquid, convalescent and normal diets for a boy of five years on a diet of 150 g of CHO daily are appended *(Table 14.1)*.

SOME SPECIAL SITUATIONS 291

TABLE 14.1

	Liquid	CHO	Convalescent	CHO	Normal	CHO
Breakfast	Lucozade 180ml (6oz)	30	45g (1⅓oz) bread, as toast	20	Cornflakes 15g (½oz)	10
			Milk 200ml (7oz)	10	Milk 200ml (7oz)	10
					Bread 20g (⅔oz)	10
Mid-morning	Milk 200ml (7oz)	10	Milk 100ml (3½oz)	5	Diabetic squash	
			1 Rich Tea biscuit	5	2 Rich Tea biscuits	10
Lunch	Tinned unsweetened orange juice 230ml (8oz)	20	Tomato soup, 100ml (3oz)	10	Mince	
			Custard 120g (4oz)	20	Cabbage	
			Milk 200ml (7oz)	10	Potatoes 60g (2oz)	10
	20g (⅔oz) glucose (4 level teaspoons)	20			Stewed apple, 120g (4oz)	10
					Custard 60g (2oz)	10
					Milk 200ml (7oz)	10
Mid-afternoon	Milk 200ml (7oz)	10	Milk 100ml (3½oz)	5	Packet of crisps	10
			1 Rich Tea biscuit	5	Diabetic squash	
Tea	Lucozade 230ml (8oz)	40	Poached egg on bread 20g (⅔oz) as toast	10	Fish fingers 60g (2oz)	10
					Chips 30g (1oz)	10
			Jelly 60g (2oz) plus evaporated milk 100ml (3oz)	10	Tomato	
					Bread 40g (1⅓oz)	20
				10		
			Milk 200ml (7oz)	10		
Supper	Milk 200ml (7oz)	10	Milk 200ml (7oz) as cocoa	10	Bread 20g (⅔oz)	10
	Ovaltine 15g (½oz)	10	Bread 20g (⅔oz) as toast	10	Milk 200ml (7oz)	10

Note (1) The liquid diet can be spread out from one meal to the next. 'Lucozade 230 ml' looks a lot, but is less than a tumblerful and can be taken over two to three hours.

Note (2) Much milk is suggested during convalescence because of its food value. If a child cannot take it all, other drinks can be substituted. These diets are only examples.

CARBOHYDRATE EXCHANGES

Unrestricted foods (free)

The following foods are allowed without restriction, if taken in normal amounts:

Bacon, beef, brains, corned beef, cheese, egg, frankfurters, ham, hare, heart, kidney, lamb, liver, ox tongue, pork, poultry, rabbit, sweetbreads, tripe and veal. Fish of any kind, cooked without batter, breadcrumbs or sauce. Butter, cooking oil, cream, dripping, ghee, lard, margarine, olive oil, suet.

Fresh fruit: Blackberries, blackcurrants, gooseberries, grapefruit, lemons, loganberries, melon, rhubarb.

Vegetables: Artichokes, asparagus, aubergine, avocado pear, beans (French or runner), broccoli, Brussels sprouts, cabbage, carrots, cauliflower, celery, chicory, cress, cucumber, endive, green peppers, leeks, lettuce, marrow, mushrooms, nuts (except chestnuts and peanuts), onion, parsley, radish, seakale, spinach, spring onions, tomato, turnips, watercress.

Gelatin, essences, chives, mustard, pepper, mint and other herbs and spices, clear mixed pickles, pickled onions, Worcester sauce, Bovril, Marmite, Oxo.

Coffee (ground or instant—no milk), tea, cocoa powder.

Clear soups, unthickened gravy.

Lemon juice, tomato juice.

Low calorie squash, diabetic squash, soda water.

Hermesetas, saccharin, Saxin, and Sweetex tablets or liquid sweeteners.

Foods to be avoided

Glucose, honey, jam, marmalade, sugar, syrup, treacle.
Mineral waters: ginger beer, lemonade, Lucozade, Ribena, squash (some of these can be used if taking extra exercise in hot weather, for example, on holiday). Gravy thickeners, sauces, batters, salad dressing, mayonnaise, fruits tinned in syrup, chocolates, boiled sweets, toffees, sweetened condensed milk.

Restricted foods

Each of the following contains about 10 g carbohydrate i.e. one portion. These may be exchanged one for another to give variety to the diet:

Cereal foods

All Bran	20 g (⅔ oz)
Plain biscuits	15 g (½ oz)
Bread* (white or brown or rolls)	20 g (⅔ oz)
Breakfast cereals	15 g (½ oz)
Cornflour, custard powder, flour, rice, sago, semolina, tapioca, oatmeal, cornmeal	15 g (½ oz)
Macaroni, noodles, spaghetti—before cooking	15 g (½ oz)
Chapati (1 thin) using ½ oz of wheat flour	15 g (½ oz)
Cooked porridge	120 g (4 oz)
Boiled rice	30 g (1 oz)
Crispbread	15 g (½ oz)

Fruit

Apples, raw with skin and core	120 g (4 oz)
Apples, stewed	150 g (5 oz)
Apples, baked with skin	120 g (4 oz)
Apricots, fresh with stone	180 g (6 oz)
Apricots, dry, raw	30 g (1 oz)
Banana, without skin	60 g (2 oz)
Cherries, with stones	120 g (4 oz)
Currants, raisins, dried sultanas	15 g (½ oz)
Damsons, with stones	150 g (5 oz)
Dates, with stones	20 g (⅔ oz)
Figs, green, raw	120 g (4 oz)

* Parents should weigh, on diabetic scales, a slice of the bread commonly used in the household, to check whether or not it is 20g (⅔ oz).

Figs, dried, stewed   45 g (1½ oz)
Grapes   60 g (2 oz)
Greengages, stewed with stones   120 g (4 oz)
Green banana   120 g (4 oz)
Nectarines, with stones   90 g (3 oz)
Oranges   120 g (4 oz)
Peaches, fresh with stones   120 g (4 oz)
Pears   120 g (4 oz)
Pineapple   90 g (3 oz)
Plums, with stones   120 g (4 oz)
Prunes, stewed with stones   60 g (2 oz)
Raspberries, fresh   180 g (6 oz)
Strawberries   180 g (6 oz)
Tangerines   120 g (4 oz)

Vegetables

Beans, baked, tinned   60 (2 oz)
Beans, broad   150 g (5 oz)
Beans, butter, boiled   60 g (2 oz)
Beans, haricot, boiled   60 g (2 oz)
Beetroot, boiled   120 g (4 oz)
Lentils, raw   20 g (⅔ oz)
Parsnips, boiled   90 g (3 oz)
Peas, fresh, frozen, boiled   135 g (4½ oz)
Peas, tinned   60 g (2 oz)
Potatoes, boiled or mashed   60 g (2 oz)
Potatoes, chips   30 g (1 oz)
Potatoes, roast or sauté   45 g (1½ oz)
Potato crisps, 1 packet   25 g (¾ oz)

Sweet corn	45 g (1½ oz)
Sweet potato, boiled	45 g (1½ oz)
Yam, boiled	45 g (1½ oz)

Nuts, shelled

Almonds	Allowed free in small quantities	240 g (8 oz)
Brazils	,, ,, ,, ,, ,,	240 g (8 oz)
Chestnuts	,, ,, ,, ,, ,,	30 g (1 oz)
Hazel nuts	,, ,, ,, ,, ,,	150 g (5 oz)
Peanuts	,, ,, ,, ,, ,,	120 g (4 oz)
Walnuts	,, ,, ,, ,, ,,	200 g (7 oz)

Milk

Fresh or sterilized	200 ml (7 oz)
Evaporated (unsweetened)	90 ml (3 oz)

Miscellaneous foods

Ice cream, any flavour	60 g (2 oz)
Plain yoghurt	200 ml (7 oz)
Mousse	60 g (2 oz)
Ordinary jelly, made up as directed on packet	60 g (2 oz)
Tinned spaghetti	90 g (3 oz)
* Sausages (prepacked or butcher's)	90 g (3 oz)

* Most children like sausages, but a doctor may be unwilling to allow them because of their doubtful CHO content. Butchers' sausages may contain 50–90 per cent meat, depending on quality, but a good butcher's sausages will contain about 75 per cent meat, the rest carbohydrate. According to my own butcher, who may be biased but who has a pleasant turn of phrase, *skinless* sausages contain 'an awful lot of emulsified cahoochie—sinew, skin and snouts' all of which count as meat on analysis. ('Cahoochie', is a Scottish dialect word for 'rubber'.) It appears that, were it not for the adhesive properties of emulsified cahoochie, a skinless sausage would disintegrate at a touch. Presumably they differ from ordinary sausages in fat and amino acid balance.

In Germany, the law demands 97 per cent meat in a sausage, so Frankfurters are allowed 'free'. 'They lie like lead on your stomach' says my butcher, loyal to his homeland, but children seem to like them.

Black pudding	90 g (3 oz)
Cream of chicken, mushroom, oxtail	250 ml (10 oz)
Cream of tomato soup	90 g (3 oz)
Fish finger	60 g (2 oz)
Unsweetened orange juice	120 ml (4 oz)
Unsweetened pineapple juice	90 ml (3 oz)

Other proprietary foods

In the book *Carbohydrate Countdown* a wide selection of proprietary food and drink is given, with the carbohydrate content of each. These foods should be used with discretion and two bars of chocolate should not be regarded as an acceptable lunch. Chocolate could, however, be carried as a sugar substitute on a journey or at a picnic.

If a child is very active on holiday in hot weather extra carbohydrate and fluids can be given together as mineral water. Roughly speaking, 3 oz of any of these contain 10 g of carbohydrate.

Appendix

General recipes

It may seem odd to ask a physician to read through a few recipes, but he may find it an advantage to be able to show an intelligent interest when the mother and the dietitian are discussing kitchen matters. The recipes which follow are few in number, but show the range available in home cooking for the diabetic. Children like fish cakes and rissoles, the kind of food which is perhaps better avoided in restaurants because of the unknown carbohydrate content, but there is no reason why they should not have them at home. Puddings and sweets based on fruit are usually popular with children, so two such recipes are given.

Mothers should be encouraged to do their own cooking. The carbohydrate content and nutritional value of each dish will then be known. One can thicken a gravy if one knows the amount of flour used, and one can calculate the precise amount of carbohydrate used in the pastry on a pie. The difficulty for a child in assessing the amount of carbohydrate in the pastry he gets at a school meal has been mentioned, but if a pie, or a pudding based on pastry, is made at home this difficulty is obviated. 'Compound foods' like pies, pastries, thick sauces, fish in batter and fancy puddings are best left alone if encountered outside, but can be taken in the home.

Lentil soup

180 g (6 oz) lentils; 1 litre (2 pints) stock or hambone + 1 litre (2 pints) water; 120 g (4 oz) potato; 30 g (1 oz) margarine; carrots, turnip; onion; 200 ml (7 oz) milk.

Sauté vegetables and lentils in fat for 20 min. Add stock and cook for two hours. Sieve or liquidize soup and add milk. Serve with chopped parsley. 8 servings each 15 g CHO.

Tomato soup

1 litre (2 pints) stock; 30 g (1 oz) butter or margarine; 1 onion; 1–2 carrots; stick celery; 450 g (15 oz) tin tomatoes; 45 g (1½ oz) cornflour; 200 ml (7 oz) milk.

Sauté vegetables in fat. Add stock and tin of tomatoes. Season and cook for half an hour. Mix cornflour and milk to a paste and add to soup. Cook for a quarter of an hour. 8 servings each 5 g CHO.

Note: Commercial tomato soup is considerably thickened, this recipe is not.

Fish cakes or rissoles

250 g (8 oz) mashed potato; 250 g (8 oz) flaked fish or 250 g (8 oz) minced meat; egg to bind; mixed herbs; salt and pepper: tomato pureé.

Mix all together to form four large or eight small cakes. Fry, grill or bake. Each large cake=10 g CHO; each small cake=5 g CHO.

Kedgeree

250 g (8 oz) fish; 60 g (2 oz) boiled rice; 1 egg hard boiled; 30 g (1 oz) butter.

Remove bones and skin. Flake the fish. Mix with rice, add butter and seasonings. Decorate with chopped egg.
One serving=20 g CHO. A white sauce can be added, but the amount of flour and milk in the sauce must be calculated.

Pies

In making steak and kidney pie, bacon and egg pie, etc. one needs to know only the carbohydrate content of the pastry and the amount of flour used in thickening any gravy. The pie can then be divided into equal portions to allow the diabetic his carbohydrate ration.

Ready made frozen puff pastry contains about 10 g of CHO per 30 g (oz), and short crust 12 g per 30 g (oz).

Fresh fruit salad

1 apple; 1 orange; 1 pear; 1 banana; melon; few grapes to decorate.

Chop all ingredients and place in bowl. Cover with Trim. Serve with cream, 4 servings each 10 g of CHO.

Fruit mousse

60 g (2 oz) ordinary jelly taken just before it sets; 45 ml (1½ oz) evaporated milk; ½ portion fresh fruit.

Liquidize all together. 1 portion=20 g of CHO.
(For a 'diabetic jelly', dissolve 15 g (½ oz) of gelatine in a little water, and add diluted diabetic squash to make ½ litre; one pint).

Sponge cakes

180 g (6 oz) flour; 120 g (4 oz) butter; 2 eggs; 1 teaspoon baking powder; 60 g (2 oz) sugar.

Cream fat and sugar. Sieve flour and baking powder. Beat in flour and eggs alternately. Divide mixture into 18 small paper cases and bake 15 min, No. 4 or 350°F. Cake=10 g of CHO.

Basic vegetable curry

1 level teaspoon red chilli (5 g); 1 level teaspoon coriander (5 g); ½ level teaspoon turmeric (2 g); ½ level teaspoon garlic powder (2 g); ½ level teaspoon ground ginger (2 g); 2 large onions (300 g); 1–2 cloves garlic; 2 tablespoons tomato pureé (50 g); 2 tablespoons oil (30 g) or 2 oz butter (60 g); salt to taste; plus any selection of chopped vegetables.

Chop onions and garlic finely together with fresh ginger if liked. Fry in oil until soft but not brown. Add 2 tablespoons water. Add spices and cook gently (2 minutes). Add tomato pureé and cook gently (2 minutes). Add salt and chopped vegetables and cook gently (2 minutes). Add 1 teacup of water. Simmer until vegetables are cooked. Total CHO=0. Serves 4.

Lentil curry (dhal)

90 g (3 oz) lentils; 2 small onions (100 g); 1 clove garlic; 5 small whole red chillies or a little chilli powder; 2–3 bay leaves; 1 teaspoon cummin powder (2 g); 1 teaspoon salt (5 g); 1 tablespoon oil (15 ml).

Chop one onion and garlic. Add lentils to ½ pint water with a little salt, the chopped onion and garlic, and bring to the boil. Simmer gently for at least 30 minutes, until mushy, adding more water if necessary. Chop the remaining onion. Fry in oil until soft. Add bay leaves, chillies and cummin and fry lightly. Add mashed lentils and mix thoroughly while re-heating. Total CHO=45 g. 1 portion=20 g CHO. Serves 2.

Sweet and sour pork balls

Sauce

1 medium sized onion (120 g); ½ green pepper (90 g); margarine (15 g); 2 teaspoons cornflour (10 g); 2 tablespoons chutney (50 g); 3 teaspoons tomato pureé (15 g); 2 teaspoons soy sauce (10 g); 2 teaspoons castor sugar (10 g); 1 tablespoon vinegar (15 ml); ½ pint water (300 ml).

Batter

120 g (3 oz) self-raising flour; ½ egg (30 g); ¼ pint water (150 ml); ½ teaspoon oil (5 ml); 180–240 g (6–8 oz) pork.

Make batter in the normal way. Slice onion and pepper and fry gently in oil. Add the chutney, cornflour, tomato pureé, soy sauce, sugar, vinegar and water. Bring to the boil and simmer for 10 minutes. Cut pork into one inch cubes. Dip in the batter and deep fry six minutes until golden and crisp. Pour sauce into a dish and arrange pork on top. Total CHO=80 g. 1 portion=20 g CHO. Serves 4.

BOOKS

From the British Diabetic Association, 10 Queen Anne Street, London W1M 0BD, one may obtain the following.

'I am a Diabetic' (white plastic disc), six for 50p.
Insulin identity card in plastic case, 8p.

The following books are also available from the BDA.

Carbohydrate Countdown (65p)
A guide to the carbohydrate content of proprietary products.

Measure for Measure (£2.10) Elizabeth O'Reilly.
Calorie and carbohydrate-controlled recipes. Attractive book aimed more at adults or teenagers.

Successful Diabetic Cooking (£1.25) Pamela Robinson and Audrey Francis.

Food exchange cards (75p)
Set of playing cards useful for teaching children food values.

Other helpful books are:

The Composition of Foods by R. A. McCance and E. M. Widdowson. Medical Research Council, London, Her Majesty's Stationery Office (£12)

Tables of Representative Values of Food Commonly Used in Tropical Countries by B. S. Platt. Medical Research Council (£3.50)

Cooking for Special Diets by Bee Nilson. Penguin (£1.25)

Index

Abdominal pain, 7
  in pancreatitis, 12
Acceleratory polypeptide, 138
Acetest, 53, 55
Acetone,
  formation, 158
  in ketoacidosis, 176
Acetyl coenzyme-A, 147
Acidosis,
  in ketoacidosis, 172, 173
  lactic, 187
Acromegaly, 146, 236
Actrapid MC, 38, 45
Addison's disease, 224
Adolescence,
  behaviour in, 60
  career prospects, 135
  education during, 73
  growth at, 202
  growth lag during, 206
  inducing ketoacidosis, 181
  insulin requirements during, 207
  Prader–Willi syndrome in, 245
  prognosis and, 269
  suicide and, 162, 181
  weight during, 105, 106
Adrenal cortical hyperglycaemia, 16
Adrenal glands,
  diabetes and, 237
Adrenaline, 153
  blood glucose and, 144
  effect on blood sugar, 153
Aetiology of diabetes, 209–232
  autoimmunity and, 224, 237

Aetiology of diabetes, (*cont.*)
  environmental factors, 213
  heredity and, 209
  high risk families, 213, 225
  HLA system, 213, 222, 230
  host susceptibility and, 222
  infection and, 219
  maturity onset, 210, 211
  racial factors, 228
  recessive gene theory, 211
  stress and, 220
  viruses and, 221
Age, *see also* Adolescence, Babies,
    Infants, Schoolchildren etc.
  bone- and height- and, 203
  choice of insulin and, 46
  complications and, 248, 268
  compulsive water drinking and, 6
  convulsions and hyperglycaemia and, 12
  dependence and independence and, 131
  diet and, 23
  education and, 72, 87
    hypoglycaemic attacks, 73
  fluids in ketoacidosis and, 166, 167
  glucose tolerance test and, 13, 14
  height and, 100
  hypoglycaemia and, 8
  incidence and, 220
  initial dose of insulin and, 38
  insulin dosage in ketoacidosis and, 169
  insulin requirements and, 206

Age, (*cont.*)
  pancreatitis and, 236
  polyuria and, 6
  prognosis and, 267, 268, 269
  recurrent ketoacidosis and, 176
  retinopathy and, 265, 268, 269
  type of insulin and, 43
Alanine, 139, 156
  cycle, 140
Alanine/pyruvate ratio as indication of control, 34
Alimentary signs, 7
Alstrom's syndrome, 242, 244
Amino acids,
  effect on plasma insulin, 143
  transport, insulin facilitating, 142
Anorexia, 7
Antidiuretic hormone,
  deficiency, 244
Anxiety,
  among parents, 77, 95
  causing diabetes, 153
  causing hypoglycaemia, 128
Arteriosclerosis, 21
Aspirin poisoning, 10, 161
Ataxia telangiectasia, 246
Autoimmunity, 224, 237

Babies,
  carbohydrate intake, 195
  cholesterol intake, 273
  urine testing in, 52
Bed-sores, 252
Behaviour, 58–71
  adolescent denial, 60
  case histories, 59, 65, 70
  disorders, 59, 68, 70
    symptoms, 61
  family reaction and, 63
  interplay of persons in, 58, 66
  types of parents, 66, 67
Blindness, 132
Blood,
  osmolality of, 181
  testing for ketones, 55
Blood sugar,
  action of exercise on, 41
  correlation with urine sugar, 204
  effect of adrenaline, 153
  effect of bread and potatoes, 275
  effect of stress on, 115, 116
  emotions and, 69

Blood sugar, (*cont.*)
  estimations, 54
    in outpatients, 112
  glycosylated haemoglobin and, 29
  growth hormone affecting, 147
  hyperthyroidism affecting, 69
  monitoring, 28, 29
    in home, 30
    in hospital, 33
  sources of, 141
  surgical operations and, 134
  testing for, 54
Bone-age, 103
  height-age and, 203
  in diabetic children, 203
Books, 300
Brain,
  oedema, 184, 185, 270
  in ketoacidosis, 164, 167
Bran, 281
British Diabetic Association,
  books published, 300–301
  meetings of, 98
  pamphlet, 78
Burns,
  glycosuria in, 10
  transient diabetic state following, 16
Burn-stress pseudo-diabetes, 16

Calories, 274–275
Carbohydrate,
  distribution in foods, 280
  exchanges, 292
  exercise and, 275
  high intake, 24
  infant intake of, 195
  in food, 275
  intake of, 283
  limited, 23, 25
    on first admission to hospital, 39
  metabolism, 138–141
    absorptive phase, 139
    fasting stage, 140, 141
    hormones involved in, 145
    relation to protein and fat metabolism, 139, 147
Car driving, 136
Careers, 135
Cataracts, 265
Catecholamines, 153–154
  in growth hormone control, 149
  in ketoacidosis, 154

INDEX 305

Central nervous system,
  damage to, 264, see also Neuropathy
Cereal foods, 293
Cerebral damage from hypoglycaemia, 128
Cerebral oedema, 184, 185, 270
  in ketoacidosis, 164, 167
Cerebrosides, 277
Cerebrospinal fluid,
  in ketoacidosis, 164
  sugar in, 11
Chemical diabetes, 4, 13, 15
  definition, 210
  screening for, 225
Child of one diabetic parent, 212
Childhood,
  complications during, 256
  growth during, 201
  prognosis and, 269
Chinese food, 288, 289, 300
Chlorpropamide,
  in neonatal diabetes, 194
Cholesterol, 273
  amounts of, 278, 279
Civilization, diabetes and, 228
Clinistix, 9, 51, 52, 53
Clinitest, 9, 51, 52
Cockayne syndrome, 246
Codeine poisoning, 17
Coeliac disease,
  combined with diabetes and hyperthyroidism, 240
  diabetes and, 238
Colour blindness, urine testing and, 53
Coma, see also Pre-coma, 160
  classification of, 160
  diabetic uraemic, 161
  hyperglycaemic, 160
  ketoacidotic, 160, see also under Ketoacidosis
  non-ketotic, 160
  non-ketotic hyperosmolar, 160, 181, 235
Communication, 72–92, see also Education
  adolescents, 73
  among parents, 97
  at time of discharge, 77, 78
  books, 300
  consultant's role, 76, 77
  dietitian's role, 76
  family doctor's role, 78
  holiday camps, 82

Communication, (cont.)
  home visiting, 79
  house-officer's role, 75, 76
  in outpatient clinic, 79
  nurse's role, 74
  on first admission to hospital, 37
  pre-school child, 72
  school medical service and, 78
  school teacher and, 79
  social worker's role, 79, 97
  teach-ins, 81
  ward sister's role, 75, 76
  with mother, 74
  with parents, 74
  with the child, 72
Completely free diet, 24
Complications of diabetes, 248–272
  age and, 248
  control of diabetes and, 23
  early, 248
  later, 256
Confusion in hypoglycaemia, 126, 127
Congenital rubella, 222
Consultant,
  in outpatient clinic, 96
  role in communication, 76, 77
Control of diabetes, 20–36, see also under Management of diabetes
  alanine/pyruvate ratio in, 34
  classification, 28
  complications and, 23
  definition, 26
  diurnal levels of growth hormone in, 34
  dwarfing in, 101
  emotions and, 70
  growth and, 204
  height and, 206
  infection affecting, 163
  infusion pumps, 33
  liberality in, 20, 25, 27
  liver size in, 34
  long-term, 29
  monitoring, 28, 29
    in home, 30
    in hospital, 33
  social background and, 94
  stabilization during first admission to hospital, 40
  standards, 27
  strictness in, 20, 22, 27, 43
  urine testing, see under Urine testing

INDEX

Control of diabetes, (cont.)
  use of glycosylated haemoglobin, 29, 30
  weight in, 107, 108
Convulsions, 12
Cortisol,
  causing hyperglycaemia, 145
  levels in ketoacidosis, 154
Counselling, 229
Course of diabetes, 193–208
Coxsackie B viruses,
  precipitating diabetes, 221, 222, 230
C-peptide, 142
  during remission, 200
Creatinine, 33
Curries, 289, 299, 300
Cushingoid features, 41
Cushing's syndrome, 10, 237
Cysteine, 156
Cystic fibrosis, 234, 270
Cytomegalovirus infection precipitating diabetes, 222

Deafness, diabetes and, 242, 243
Death,
  in diabetes, 270
  in very young, 268
Definitions, 210
Dehydration,
  hypernatraemic, 11
  of lens, 8
Dental extractions, 133
Dependence and independence, 131
Desamido-insulins, 45
Developing countries, diabetes in, 227
Dextrostix, 54
Diabetes insipidus, 6, 243
  with diabetes mellitus, 210, 243
  with Friedreich's ataxia, 243
Diabetic encephalopathy, 264
Diabetic products, 283
Diagnosis, 5
  delay in, 5
  differential, 9
  symptoms and signs, 6
Diarrhoea, 7, 8
Diastix, 9, 52
DIDMOAD syndrome, 210, 243
Diet, 277–296, see also Food
  adjustments to, 283
  age and, 23
  calories, 274

Diet, (cont.)
  carbohydrates in, 275
  completely free, 24
  diabetic products, 276
  during illness, 290
  dwarfism and, 22
  eating out, 287
  family participation in, 64
  fibre in, 281
  free, 24, 25
  growth and, 22
  high carbohydrate, 24
  history of, 21
  insulin and, 25
  investigation of, 114
  Lawrence Line, 21, 274
  limited carbohydrate, 23
    on first admission to hospital, 39
  lipids in, 277
  national habits, 282
  on first admission to hospital, 39
  parties, 289
  picnics, 290
  protein in, 280
  recipes, 297–300
  school meals and, 286
  social aspects of, 283
  special situations, 286
  strictness in, 20
  'take away' meals, 288
Diet-breaking, 108
  causing ketoacidosis, 162
Dietitian,
  in communication, 76
  in outpatient clinic, 96
Differential diagnosis, 9
Diffuse intravascular coagulation, 190, 264
Doctor–parent relations, 64
Doctors, in outpatient clinic, 96
Drinks, 295
Drop-foot, 252, 255
Ductless glands, diabetes and, 236–237
Dwarfism, 22, 41, 101, 201, 206, 256–258

Education, 72, see also Communication
  age of child and, 87
  amount of information given, 74
  booklets, 78, 89
  further, 80
  holiday camps, 82

Education, (*cont.*)
  home visiting and, 79
  on insulin increase, 120
  parents' groups, 80
  schoolchild, 72
  school medical service in, 78
  school teacher in, 79
  subjects involved, 77
  teach-ins, 81
  towards self-care, 85
Electroencephalography, 264
Electrolyte therapy in ketoacidosis, 172
Emotions,
  blood sugar and, 69
  diabetic control and, 70
  disturbances, 68
  effects of, 119
    on insulin action, 120
  injections and, 58
Encephalomyocarditis virus, 221
Encephalopathy, 264
Endocrine system, diabetes and, 236–237
Entero-insular axis, 152
Environmental factors in diabetes, 213
Enzyme tests, 9
Epilepsy, 129, 268
Erythema at injection sites, 250
Euglycaemic diabetic ketoacidosis, 186, 188
Exercise,
  action on blood sugar, 41
  carbohydrates and, 275
  instructions to parents, 92
  investigation of, 114
  response to, 144
Eyes, 132
  dehydration of lens, 8
  diabetes and, 242, 265

Family, 69
  failure to cope, 65
  high-risk, 213
  low intelligence, 65
  reaction to diabetes, 63
  role of, 85
Family doctor, role of, 78
Fat atrophy, 260, 261
Fat metabolism,
  relation to carbohydrate metabolism, 147

Fat, metabolism, (*cont.*)
  relation to protein metabolism, 139
Fats, 277
  animal, 279
  in diet, 273, 277, 280
  intake of, 283
  ketoacidosis and, 154
  protein and, 280
  saturation, degree of, 277, 279
Fatty acids, 154
  insulin action on, 144
Fatty tumours, 260
Fibre, 281
Fibrinogen, 190
Finger joints, contractures of, 263
Fish cakes, 298
Fish fingers, 287
Fluids in ketoacidosis, 164
Food, *see also* Diet
  calories, 274
  carbohydrates in, 275
  diabetic products, 276
  national habits, 282
  restricted, 292
  social aspects of, 283
  to be avoided, 292
  unrestricted, 292
Free diet, 24, 25
Free fatty acids, 154
  insulin action on, 144
Friedreich's ataxia, 210, 242, 243
Fructose, 275
  in ketoacidosis, 175
Fruit, 292, 293
  in diet, 282
  salad, 299

Gastric lavage in ketoacidosis, 174
Gastric parietal cells, antibodies to, 237
Gastrointestinal function in diabetic, 238
Gastrointestinal polypeptide, 152
Genetics of diabetes, 209, 223
  child of one diabetic parent, 212
  counselling, 229
  high-risk families, 213, 225
  of insulin antagonists, 212
  maturity onset diabetes in young, 5
  neonatal diabetes, 193
  of optic atrophy and diabetes, 242
  siblings, 212

INDEX

Gerhardt's ferric chloride test, 53
Gigantism, 236
Glandular fever, diabetes and, 222
Glibenclamide, 199
Glomerulosclerosis, 266
Glucagon, 149–151
  blood glucose and, 144
  in islet cells, 149
  levels in ketoacidosis, 154
  receptor sites, 150
  response of, 150
  stress and, 150
Glucagon-like immunoreactivity, 152
Glucocorticoids, carbohydrate metabolism and, 145
Gluconeogenesis,
  basis of, 155
  in non-ketotic hyperosmolar coma, 186
  insulin depressing, 155
Glucoregulatory state, 147
Glucose,
  entry into cells, 141
  growth hormone and, 144
  metabolism, 139
    adrenaline and, 144
  muscles as source of, 141
  uptake, 138
Glucose-6-PD deficiency, 246
Glucose tolerance test, 13–15
  age and, 13, 14
  errors in, 14
  interpretation of, 14, 16
  in transient diabetic state, 15
  obesity and, 226
  reliance on, 227
Glycerol, utilization, 154
Glycogen,
  in liver, 258
  synthesis, 141
Glycogen nephrosis, 266
Glycogen storage disease, 246, 258
Glycosuria,
  differential diagnosis, 10
  fluctuations in,
    insulin and, 116, 119
  growth and, 204
  in Cushing's syndrome, 237
  in salicylate poisoning, 10
  renal, 12
  tests for, validity of, 9
Glycosylated haemoglobin, 29–30
  estimation of, 29

Growth hormone, 138, 146–149, 196, 236
  action of, 147
  blood glucose and, 144
  catecholamines and, 149
  causing hyperglycaemia, 148
  deficiency, 246
  diurnal levels of, 34
  effect on blood sugar, 147
  emotional effects on levels, 69
  glucoregulatory state and, 147
  in ketoacidosis, 170
Growth hormone release inhibiting hormone, *see* Somatostatin
Growth of diabetic children, 200–206
  annual lag, 202, 206
  at puberty, 202
  control of diabetes and, 204
  diet and, 22
  glycosuria and, 204
  hepatomegaly and, 205
  in childhood, 201
  ketosis and, 204
  maturation and, 203
  pre-pubertal spurt, 202
  social factors in, 205
Guar, 288
Guilt, among parents, 125
Gun, 50

Haemochromatosis, 10, 26, 235
Haemoglobin, glycosylated (HbA_1), *see* Glycosylated haemoglobin
Haplotypes, 223
Height, 99–104, 268
  adult, of diabetic children, 200
  at onset of diabetes, 196
  bone-age and, 103, 203
  diabetes and, 258
  diabetic control and, 206
  velocity charts, 103
Hepatitis, diabetes following, 222
Hepatomegaly, 41, 256
  causes of, 258
  growth and, 205
  indicating control, 34
Heredity in diabetes, 209, *see also* Genetics
  counselling, 229
  HLA system and, 213, 223
  insulin antagonists, 212
  pancreatitis, 236

INDEX 309

Heredopathia atactica polyneuritiformis, *see Refsum's syndrome*
History, 1–19
  length of, 1
  long duration, 3
  short, 2
  speed of onset, 3
  taking, 5
HLA system,
  diabetes and, 213, 222, 230, 239, 240, 266
  infection and, 224
Holiday camps, 82
Holidays, 129
  abroad, 130
Home visiting, 79
Hospital,
  admission for recurrent ketoacidosis, 176
  discharge from, communication and, 77, 78
  first admission to, 37–57, 248
    choice of insulin, 40
    communication and, 37
    diet in, 39
    discharge, 56
    education of mother during, 74
    emotional aspects, 61
    initial dose of insulin, 38
    stabilization during, 40
    urine testing, 51
  first day in, 37
  readmission,
    for prolonged vomiting, 163
    reasons for, 122
    social factors, 122
House-officers, role in communication, 75, 76
Huntington's chorea, 246
Hyperglycaemia,
  adrenal cortical, 16
  convulsions producing, 12
  cortisol causing, 145
  glucagon producing, 149
  growth hormone causing, 148
  in Cushing's syndrome, 237
  non-ketotic coma, 4
  transient, emotional causes, 69
Hyperglycaemic coma, 160
Hyperlipidaemia, 245
  in ketoacidosis, 11
Hyperlipoproteinaemias, 246

Hypernatraemia,
  in hyperosmolality, 185
  in ketacidosis, 165
Hypernatraemic dehydration, 11
Hyperosmolality, treatment of, 183
Hypertension, 269
Hyperthyroidism, blood sugar and, 69
Hypertrophy, 260
Hyperventilation, 8
  causing pneumomediastinum, 256
  in ketoacidosis, 161
Hypoglycaemia, 8, 26, 126–129
  anxiety causing, 128
  causing brain damage, 128
  confusion in, 126, 127
  dangers of, 128
  deliberate causing of, 38
  differential diagnosis, 127
  distinguishing from ketoacidosis, 162
  from insulin excess, 118
  in infants, 194
  in outpatient clinic, 129
  irritability and, 126
  nocturnal, 127
  visual disorders during, 265
Hypoglycaemic attack,
  faking, 128
  instruction for, 73, 91
  patterns of, 126
  signs of, 126
  unexplained, 121
Hypoglycaemic coma,
  glucagon in, 149
  glucocorticoids in, 145
Hypogonadism, 256
Hypoguard, 50
Hypopituitarism, 146
Hypotension, ketoacidosis and, 168
Hypothermia in ketoacidosis, 189
Hypothyroidism, 224, 241

Illness, diet during, 290
Immunoglobulin deficiency, 240
Incidence of diabetes, 214
  age and, 220
  racial factors, 228
  rises in, 216
  seasonal, 216
Infants,
  carbohydrate intake, 195
  diabetes in, 194–196
  insulin for, 46
  prognosis and, 268

Infection,
  causing ketoacidosis, 163
  effects of, 115
  HLA system and, 224
  insulin dosage and, 121
  precipitating diabetes, 219
  terminating remission, 198
Infectious mononucleosis, diabetes and, 222
Infusion pumps, 33
Inhibitory polypeptide, 138
Injections,
  emotional impact of, 58
  Hypoguard, 50
  needles, 49
  Palmer injector, 50
  syringes, 48–49
  technique of, 51
Injection sites,
  choice of, 51
  erythema at, 250
  fat hypertrophy at, 260
  importance of, 40
  problems, 114
Insulin, 21, 22, 141–154
  action of, 141
    exercise and, 144
    on free fatty acids, 144
    Somogyi effect and, 116
  adjustment of, 56, 114, 120
    instructions for parents, 91
    on readmission, 122
  amino acids affecting, 143
  antagonists, 144–154, *see also under specific compounds*
    catecholamines, 153
    gastrointestinal hormones, 152
    glucagon, 149
    growth hormone, 146
    inheritance of, 212
    insulinase, 146
    islet cells, 149
  attitude towards, 25
  beef or pork?, 44
  body stores, 142
  breakdown, 146
  care of equipment, 48
  choice of, 40
    summary, 46
  choice of old and new, 44
  depot, 38
  depressing gluconeogenesis, 155
  diet and, 25

Insulin, (*cont.*)
  dosage, 169
    for infants, 195
    infection and, 121
    initial, 38
    old and new compared, 46
    modifications in, 121
  during remission period, 199
  facilitating amino acid transport, 142
  for infants, 46
  impurities, 44, 45, 262
  in babies, 194
  infusion during surgery, 135
  in islet cells, 149
  injection,
    emotional impact of, 58
    failure causing ketoacidosis, 163
    Hypoguard, 50
    needles, 49
    Palmer injector, 50
    problems, 114
    syringes, 48–49
    technique of, 51
    instructions, 90
  injection sites, 51
    erythema at, 250
    fat hypertrophy at, 260
    importance of, 40
  in ketoacidosis, 169–172, 174
  in liver, 143
  in pre-coma, 169
  intravenous in ketoacidosis, 172
  length of action, 40
    injection site influencing, 40
    variation in, 41
  Lente (IZS), 25
  long-acting (PZI), 41
  medium-acting, 42
  metabolism and, 138–159
    renal factors, 146
  mixed, 43, 48
  newer, 44
    benefits of, 44
  overtreatment with, 117
    causes of, 119
    causing ketoacidosis, 180
    control of, 119
    signs of, 118
  pork, 262
  pure or impure, 44
  purified, 45
  receptors, 152–153

Insulin, *(cont.)*
  release of, 143
  requirements, 206–207
  resistance, 118
  response, 150
  secretion during remission, 199, 200
  short-acting, 38, 40, 41
  Somogyi effect and, 115
  starvation and, 144
  stimulating triglyceride formation, 142
  storage, 50
  synonyms, 42
  synthesis and secretion, 142
    stimulus to, 143
  types, 41, 42, *see also under names*
Insulinase, 146
Insulitis, 221
  perivascular cuffing, 238
Insulinomas, 142, 235
Insulinopenia, 234
Insurance, 130
Intelligence, 268
Intrinsic factor, antibodies to, 238
Iron metabolism, in haemochromatosis, 235
Irritability, hypoglycaemia and, 126
Islet cells, 149
  antibodies to, 224, 227, 238
Isoproterenol, in ketoacidosis, 181, 188

Joint contractures, 263

Karela, 281
Kedgeree, 298
Ketoacidosis, 160–192
  acetone levels in, 176
  biochemistry of, 154
  catecholamine levels in, 154
  causes of, 156, 162
  cerebral intravascular coagulation and, 264
  cerebral oedema in, 167
  CSF pressure in, 164
  clinical, 161
  coma in, 160
    definition, 160
  cortisol levels in, 154
  diagnosis of, 161
  diet-breaking causing, 162

Ketoacidosis, *(cont.)*
  diffuse intravascular coagulation in, 190
  distinguishing from hypoglycaemia, 162
  euglycaemic, 186, 188
  failure in insulin administration causing, 163
  fat and, 154
  fluids in, 164–169
    age affecting, 166, 167
    quantity of, 165
    total amount, 167
    type of, 164
  glucagon causing, 149
  glucagon levels in, 154
  growth hormone levels in, 170
  hyperlipidaemia in, 11
  infection causing, 163
  lactate in, 170
  management of, 37
  manifestations of, 188
  non-diabetic, 161
  over-treatment and, 180
  pneumomediastinum and, 255
  production of, 154–157
  protein and, 155
  psychiatric factors, 124
  recurrent, 176–181
    deliberate production of, 180
    differential diagnosis, 180
    speed of onset, 179
    treatment of, 181
  signs of, 161
  stress causing, 164, 179, 181
  treatment of, 164
    electrolyte therapy, 172
    fluids, 164
    fructose, 175
    gastric lavage in, 174
    insulin in, 169–172, 174
    intravenous insulin in, 172
    monitoring, 175
    on a shoestring, 175
    oral fluids in, 168
    phosphate in, 175
    potassium, 174
    saline in, 165
    sodium bicarbonate, 172
  vomiting causing, 163
Ketoacidotic coma, 4
Ketodiastix, 51, 52, 54
Ketogenesis, lack of, 185

Ketone bodies, 155
Ketones, testing for, 53, 55
Ketosis, 7
  growth and, 204
  in cystic fibrosis, 234
  in haemochromatosis, 235
  in neonatal diabetes, 193
  in pancreatic diabetes, 233
Ketostix, 52, 53, 55
  in diagnosis of ketoacidosis, 161
Kidney,
  gluconeogenesis in, 158
  in diabetes, 266
  in insulin degradation, 146
Kimmelstiel-Wilson glomerulosclerosis, 266
Klinefelter's syndrome, 246

Lactate, in ketoacidosis, 170
Lactic acid,
  production, 187
Lactic acidosis, 161, 187
Laurence-Biedl syndrome, 242, 244
Lawrence Line diet, 21, 274
Lens, dehydration of, 8
Lente insulin, 41, 127
Lentil curry, 300
Lentil soup recipe, 297
Leo Neutral RI, 38, 45
Lethargy, 6, 7
Leucine, 143
Leucoderma, 246
Liberality in management, 20, 25, 27
Life expectancy, 267
Lipids, *see* Fats
Lipoatrophic diabetes, acquired, 245
Lipoatrophy, 245
Liver,
  enlargement, 41, 205, 256, 258
  fatty acid conversion in, 141
  glucose synthesis in, 141
  glycogen accumulation in, 258
  height, 257
  insulin degradation in, 146
  insulin secretion and, 143
  size of, 257
    indicating control, 34
    scratching test, 257*n*
Lung infection, in cystic fibrosis, 234
Lymphocytes, 224
Lysine, 143

Malabsorption, 238, 239, 240
Management of diabetes, 20–36, *see also* Control of diabetes
  booklets on, 78, 89
  care of equipment, 48
  diet in, *see under* Diet
  during remission, 199
  emotional problems, 58
  first admission to hospital, 37–57
    choice of insulin, 40
    communication and, 37
    diet in, 39
    discharge, 56
    emotional aspects, 61
    initial dose of insulin, 38
    stabilization during, 40
    urine testing, 51
  infusion pumps, 33
  injection of insulin, *see under* Insulin or Injection
  insulin, *see under* Insulin
  ketones in urine, 53
  liberality in, 20, 25, 27
  long-term therapy, 29, 40–57
  overtreatment, 117
    hepatomegaly and, 259
    oedema and, 253
  strictness in, 20, 22, 27, 43
  testing blood sugar, 54
  urine testing, *see under* Urine testing
Marriage, 229
Maturation, 203
Maturity onset diabetes,
  compared with juvenile onset diabetes, 210, 211
  detection of, 225
  genetic factor, 209
Maturity onset diabetes in young (MODY), 4–5, 198
  genetics of, 210
  true form, 5
Mauriac syndrome, 41, 206, 256, *see also* Dwarfing
Meat, 282, 287, 292
Menarche, insulin requirements, 207
Milk, 284, 295
Moniliasis, 250
Monotard MC, 45
Morbidity of diabetes, 214
Mortality rates, 213, 270
  in very young, 268
Mothers, communication with, 74
Mumps, diabetes following, 222

Muscles, as source of glucose, 141
Muscular dystrophy, 246
Myasthenia gravis, 153
Myopia, 8

Necrobiosis lipoidica diabeticorum, 250
Necrosis of skin, 250
Needles, 49
Neonatal diabetes, 193–194
Nephropathy,
  complicating diabetes, 266
Neuropathy,
  age incidence of, 268
  autonomic, 255
  during childhood, 263
  in diabetes, 253
Nightmare, hypoglycaemia and, 127
Non-coeliac steatorrhoea, 238
Non-hyperosmolar coma, 160
Non-ketotic diabetic coma, 160
Non-ketotic hyperosmolar coma, 151, 235
  osmolality, 181
  prognosis, 185
  treatment of hyperosmality, 183
Noradrenaline, 153
Nurses,
  communication with parents, 74
  in outpatient clinic, 96
Nuts, 294

Obesity, 108, 226, 237, 256
  glucose tolerance tests and, 226
  in Prader-Willi syndrome, 245
Occupations barred to diabetics, 135
Oedema, 253
Oils, vegetable, 278
Optic atrophy,
  diabetes and, 242
    with deafness, 243
    with Friedreich's ataxia, 243
Oral antidiabetic agents, 47
  benefits of, 47
  during remission period, 199
Oral hygiene, 132
Osmolality, in non-ketotic coma, 181
Outpatient clinic, 93
  backing for, 98
  communication and, 79

Outpatient clinic, (*cont.*)
  constitution of, 95
  dietitian in, 96
  doctors in, 96
  general considerations, 93
  hypoglycaemic attacks in, 129
  nurse-technician in, 96
  patients in, 95
  social workers in, 96
  staffing, 96
  talking points, 129
    car driving, 136
    careers, 135
    dependence and independence, 131
    eyes, 132
    holidays, 129
    smoking, 132
    teeth, 132
  'trusties', 97
  typical morning in, 99
  urine charts, *see* Urine charts
Over-protection, 59

Pain,
  abdominal, 7
  in pancreatitis, 12
Palmer injector, 50
Pancreatectomy, 142, 233, 234
Pancreatic diabetes, 233–236
  classification, 234
Pancreatic hormones, as impurity in insulin, 45
Pancreatic insufficiency, 148
Pancreatic polypeptide, 149, 152
Pancreatitis,
  acute, 12
  chronic, 26, 235
    producing diabetes, 12
  hereditary, 236
  virus induced, 221
Pancreozymin, 152
Parents,
  advice to, 94
  anxiety of, 77, 95
  as psychological problem, 124
  attitudes of, 94
  communication with, 64, 74
  first day in hospital, 37
  dependence and independence and, 131
  doubting, 125, 126
  failure to cope, 65

Parents, (*cont.*)
  feckless, 68
  guilt feelings, 125
  instructional booklets for, 78, 89
  instructions on raising insulin, 120
  obsessional, 67
  of low intelligence, 65
  over-anxious, 67
  over-protection by, 59
  reaction to diabetic child, 63
  rejecting, 67
  role of, 85
  self-pitying, 67
  types of, 66, 67
Parents' groups, 80
Pastry, 287, 298
Perineal rash, 250
Perivascular cuffing, 238
Pernicious anaemia, 224
Personality defects, 123
Phaeochromocytoma, 10, 237
Phenformin, causing lactic acidosis, 188
Phenylalanine, 143
Phosphate, in ketoacidosis, 175
Phospholipids, 277
Picnics, 290
Pies, 298
Pineal hyperplasia, 246
Piqûre diabetes, 162
Pituitary gland,
  diabetes and, 236
  dysfunction of, 244
Pneumomediastinum, 255
Polydipsia, 6
Polyneuritis, 244
Polyuria, 6, 161
Porphyria, 246
Portal system, insulin secretion into, 143
Potassium in ketoacidosis, 168, 171, 174
Potential diabetes, *see Pre-diabetes*
Prader-Willi syndrome, 245
Pre-coma, 160
  instructions for parents, 91
  treatment of, 169
Pre-diabetes,
  terminology, 13
  vascular changes in, 26
Pregnancy, diabetes in, 220
Prevention of diabetes, 230

Prognosis of diabetes, 267–270
  before age of ten, 269
  before age of 15, 269
  very young diabetic, 268
Proinsulin, 45
  conversion of, 142
Prostaglandins, 277
Protein,
  distribution in foods, 280
  in diet, 280
  in ketoacidosis, 155
  metabolism in relation to fat metabolism, 139
Proteinuria, 266, 268, 269
Pruritis, 250
  in Cushing's syndrome, 237
Psychiatric opinion, need for, 123
Psychological factors,
  and glucagon control, 151
  in ketoacidosis, 178
Psychoneurosis, 62
Puberty,
  delayed, 206
  insulin requirements, 207
  significance of, 267
Pyelonephritis, 115

Rapitard, 41
Recessive gene theory, 211
Recipes, 297–300
Reflectance meters, 54, 112
Refsum's disease, 242, 244
Registrar, role in communication, 75
Remission, 197
  definition of, 198
  hypothyroidism and, 241
  infection terminating, 198
  insulin during, 207
  insulin secretion during, 199, 200
  oral hypoglycaemic agents during, 199
Renal failure, chronic, 7
Renal glycosuria, 12
Retard RI, 45
Retinitis, 268
Retinitis pigmentosa, 244
Retinopathy, 264, 269
  definition of, 265
  hypopituitarism and, 146
Rothera's nitroprusside test, 53
Royal Hospital for Sick Children, Glasgow, booklet, 89

Rubella precipitating diabetes, 222

Saccharin, 276
Salicylate poisoning, glycosuria in, 10
Saline in ketoacidosis, 165
Saxin, 276
Schmidt's syndrome, 246
Schoolchildren,
 growth of, 201
 progress of, 62
School meals, 286
School medical service, 78
School teacher, role of, 79
Screening for diabetes, 225
 methods, 226
Secretin, 152
Seizures, 264
Self-care in diabetes, 85
Semilente insulin, 41, 42, 44, 127
Semitard, 41
Semitard MC, 45
Serine, 156
Serotonin, 149
Sex incidence,
 of height loss, 268
 of oedema, 253
Siblings of diabetics, 212
Signs and symptoms, 6
Skin lesions, 250
Skin sepsis, 8
Smoking, among diabetics, 132
Social background, role of, 93
Social behaviour, disturbances in, 62
Social eating, 283
Social factors, 70
 for readmission, 122
 growth and, 205
Social workers,
 in outpatient clinic, 97
 role of, 79
Sodium bicarbonate in ketoacidosis, 172
Somatostatin, 149, 151–152
 effect on insulin, 151
Somogyi effect, 41, 115–117, 120, 121, 122
 overtreatment with insulin and, 117
 recognition of, 116
Sorbitol, 276
Starch, 275
Starvation, insulin in, 144
Steatorrhoea, 238, 239, 240

Steroids, carbohydrate metabolism and, 145
Sterols, 277
Stress,
 blood sugar and, 116
 causing diabetes, 153
 causing ketoacidosis, 164, 181
 effect on blood sugar, 115
 glucagon and, 150
 ketoacidosis and, 179
 precipitating diabetes, 220
 urine and, 115
Strictness in management, 20, 22, 27, 43
Subcutaneous tissue, necrosis of, 250
Sucrose, 276
Sugar, urine testing for, 51–53
Suicide, attempted, 124, 162, 181
Sulphonylureas, delaying onset of diabetes, 226
Surgical operations, 134–135
 effect on blood sugar, 134
Sweeteners, 276
Syringes, 48
 boiling, 49
 disposable, 49
 instructions on, 90

Teach-ins, 81
Technician in outpatients, 96
Teeth,
 care of, 132
 extraction of, 133
Terminology, 13
Tes-Tape, 53
Third world, diabetes in, 227
Thyroid antibodies, 241
Thyroid gland, diabetes and, 237
Thyroiditis, diabetes and, 241
Thyrotoxicosis, 10, 145
Thyroxin, 145, 237, 241
 in maturation, 203
Tomato soup, 298
Transient diabetic state, 12, 15–16
 case history, 17
 following burns, 16
Triglyceride formation, 142
Tuberculosis, in diabetes, 115
Turner's syndrome, 246
Twin studies, 212, 223, 229

Uraemic coma, 161
Urea, formation, 158
Urinary infection, diagnosis of, 7
Urine,
  in Somogyi effect, 115
  salicylate in, 10
Urine charts, 109, 121
  faking, 113
  problems, 131
    bad chart and falling weight, 113
    good chart and falling weight, 112
  suspicious looking, 109, 110
Urine testing, 5, 51–54
  at home, 55
  colour blindness and, 53
  five drop, 52, 109
  in control, 28
  in infants, 195
  instruction in, 51, 90
  investigation of, 114
  ketones, 53
  sugar, 51
  24-hour fractional, 31
  two-drop, 52

Vasoactive intestinal polypeptide, 149 152
Vegetable curry, 299
Vegetables, 294
Viruses precipitating diabetes, 221
Vision, transient disorders of, 265
Vomiting, causing ketoacidosis, 163

Ward sisters, role in communication, 75, 76
Wartime, diabetic mortality rates during, 214
Water, compulsive drinking, 6
Weight, 104–109
  excessive gain, 107, 118
  excessive loss of, 108
  gain, 106
  loss of, 7, 112, 113
  seasonal variation in, 105
Werner's syndrome, 246

Xanthoma, 245